# BIOGRAPHIES OF REMEDIES: DRUGS, MEDICINES AND CONTRACEPTIVES IN DUTCH AND ANGLO-AMERICAN HEALING CULTURES

# THE WELLCOME SERIES IN THE HISTORY OF MEDICINE

**Forthcoming Titles:**

*The Road to Medical Statistics*
Edited by Eileen Magnello and Anne Hardy

*The Home Office and the Dangerous Trades*
By P. W. J. Bartrip

*The Regius Chair of Military Surgery
in the University of Edinburgh, 1806-55*
By Matthew H. Kaufman

The Wellcome Series in the History of Medicine editors are
H. J. Cook, C. J. Lawrence and V. Nutton.
Please send all queries regarding the series to Michael Laycock,
The Wellcome Trust Centre for the History of Medicine at UCL,
24 Eversholt Street, London NW1 1AD, UK.

# BIOGRAPHIES OF REMEDIES: DRUGS, MEDICINES AND CONTRACEPTIVES IN DUTCH AND ANGLO–AMERICAN HEALING CULTURES

*Edited by*
*M. Gijswijt-Hofstra, G. M. Van Heteren*
*and E. M. Tansey*

First published in 2002
by Editions Rodopi B. V., Amsterdam – New York, NY 2002.

M. Gijswijt-Hofstra, G. M. Van Heteren
and E. M. Tansey © 2002.

Design and Typesetting by Michael Laycock,
The Wellcome Trust Centre for the History of Medicine at UCL.
Printed and bound in The Netherlands by Editions Rodopi B. V.,
Amsterdam – New York, NY 2002.

Index by Dr Laurence Errington.

All rights reserved. No part of this book may be reprinted or reproduced or utilised in any form or by any electronic, mechanical, or other means, now known or hereafter invented, including photocopying and recording, or in any information storage or retrieval system, without permission in writing from The Wellcome Trust Centre for the History of Medicine at UCL.

**British Library Cataloguing in Publication Data**
A catalogue record for this book is available from the British Library.
ISBN 90-420-1577-2 (Paper)
ISBN 90-420-1587-X (Bound)

Biographies of Remedies
Drugs, medicines and contraceptives in
Dutch and Anglo–American healing cultures
Amsterdam – New York, NY
Rodopi. – ill.
(Clio Medica Series No. 66/ ISSN 0045-7183;
The Wellcome Series in the History of Medicine)

Front cover:
'Mannikin of an apothecary composed of the attributes of the trade.'
Courtesy: Wellcome Library, London. Design by Michael Laycock.

© Editions Rodopi B. V., Amsterdam – New York, NY 2002
Printed in The Netherlands

All titles in the Clio Medica series (from 1999 onwards) are available to download from the CatchWord website: http://www.catchword.co.uk

# Contents

Contributors     i

Introduction
*Godelieve van Heteren;
Marijke Gijswijt-Hofstra; Tilli Tansey*     1

1. Changing places:
Illicit drugs, medicines, tobacco and nicotine in the nineteenth and twentieth centuries
*Virginia Berridge*     11

2. Pharmacists, druggists and the spirit of Thorbecke:
The shaping of the Dutch pharmacy, 1865–c.1920
*Frank Huisman*     35

3. The 'Dutch drugstore' as an attempt to reshape pharmaceutical practice:
The conflict between ethical and commercial pharmacy in Dutch cultures of medicines
*Rein Vos*     57

4. Community pharmacy in Great Britain:
Mediation at the boundary between professional and lay care 1920 to 1995
*Stuart Anderson*     75

5. Homoeopathy and its concern for purity:
The Dutch case in the early-twentieth century
*Marijke Gijswijt-Hofstra*     99

6. Drugs for healthy people:
The culture of testing hormonal contraceptives for women and men.
*Nelly Oudshoorn*     123

7. Contrasting cultures of contraception: Birth control clinics and the working-classes in Britain between the wars
*Kate Fisher*     141

8.  'Public spirited and enterprising volunteers':
    The Council for the Investigation of Fertility Control and the
    British clinical trials of the contraceptive pill, 1959–1973
    *Lara Marks*     159

9.  'Hygienic articles, patent medicines and rubber goods':
    Markets and meanings in early twentieth century Netherlands
    *Willem de Blécourt*     183

10. Streptomycin in postwar Britain: A cultural history of a
    miracle drug
    *Alan Yoshioka*     203

11. About media, audiences and marketing medicines:
    The interferons
    *Toine Pieters*     229

12. The billion dollar molecule:
    Taxol in historical and theoretical perspective
    *Vivien Walsh & Jordan Goodman*     245

13  Afterword:
    Remedies: Who Cares? Remedies, care and cultures of healing
    in the twentieth century
    *Godelieve van Heteren*     269

    Index     283

## Contributors

**Stuart Anderson** is senior lecturer in the history of pharmacy at the London School of Hygiene and Tropical Medicine, University of London. He has recently completed an oral history of British community pharmacy. He is currently working on an oral history of British hospital pharmacy, and a book on the social history of pharmacy.

**Virginia Berridge** is professor of history at the London School of Hygiene and Tropical Medicine, University of London. She is head of the Health Promotion Research Unit and directs a group of historians, including the 'Science speaks to Policy' programme. Her most recent book is *Health and Society in Britain since 1939* (Cambridge: Cambridge University Press, 1999).

**Willem de Blécourt** is a historian of medicine. He holds an Honorary Research Fellowship at the Huizinga Institute, Amsterdam, and is an Associate Fellow in the Department of History at the University of Warwick. His current research interests are lay healers and the twentieth-century cultural history of abortion and contraception.

**Kate Fisher** was awarded her doctorate in 1998 for a thesis entitled: *An Oral History of Birth Control Practice c.1925–1950. A Study of Oxford and South Wales*. She is a lecturer in history at Exeter University. Her current research is an oral history of marriage, fertility and sexuality, 1900–1950.

**Marijke Gijswijt-Hofstra** is professor of social and cultural history at the University of Amsterdam and is particularly interested in the social history of medicine, homeopathy and psychiatry in the nineteenth to twentieth centuries, and witchcraft, deviance and tolerance in the fifteenth to twentieth centuries.

*Contributors*

**Jordan Goodman** is senior lecturer in history at the University of Manchester Institute of Science and Technology. His current research interests are in the history of twentieth-century medicine and science. He is currently completing a book on the anticancer drug taxol with Vivien Walsh.

**Godelieve van Heteren** is a university lecturer in the history of medicine at the Catholic University of Nijmegen. She has a special interest in the comparative history of European healthcare systems and in the history of Dutch colonial medicine in the Dutch East Indies between 1870–1942.

**Frank Huisman** is assistant professor at the Department of History of the University of Maastricht. He has published on early modern and modern Dutch health care and on medical historiography, and is currently working on two projects: the history of medical historiography and the culture of medicines in The Netherlands, 1880-1940.

**Lara Marks** is a visiting senior research associate at the Cambridge Group for the History of Population and Social Structure, Cambridge University and an honorary senior lecturer at the London School of Hygiene and Tropical Medicine. She has published widely on the history of maternal and child health and questions of ethnicity and health. Her latest book is *Sexual Chemistry: A History of the Pill* (New Haven: Yale University Press, 2001). She is currently working on the discovery and development process in the pharmaceutical industry.

**Nelly Oudshoorn** is a professor in the Department of Philosophy of Science and Technology at the University of Twente and a lecturer in the Department of Science and Technology Dynamics at the University of Amsterdam. Her research interests include the social and material shaping of gender, bodies and technologies. She is the author of *Beyond the Natural Body: An Archaeology of Sex Hormones* (London: Routledge, 1994).

**Toine Pieters** is assistant professor of the history of medicine at the Vrije Universiteit Amsterdam School of Medicine. He has written a number of articles on the history of twentieth - century science and medicine and is completing a study of a specific 'family' of therapeutic drugs, the interferons, examining the intricate relations that have emerged in this century between medicine, academic research, industry and health politics. He is currently working on a study of the co-

## Contributors

development of psychiatric drugs and psychiatric practices in Dutch mental health (1950–2000).

**Tilli Tansey** is historian of modern medical science at the Wellcome Trust Centre for the History of Medicine at UCL and convenor of the History of Twentieth Century Medicine Group. Her research interests include the history of the modern medical research laboratory, focusing especially on physiology and pharmacology.

**Rein Vos** is professor in health ethics and philosophy at the University of Maastricht, The Netherlands. His special interest are normative issues and historical developments regarding health care and medical-pharmaceutical technology in the twentieth century.

**Vivien Walsh** is reader in innovation at the University of Manchester Institute of Science and Technology. Her PhD was about the interactions between academic and industrial research in the development of oral contraceptives. Her current research includes the recent and on-going history of pharmaceuticals, food, biotechnology and chemicals, focusing on such themes as globalization, innovation networks, the changing boundaries of industry and the behaviour of firms.

**Alan Yoshioka** was awarded a PhD from the University of London in 1998 for his thesis on the introduction of streptomycin into Britain. He was then at the Centre for History of Science, Technology and Medicine, Imperial College, London, and has lectured in humanities at York University in Toronto. He currently works in the pharmaceutical industry and remains interested in the role of scientific expertise within the welfare state.

## Introduction

*Godelieve Van Heteren
Marijke Gijswijt-Hofstra
Tilli Tansey*

What constituted healing in the twentieth century? What are the most insightful ways in which one could study the relationship between remedies and healing practices historically? In which cultural environments did specific drugs, remedies, and therapeutic strategies emerge, which social circumstances helped to encourage them, and – in turn – which social effects did they engender? These are but a few of the numerous questions that arose when the subject of 'healing in the twentieth century' was put on the agenda at the Anglo-Dutch Workshop on *Remedies and Healing Cultures in Britain and the Netherlands in the Twentieth Century*, convened by the editors at the Wellcome Institute for the History of Medicine in June 1998. The articles in this volume are based on reworkings of the papers presented at that workshop.

Few of the medical practitioners who proudly experimented with tuberculin or aseptic surgery at the end of the nineteenth century could have predicted the radical transformations in Western healing cultures that the twentieth century has witnessed. These include the rise of a high tech hospital system for all, a variety of specialized care institutions, the explosive growth of new pharmaceutical regimes, the successful introduction of organ transplantations and artificial organs, and the arrival of biomaterials, genetic engineering and microchips.

These changes have not occurred in isolation. Healing cultures have been profoundly affected by the socio-economic and political developments of the century. They too have experienced a clash of ideologies, the final stages of Western secularization, the many social effects of two World Wars. Healing practices both developed from, and have fed into, the shifting configurations of Westerners' sense of self and social responsibility.

In the course of the twentieth century biomedicine assumed a dominant role in many healing cultures. It deeply affected the institutional landscape of healing, which was modified several times, not least as a consequence of the explosive growth of biomedically-inspired diagnostic and therapeutic technologies. A whole range of new professionals had arrived on the scene. Sophisticated health insurance systems have now been constructed, making medical care more widely accessible. Not surprisingly, popular expectations, of the do-able and the desirable in health care, have shifted as well.

Some developments in the twentieth century have been characterised as part of a process of medicalization of large segments of social life. Branches of medicine have ventured into family, school and factory. They have helped to promote new ideals of body and mind, although not without opposition. Since the 1960s especially, this medicalization has been subjected to an energetic critique that stresses the social problems and moral dilemmas resulting from biomedical expansionism. Simultaneously, new interest has arisen in traditions of healing other than Western biomedicine, forms of healing that biomedicine had supposedly left behind.

### From history of therapy to history of remedies

The broadening awareness of the heterogeneity of needs and expectations, social relationships and healing strategies, has been reflected in a translation from a historiography of 'therapy' to one of 'remedies'.

At the beginning of the twentieth century, historical interest in therapies tended to be confined to professional medical curiosity. Historical studies often focused on previously dominant ideas of how to fight disease. Such histories frequently amounted to historical descriptions of past systems of pathology that were supposed to underpin particular therapeutical endeavours. They tended to portray creative scientists heroically struggling against death and disease (for example, Koch against tuberculosis, Ehrlich against syphilis, Banting and Best against diabetes).[1] They stressed the efficiency of new therapeutic techniques and praised the supposedly beneficial relations such techniques forged between doctors and patients.

This therapeutic work underwent radical historical transformation at the hands of scholars such as Erwin Ackerknecht, Charles Rosenberg, John Harley Warner and others.[2] These authors paid greater attention to the wider spectrum of therapeutic practices and their heterogeneity; and moved from monolinear treatments of the connections between etiological models and healing strategies into a social history of healing practices.³

Whilst the historiography of therapies has gained enormously in breadth and sophistication, the call for a history of 'remedies' signals yet another important shift: 'remedies' evokes other semantic registers than those produced by 'therapies'. The term 'remedies' focuses interest on concrete objects of healing. It evokes notions of production. It directs attention to the buzz of productivity and commerce linked to the worlds of healing. This may result in rather different historical pictures. In modern times 'therapy' tends to stir images of professionally sanctioned care and cure, set in consulting rooms and clinics, operating theatres and hospitals, whilst reference to 'remedies' suggests a broader cultural range in which more divergent sets of rites and rituals are performed to heal a person's ailments. The terminological shift to remedies, we would suggest, can bring us closer to the whole range of culturally accepted ways to deal with disease and suffering, not merely the professional ones.

### Remedies: healing and forms of production

Of course, we do not wish to overstate the distinction between histories of therapies and those of remedies. It goes without saying that many overlapping interests exist between historians engaged in either endeavour. Nonetheless, when one reflects upon remedies, two related topics surface readily: the status of remedies as medical, economic, social, and cultural objects; and their particular forms of production.

Connections between remedies, healing and forms of production became exceedingly complex in the twentieth century. As a consequence, there is a variety of ways in which remedies can be related to production. With some anthropologists, we would discriminate between economic, social, political and cultural forms of production.⁴

There are, for instance, researchers who examine the changing ways in which remedies are physically produced and processed. They follow the scaled enlargement of manufacturing from research processes, the diversity of implementation strategies of remedies, the impact of new professionals, the 'scientification' of production, and also the growing sophistication of marketing and advertising techniques.

This is, of course, only one set of ways in which healing and production can be seen to interrelate. Other research, for example, has been devoted to how particular remedies were favoured because they affected workers and the 'economically productive'. Over and above studying the preferential support of the 'economically viable', such studies usually examine also the multifarious social and political links between health and wealth.[5]

A further, growing, body of literature addresses healing practices in their relation to the production of social and moral categories. Remedies are seen not as the mere consequences of particular senses of disorder or disease, but as instrumental in defining individual and social ills. For instance, genetic therapies of today are likely to have a strong impact on peoples' idea of the kind of life worth living. Remedies have redrawn the map of what people consider 'normal' and 'abnormal'. Remedies can produce new dependencies by turning formerly 'healthy' people into persons dependent on one or other medical regime. The several articles on contraceptives in this volume testify to the richness of this latter approach. Remedies can be influential in defining and shifting control over people's lives. For instance, psychopharmacological developments in the 1950s were of paramount importance in supporting the deinstitutionalization of many psychiatric patients all over the Western world.[6]

Twentieth century remedies, in short, are embedded in the complex relationships of production that characterise the last hundred years. Not only do they embody key features of a given era's production ideology, (such as genetics in the era of informatics), but also they help to make certain forms of production possible. Thus, studying the remedies of a particular period relates closely to analysing contemporary forms of production.

## This volume

Several of the heterogeneous forms of productivity in which twentieth century remedies act become apparent in this volume.

Virginia Berridge opens by confronting the key issue of what 'defines' a remedy, by addressing the sociocultural production of 'what exactly counts as a drug, a medicine, or even a food'. She tries to answer the question of why, in the case of opium and nicotine, boundaries have shifted between licit and illicit use, medicinal applications or other forms of consumption. Berridge relates the changing attitudes to both substances to emerging systems of medical and pharmaceutical regimentation, and to new technological and political developments.

Frank Huisman, Rein Vos and Stuart Anderson are more interested in articulating the factors that have been decisive in the production of various professional identities for the distributors of remedies, the chemists and pharmacists. Huisman looks at the creation of a new pharmaceutical profession in the Netherlands, following the passing of several medico-legal Acts in the 1860s and 1870s. Negotiations about the construction of an academic, scientific profile for pharmacists figure strongly in Huisman's article. Vos extends these discussions into the post Second World War era, and critically analyses attempts in the 1950s and 1960s to reconfigure the Dutch pharmacist, a process culminating in a series of clashes between a more traditional professional attitude and a more commercially-oriented ethos. Stuart Anderson draws on interviews to recapture the various cultural positions that British community pharmacists have occupied since the 1920s. His choice of the British community pharmacist as a clear 'mediator at the professional-lay care boundary' underpins his tracing of four phases since the 1920s during which the profile of the British pharmacist changed. Anderson links these shifts primarily to changing health care costs and accessibility. Particularly telling are his remarks about the delicate balance between the pharmacist's dispensing and advisory roles: pharmacists as dispensers quadrupled in the wake of the founding of the NHS in 1948, but their traditional advisory role declined. Some was regained through active campaigning by community pharmacists in the 1980s, but previous levels of personal communication have been hard to re-establish.

Marijke Gijswijt's paper on Dutch homoeopathy illustrates that concern about the production of professional identities was not confined to 'orthodox' healers. Focusing on the early-twentieth century, she analyses many disputes amongst Dutch homoeopaths concerning the key question of 'homoeopathic purity', of how flexibly the teachings of Samuel Hahnemann could be interpreted. She recalls bitter quarrels on the matter in the international homoeopathic community, before sketching the severe identity crisis of the relatively small group of Dutch homoeopaths at the beginning of the twentieth century. Gijswijt conveys the difficulties that faced homoeopaths trying to find their niche in the world of healers, pointing in her discussion to the failed attempt by some Dutch homoeopaths to add a homoeopathic supplement to the regular Dutch Pharmacopoeia in order to gain 'respectability'.

In their studies of contraceptives and contraception, Nelly Oudshoorn, Kate Fisher and Lara Marks take up various issues that surround the production and distribution of 'drugs for healthy people'. They pose a range of questions related to the testing and application of medicinal substances for people 'who are not ill'. Here, one could argue, the production of expert systems and research guidelines, 'healthy volunteers', and new forms of medical and social regimentation, are the central themes.

Nelly Oudshoorn describes various difficulties associated with the clinical testing of hormonal contraceptives for women in the 1950s and 1960s. She compares these with the rather different problems encountered when a contraceptive injection for men became available thirty years later. Oudshoorn is interested in factors that determine the production of drugs for people who are not ill. Her discussion of the quest for female volunteers in the 1950s and 1960s touches on all the taboos surrounding contraceptives during those years. She presents an intriguing story of the many attempts to find 'politically acceptable' testing environments and to circumventing licensing authorities. Oudshoorn demonstrates how in practice this involved taking testing out of established medical research settings into external locations such as family planning clinics. Oudshoorn's comparison of female contraceptive testing in the 1950s with that carried out amply demonstrates how various cultural and gender biases shape the testing and production of remedies.

Kate Fisher exposes the deep conflicts that were present when people were first exposed to birth control clinics during the interwar years in Britain. Her interviews with working class men and women in South Wales and Oxford who married during those years, shows the complicated adherence that many of her respondents continued to maintain to more traditional forms of birth control. Fisher's study challenges any lingering belief that new remedies are simply and automatically adopted by people when first produced.

Lara Marks details the first stages in the development of control mechanisms on testing of pharmaceutical products in Britain. She examines the peculiar status of the Council for the Investigation of Fertility Control (CIFC) in the supervision of clinical trials of the contraceptive pill in the 1960s. The Committee on Safety of Drugs was not founded in Britain until 1964, and the CIFC, a voluntary agency established under the auspices of the British Family Planning Association, undertook trials on many different types of contraceptive pills from the early 1960s onwards. Marks' story is another significant example of the importance of voluntary efforts in British medical life. The CIFC filled a vacuum and prevented the pharmaceutical industry from releasing the pill on the British markets without further controls.

Willem de Blécourt takes the reader from the world of licensed distributors of contraceptives to the darker corners of

## Introduction

Dutch 'hygiene shops' at the beginning of the century. He explores the half-veiled 'marketing' methods employed by suppliers of 'hygienic articles', contraceptive products and abortificants, sold from a variety of establishments before the Second World War. Drawing on newspaper advertisements, lawcourt records, and articles in the *Monthly Journal of the Dutch Society for the Repression of Quackery* (*Maandblad tegen de Kwakzalverij*), de Blécourt provides a reconstruction of a variety of these 'hygienic' establishments in which 'hygienic objects', 'patent remedies' and 'rubberware' were on offer. The coded language used in marketing such devices before 1940 reminds us how rapidly the cultural meanings attached to contraceptives have changed during this century.

The final three articles of the present volume convey the richness of cultural production that has surrounded medicinal substances in this century – cultural in this context meaning produced through a series of economic, public and research practices.

Alan Yoshioka describes the fluctuating socio-cultural evaluations that surrounded streptomycin when it was first introduced. After presenting a detailed account of the debates that accompanied this process in Britain, he discusses more generally the properties commonly attributed to substances culturally configured as 'wonder drugs'. Twentieth-century wonder drugs are particularly interesting, he argues, because they involve 'scientifically manufactured' substances to which 'talismanic' properties are attached, albeit in the modernist vocabulary of innovation. They clearly demonstrate the range of cultural forces and expectations that rupon which remedies still play. Discussing in greater detail the case of streptomycin's market début in the late 1940s, Yoshioka tells the complex story of the attempt of official bodies to manage a wide range of cultural expectations.

Toine Pieters has focused his contribution on yet another so-called 'miracle' drug, interferon. Pieters discusses how interferon's identity was reshaped after its initial 'débâcle' as a cancer drug in the early 1980s. He highlights in particular the influence of networks of researchers, academics and some executive officers in pharmaceutical companies on the reconfiguration of interferon to make it representative of a new generation of biosynthetic drugs, closely linked to the new molecular biology and immunotherapy. Pieters' story is particularly revealing in its details about the roles of research control agencies, industrial capital, and the media in keeping interferon afloat.

Jordan Goodman and Vivien Walsh introduce the notion of 'a remedy's biography' in their description of the heterogeneous milieux through which taxol travelled on its way to become a medicinal substance. The authors emphasize this plurality of practices and routes taken in the process which leads to the establishment of a particular drug. At the same time they argue strongly for greater awareness of contingency: none of the roads that were taken were 'inevitable'. Equally, none of the controversies which surrounded the production and distribution of taxol (such as environmentalists contesting the harvesting of its natural source material) involved any absolute 'necessity'. This article pleads for the introduction of a more 'ethnographic methodology' into historical research on twentieth-century medicine, combined with an actor-network perspective on historical developments that is sophisticated about ownership and property relations. The authors successfully follow taxol 'as it wound its way through the procedures of science and the decision networks of state agencies and into the political arena, finally being appropriated by a pharmaceutical company'.

In her afterword, Godelieve Van Heteren suggests five possible avenues for further research on the basis of the methods and findings of the articles in this volume. Remedies deserve to be studied further as indicators of changing healing powers and dependencies. They can also be analysed as indicators of the changing role of economic forces in health care. They can be examined as indicators of the growing impact of technology, as representing material interactionism in health care, or as indicators of a weakening of national boundaries of health cultures. And finally, they can be researched with regards to their role in changing systems of care.

One aim in drawing together the work of British and Dutch scholars was to make available materials for future comparative research. Although most of the authors in this volume have not explicitly engaged in such comparisons themselves, we feel confident that their rich contributions will be of use to researchers who wish to do so.

### Acknowledgements

We are grateful to the Wellcome Institute for the History of Medicine for hosting and funding this workshop, to Mrs Lois Reynolds in particular for her editorial assistance, and Mr Michael Laycock for his design assistance. We thank the anonymous Rodopi referees who made many helpful comments on the chapters in this volume.

January 2001

## Introduction

### Notes

1. Erwin Ackerknecht, *Therapie. Von den primitiven bis zum 20 Jahrhundert* (Stuttgart: Ferdinand Enke Verlag, 1970), despite its date, is still an example of the 'old school'. The same could be said of works such as: Esmond L. Long, *A History of the Therapy of Tuberculosis and the Case of Frederic Chopin* (Lawrence, KS: University of Kansas Press, 1956); F. Neil Johnson, *The History of Lithium Therapy* (London: Macmillan, 1984); D. F. Scott, *The History of Epileptic Therapy: An account of how mediation was developed* (Carnforth, Lancs: Parthenon Publishing, 1993) or even Thomas W. Feeley (ed.), *A History of Critical Care and Hyperbaric Oxygen Therapy as Documented in the International Anesthesiology Clinics* (Philadelphia, PA: Lippincott Williams & Wilkins, 1999).
2. See, for example, Erwin H. Ackerknecht, *Medicine at the Paris Hospital: 1794–1848* (Baltimore, MD: Johns Hopkins Press, 1967); Morris J. Vogel, Charles Rosenberg (eds.), *The Therapeutic Revolution: Essays in the social history of American medicine* (Philadelphia, PA: University of Pennsylvania Press, 1979); Charles E. Rosenberg, *The Care of Strangers: The rise of American's hospital system* (New York: Basic Books, 1987) or John H. Warner, *The Therapeutic Perspective: Medical practice, knowledge, and identity in America, 1820-1885* (Cambridge, MA: Harvard University Press, 1986). Publications which contain a mixture of old and new approaches to healing include D. von Engelhardt (ed.), *Diabetes. Its medical and cultural history* (Berlin: Springer Verlag, 1989).
3. For secondary literature on drug discovery, see, for example, M. J. Parnham and J. Bruinvels (eds) *Discoveries in Pharmacology*, vol. 1, *Psycho- and neuro-pharmacology*; vol. 2, *Haemodynamics, hormones and inflammation*; vol. 3, *Pharmacological methods, receptors and chemotherapy* (Amsterdam and Oxford: Elsevier, 1983–1986); Miles Weatherall, *In search of a Cure: A history of the pharmaceutical industry* (Oxford and New York: Oxford University Press, 1990); Walter Sneader, *Drug discovery: The evolution of modern medicines* (Chichester and New York: Wiley, 1985); Walter Sneader, *Drug Prototypes and their Exploitation* (Chichester: John Wiley, 1996).
4. See, for example, Sjaak Van der Geest, 'Pharmaceutical anthropology: perspectives for research and application', in Sjaak Van der Geest and Susan Reynolds Whyte (eds), *The Context of Medicines in Developing Countries: Studies in pharmaceutical anthropology* (Dordrecht and Boston, MA: Kluwer Academic Publishers, 1988), 329–65. See also R. Vos, *Drugs Looking for Diseases. Innovative drug*

*Research and the development of the beta blockers and the calcium antagonists* (Amsterdam: Kluwer Academics Publishers, 1991).
5. This literature develops most quickly in the context of health economics, developmental and welfare theory. See, for example, J. Muysken, I Hakan Yetkinen and Th. Ziesemer, *Health, Labour Productivity and Growth* (Maastricht: MERIT, 1999), or Gareth M. Green, Fr. Baker, *Work, Health, and Productivity* (New York: Oxford University Press, 1994). Many historians of public health have drawn attention to the relationship between health, wealth and productivity, and nations' interest in health promotion in order to stimulate national productivity. See, for instance, Dorothy Porter (ed.), *The History of Public Health and the Modern State* (Amsterdam and Atlanta, GA: Rodopi, 1994)
6. See, for example, some of the essays in Marijke Gijswijt-Hofstra and Roy Porter (eds), *Cultures of Psychiatry and Mental Health Care in Postwar Britain and the Netherlands* (Amsterdam and Atlanta, GA: Rodopi, 1998).

# 1

## Changing places:
## Illicit drugs, medicines, tobacco and nicotine in the nineteenth and twentieth centuries

*Virginia Berridge*

Historians and anthropologists have reminded us many times that what counts as a drug, a medicine, or even a food, is socially, culturally and historically constructed. The term 'drug' is now used for a category of substances taken into the body for purposes other than nutrition. 'Drug', in this sense, is quite distinct from 'food'. 'Drugs' are defined within two broad categories; either medicinal preparations or those used to bring psychological rather than physiological changes. But these categorisations are quite recent. As Andrew Sherratt has pointed out, they have arisen within the context of capitalism and the Industrial Revolution, relating specifically to societies with the technical capacity to manufacture chemically refined products and to economies within which those products circulate.[1,2]

These developments have caused a rupture with earlier folk usages, and a disjuncture between 'drugs' and other substances that also affect the mind and moods. Food and drink (coffee, tea and chocolate), and other habits such as smoking, sniffing and chewing substances, are particular examples. The boundary between drugs and other substances has varied over time, and also across cultures. Likewise the boundary between illicit and licit usage has been a shifting and negotiable one.

I have been increasingly struck by the historical contingency of these definitions in my current work on postwar British smoking policy. In this article, therefore, I want to look at two groups of substances on which I have researched, at the boundary changes that have taken place since the last century, and at what seem to be some of the complex of issues that have underpinned those changes. My two groups are the opiates and allied alkaloids (morphine, heroin and cocaine), and tobacco with its active principle, nicotine. Similar elements and definitions have been present since the nineteenth century for both substances; but they have been differently positioned at different stages in a historical continuum. Why, for example, was the concept of 'addiction' and the idea of medical ownership of opiates established at the turn of the century, while for tobacco and nicotine, those debates are in play a century later? A progressive framework could be the explanation, the onward march of scientific understanding. But I seek rather to explore some of the cultural, industrial and professional issues which, I argue, have shaped those different historical patterns of definition. The focus here is primarily on the British experience, in its international context, but the question will also be addressed as to how far these conclusions apply in different national cultures.

## The nineteenth century: opium's shifting location

The uses of opiates in the nineteenth century spanned both folk–lay and orthodox medicine. Jonathan Pereira noted in his standard text book of materia medica in 1839 that opium was used in medical practice 'to mitigate pain, to allay spasm, to promote sleep, to reduce nervous restlessness, to produce perspiration, and to check profuse mucous discharges from the bronchial tubes and gastro-intestinal canal.'[3]

Opium was one of medicine's most valuable drugs/medicines. But there was no formal medical control of the drug. Behind the advice in the medical text books and journals also lay a large, and socially acceptable, hinterland of lay control of supply and use. Until the 1868 Pharmacy Act in Britain restricted the supply of opiates over a certain strength to professionally qualified pharmaceutical chemists, opium was to be bought anywhere, from market stalls, from the corner grocer's shop, the type of errand on which a child would be sent.[4] Such usage was linked to the 'consumer revolution' of the previous century, which saw opium-based patent medicines enter the mass market; it was also linked with earlier folk usage of domestic remedies based on the poppy. Thomas Hardy's Bob Loveday fell into a stupor by using poppy heads in the time honoured way.

> ...I picked some of the poppy heads in the border, which I once heard was a good thing for sending folks to sleep when they are in pain....[5]

The boundaries between lay and medical usage were relatively unformed.

Likewise, the boundaries between what was perceived as 'non-medical' and 'medical' usage, between the subsequently pejorative category of 'drug', and that of licit 'medicine' were blurred. The British politicians, William Wilberforce, reformer of the slave trade, and Prime Minister William Ewart Gladstone, were known to take opium before speeches in the House of Commons as a form of stimulant or 'pick me up'. But such usage was rarely publicly condemned. Where condemnation of opiate use as a 'luxury' (in the terminology of the time) began was in relation to usage in the industrial towns. The public health enquiries of the 1840s began to show concern about that type of usage; and the issue of lower class consumption remained as a continuing issue, in particular in relation to the 'cotton famine' in Lancashire in the 1860s and to working class use of 'childrens' quieteners' to keep children comatose while their mothers were at work. The details and the validity of those arguments are outside the scope of the current article.[6] The main point here is that the type of user was clearly a factor in beginning to establish boundaries between licit and illicit usage. Gladstone's laudanum-laced cup of coffee carried with it none of the potential threat of the opium (or alcohol) consuming inhabitants of the industrial cities.

### Establishing the boundaries: the turn of the century

This is a very different situation to the one that prevails today in British society. How did the boundary change occur and why? I have written about this elsewhere and shall briefly summarise what seem to be the key issues to bear in mind – and which also have relevance to our other substances. The professionalisation of pharmacy and medicine was clearly associated, in newly established systems of legal regulation through the Pharmacy Acts. There were conceptual–legal changes, as expressed for medicine through the disease of inebriety, but also through proposed legal regulation in the form of expanded inebriates acts. Systems of medical and pharmaceutical discipline led to increased control of the nature and form of use. Technological developments were related to these systems, through the isolation of the early alkaloids, morphine and codeine, in the first decades of the nineteenth century, with heroin later in the century. There was also that new 'drug delivery system', the syringe, which was largely under medical control. Morphine was a drug and a medicine that fulfilled a number of different functions; a 'new drug' that formed a vehicle for the professional and cultural aspirations of its professional prescribers and middle-class users; also a refined product that suited the needs of the expanding pharmaceutical industry. Early euphoria about the value of this new 'wonder medicine' were soon tempered by unease about the possibilities of abuse. Morphine and its reception was some kind of boundary marker - both medicine and, by implication, dangerous drug. Cocaine, too, passed through this similar process of boundary reallocation at the end of the nineteenth century. The important variables in establishing new definitions were technology (alkaloids, the syringe) and industry (the increasingly important role of the pharmaceutical industry).

There was in addition an international dimension with cultural, economic and strategic ramifications. The moral agitation that arose in Britain, primarily from the 1880s through the Society for the Suppression of the Opium Trade, also emphasised, in its propaganda, the distinction between 'drug' and 'medicine', between medical and non-medical usage. This was an area of debate in the colonial context. Initially in that context, the moral arguments made little headway. The Report of the Royal Commission on Opium in 1895 pointed out that the distinction was rarely applicable in practice and was inappropriate in the context of Indian culture.

> ...opium is extensively used for non-medical and quasi-medical purposes, in some cases with benefit, and for the most part without injurious consequences. The non-medical uses are so interwoven with the medical uses that it should not be practicable to draw a distinction between them in the distribution and sale of the drug.[7]

The colonial acceptance of opium was by this time greater than in Britain. India had its state opium monopoly and its licensed opium shops. In contrast, at home opium was more marginal in both medical and general culture by the end of the century. It was this international dimension that was formalised in the first two decades of the twentieth century, boundaries that had already begun to form within Britain. International control was the vehicle, initially with a Far Eastern emphasis through the Shanghai Opium Commission and subsequently through the Hague Convention of 1912 which envisaged a worldwide control system. The Chinese opium situation, to deal with which this whole international process had started, at American instigation, was already becoming a 'non problem'. The opium trade revenue was a declining proportion of the Indian budget; and moves were already in train to end the export trade. But those arguments are beside the point. What drove international control – and the decisive boundary shift – was initially American moral entrepreneurship and an allied desire to expand her strategic interests in South East Asia; and subsequently, the economic issues involved for the morphine and cocaine industries. It was this economic issue which brought the final move to internationalism. The Shanghai Commission recognised the growth of morphine smuggling to the Far East, and the British Foreign Office raised the issue of morphine and cocaine again before the meetings at the Hague in 1911–12. Partly a delaying tactic to divert American attention from the Far East, the British proposal also arose out of genuine concern about the growth of smuggled morphine and cocaine and its effects on the industry; for Britain was the world's major manufacturer of morphine. The Hague conference decision that morphine and cocaine as well as opium be confined to 'legitimate medical purposes' was a crucial one. And it was again industrial interests that led to worldwide application. Germany, anxious to protect her cocaine industry, insisted on the adoption of a novel ratification procedure whereby no power was to be committed to carry out the convention until it had been accepted by a list of 34 others. Control was to be an all or nothing affair.[8] The report of the delegates recognised the importance of these economic interests in defining new boundaries.

> The Shanghai Commission directed itself mainly to the subject of the opium traffic in the Far East, and was primarily concerned with rendering assistance to the opium suppression movement which the Chinese government had lately initiated. The present convention goes far beyond this. It has dealt with morphine, cocaine, etc as well as with opium; and in prescribing measures for use of the two first mentioned drugs, and the others referred to in Chapter III, to legitimate medical purposes. ...It has, for the first time, laid down as a principle of international morality that the various countries concerned cannot stand alone in these measures.[9]

In looking at the nineteenth-century history of changing boundaries and definitions in relation to the opiates, it is the issues of professional power, technological change and the rise of a commodity-based international economy, including the rise of the pharmaceutical industry which stand out as defining issues.

### Drug and medicine: from the 1920s to the 1960s

The opiates retained a form of duality in the twentieth century. They were both 'dangerous drugs' and medicines, under systems of both legal proscription and medical prescription. It was the alkaloids which retained this duality, while less industrialised preparations –

most obviously opium smoking – fell within the proscription only model. The systems of professional discipline that had been established in the nineteenth century changed, but also remained of great significance in boundary definition. Let me illustrate this through three periods of policy crisis: the 1920s, the 1950s and the 1960s. The 1920s, about which I have written in detail elsewhere, demonstrated the power of medical, rather than pharmaceutical ownership.[10] The systems of control established in Britain after the First World War, most obviously the 1920 Dangerous Drugs Act, modified the prime nineteenth century position of pharmacy in this area. An increased emphasis was placed on medical prescription and on control of prescribing. This paralleled the greater general emphasis on the doctor's prescription for panel patients established in 1911 by the National Insurance Act. How the boundary would be drawn remained uncertain at a time of policy flux. The Home Office, the justice ministry, given responsibility for drug control in opposition to the newly established Ministry of Health, envisaged a draconian reaction on the American model, whereby users of narcotics and those who prescribed or dispensed them, would be criminalized. The issue, in its eyes, was essentially a short-term one; the 'problem' could be stamped out within a few years. Opiates (and allied cocaine) would become 'drugs'; they would be dangerous, pure and simple. But in the event 'dangerous drugs' retained their dual medicine/drug status. The 1926 Report of the Rolleston Committee on Morphine and Heroin Addiction firmly stated that addiction was the proper province of the profession, and crucially that prescription of such drugs to addicts who could not function without them was acceptable medical practice. Dr E. W. Adams, the secretary of the committee and a Ministry of Health medical civil servant, produced a memorandum in 1923, which accurately defined the rationale for this response. He wrote,

> ...if the addict is unwilling to enter into the relationship of patient to physician, but admits that he is merely coming to obtain supplies of a drug which he cannot otherwise get, then it is the clear duty of the doctor to refuse the case. But if the habitué desires treatment as a sick person for the relief of his pathological condition, the physician must be allowed to use his discretion.[11]

The distinction between illicit drug use and medical prescription was inevitably based on professional power and perceptions. Rolleston emphasised the power of the British medical profession and the 'system' it established, given the small number of addicts in the UK, endured until the 1960s. Medical control and prescribing operated within a framework of penal control, for the Home Office remained the ultimate policy authority. Medicine and legal systems had reached an accommodation. Alternative systems of professional regulation remained in operation, although increasingly subordinate to the medico-legal balance of power. Stuart Anderson's oral histories of pharmacists who practised in the interwar years show how pharmacists retained a role in over-the-counter sales for preparations that fell below the strength stipulated in the Acts, and also a role in the dispensing of opiate based medical prescriptions.[12]

The balance of power established in the 1920s was rarely challenged. When it was, professional and industrial interests emerged triumphant. In the 1950s, the World Health Organisation put pressure on the British government to ban the manufacture and medical prescription of heroin. Medical opposition to this United Nations, American-inspired move, was initially less than unanimous. But once the ban had been formally announced in 1955, a virtually united front of opposition emerged. The government backed down on a technicality in 1956 – it was apparently doubtful if the government could prohibit, rather than control, under the terms of the Dangerous Drugs Act. In America in the 1920s medical opinion had lined up in favour of prohibition when similar discussions had taken place. In Britain in the 1950s, traditions of clinical autonomy and the emphasis on legitimate medical prescribing held sway. Heroin was medicine and drug, and also a commodity.[13]

But the boundaries were realigned in the 1960s. Here the operative factor was the rise in numbers of addicts and the descent down the social scale that took place in the early 1960s. Again, as in the 1920s, it was a government committee, the Brain committee, that drove the change. There were in fact two Brain committees. The first, appointed in 1958 to investigate the situation, reported that there was no problem; the illicit market was small and addict numbers were low. The evidence it heard indicated that the Rolleston policy of medical prescription to stabilise addicts appeared to be one that there was no reason to overturn. But the committee's conclusions were disputed, and a further report in 1965 changed the balance. Prescribing was again the fulcrum of control. The Report commented,

> If there is insufficient control it may lead to the spread of addiction – as is happening at present. If, on the other hand, the restrictions are so severe as to prevent or seriously discourage the addict from

obtaining any supplies from legitimate sources it may lead to the development of an organised illicit traffic. The absence hitherto of such an organised illicit traffic has been attributed largely to the fact that an addict has been able to obtain supplies of drugs legally. But this facility has now been abused with the result that addiction has increased.[14]

The committee made three linked proposals; the restriction of supplies to addicts, the provision of specialist treatment centres, and a system of formal notification of addicts to the Home Office. Doctors other than those working at the treatment centres would be prohibited from involvement with prescribing 'dangerous drugs' to addicts. But these proposals applied only to heroin and cocaine and were only in respect of addicts. Other doctors would 'retain the right to prescribe, supply or administer any dangerous drugs required for other patients in the treatment of organic disease.' The medicine/drug dichotomy was maintained, but the boundaries between the two categories were realigned. The public health rationale of infectious disease (addiction was seen as a potential menace to the community at large) complemented the language of treatment and disease. At the same time, medical prescribing for addicts was removed from the ambit of general practice, from the power base of medical prescribing established after 1911, and located within the specialist competence of hospital-based psychiatry. Over-prescribing by a number of London-based general practitioners helped fuel the change, and also undermined the professional opposition that had killed the heroin ban. Some called the new Drug Dependence units 'prescribing clinics', but others involved in the change saw the aim as encouraging the cessation of drug use. Maintenance prescribing would work, according to Max Glatt, a psychiatrist, only with therapeutic or medical professional addicts.[15]

## The 1970s to the 1990s: the methadone story

The balance between 'dangerous drug' and licit medicine was maintained through medical ownership at these times of policy change. But the 1970s saw a new process of redefinition, in which the role of the opium alkaloids as forms of addiction 'treatment' through maintenance prescribing declined. A substitute 'medicine', methadone, replaced the medically prescribed 'drug'. Although the treatment clinics at the end of the 1960s originally prescribed heroin and even cocaine, such prescribing gave way in the 1970s initially to oral methadone and subsequently to short-term methadone prescribing over a defined period of time, with abstinence as the ultimate aim. Behind these changes, as Stimson and Oppenheimer have analysed, lay distinct developments in drug policy and clinic and medical culture.[16] Methadone offered more of a long lasting medicalized model of control than the shorter-term effects of prescribed heroin; this fitted with a post-1960s medical definition of addiction, which emphasised the social as well as the medical advantages of control. Prescribing had a social function – to prevent the spread of addiction into the general population – as well as an individualised medical one. It also fitted with the developing notion of active treatment among clinical psychiatrists and drug workers in the 1970s. A hiatus in the general spread of drug use encouraged beliefs that the 'epidemic' had been contained, underpinning a focus on 'proper treatment' in the clinics. Doctors did not wish to be perceived as surrogate shopkeepers, purveying heroin to long term users who had no wish for abstinence. Methadone and short-term prescribing offered a more professional role, and one that, as Stimson and Oppenheimer note, made the clinics nicer places for the staff to work in. Research by Hartnoll and Mitcheson – the controlled trial of heroin versus methadone prescribing – helped to establish a medical view of methadone as a more 'confrontational' form of treatment, although potentially leading to greater criminal involvement on the part of its users. It was 'active treatment' and fitted better with professional aspirations.[17]

The advent of AIDS saw a revived role for methadone (which fell from favour in the early-1980s), with again a social rationale to the fore. The Advisory Council on the Misuse of Drugs (ACMD) Part I report on *AIDS and Drug Misuse* in 1988 placed the potential spread of HIV into the general population through the medium of drug use as a greater threat to the health of the nation than drug use *per se*.[18] The priority was not, as with abstinence focused prescribing, to test the will of the drug user, but to entice him or her into treatment, with methadone as the bait. 'Competitive prescribing', a feature of the late-1960s and early-1970s, saw a revival. In the 1970s, prescribing was the bait to undercut the development of a black market. In the 1980s methadone was the presumed bait to undercut the spread of AIDS. Certainly methadone prescribing rocketed in the wake of AIDS. A substitute prescribed medicine has largely (although not entirely) replaced the medically prescribed drug, so far as the treatment of addiction is concerned.

The methadone story to date indicates some of the complexities of the interrelations between 'dangerous drug' and prescribed medicine. The rationale for methadone prescribing hinged, both in the 1970s and again post-AIDS, on a mixture of social, individual medical and public health perceptions. The use of the drug was defined as 'treatment', although at least initially it seemed little more than the replacement of a less medicalized drug (heroin) with a more medicalized one, which had distinct advantages in terms of social and medical control of the user. These broader issues of control and prevention were also part of the process of definition. In the 1970s methadone was a means of preventing a black market. In the late 1980s, its preventive function was more directly health focused, in terms of preventing the spread of AIDS.

It is interesting to note parallels with the Dutch situation. In the media it was commonplace to contrast the 'liberal' Dutch system with the supposedly more penal British policy in the 1980s. In reality, although social and medical systems were different in the two countries, the actual practice in relation to addiction was not so different. Methadone as medicalised 'drug' was common to both.

## Tobacco and nicotine: Technology and the mass market

As Sherratt[1] notes, the categories of 'drug' and 'food' leave no room for an important range of preparations with psychoactive properties, which form part of everyday consumption. High on this list of 'peculiar substances' he includes tobacco – and it is to the changing boundaries around this substance that I now turn.

If we compare tobacco as a substance with the forms of boundary change that have defined the medicine/drug dichotomy for the opiates, crucial differences emerge. Tobacco had its medical uses, and its lay consumption was based on a mix of health-based and recreational-'luxurious' rationales. But technological change developed a mass market, rather than a medical market. The cigarette was another new drug delivery system in the last quarter of the nineteenth century. Its success, as Brandt has remarked, marked the convergence of corporate capitalism, technology, mass marketing and ultimately the impact of advertising.[19] By 1919, cigarette sales had overtaken the sales of all tobacco products in the UK.[20]

Mass advertising in the interwar period brought claims that drew on health beliefs, on popular culture, on danger and allure. Cigarettes and tobacco were dangerous, but in terms of sexual attractiveness and seduction. But they were not under a system of medical or pharmaceutical control. Pharmacists did sell tobacco, and doctors did write about its health-giving properties – or worry about its use, in particular the turn of the century 'problem' of juvenile smoking, which led to restrictions on smoking through the 1908 Children Act.[21,22] But smoking remained a 'habit' rather than a disease, and the medical involvement in anti-tobacco movements (such as the National Society of Non-Smokers) was never as strong. Morality and health were entwined in disease categorisations; for anti-tobacco, the moral element was always to the fore. The cigarette, unlike the syringe, was a mass market technology.

### Epidemiological ownership and the marginality of treatment

Medical ownership or involvement did come – but through a different route and in a different set of circumstances. This was a post-Second World War phenomenon, through the epidemiological researches at the London School of Hygiene and Tropical Medicine (LSHTM) of Sir Austin Bradford Hill and Dr Richard Doll, published in the 1950s and through subsequent follow up studies of the original doctors' study.[23] The late nineteenth century debates on the opiates had hinged on whether the inebriate-addict was 'sick ' or 'bad', with the individual clinical case history as the model. The debates in the 1950s over smoking were over the nature of statistical inference and whether causality could be inferred from the cohort and prospective studies. Sir John Charles, the Chief Medical Officer, told Percy Stocks of the MRC:

> As regards the evidence, I am in general agreement with what you say, but what I was looking for was evidence apart from the analogous or purely statistical. So far as I am aware, there is no *purely* pathological evidence of this long incubation period in lung cancer...[24]

The nature of epidemiological explanation was initially debatable. But this was the route to the partial medicalization of tobacco, especially after the first Royal College of Physicians (RCP) report in 1962 gave the epidemiological case its medical authority and effectively raised the issue in the public and policy domain. Other medical disciplines – chest medicine, gastroenterology, the cancer specialities, for example – were associated, but this remained an area of medical heterogeneity.[25] Epidemiology, as the lead methodology, was associated increasingly with public health in its redefinition as community medicine in the 1960s.[26] This was essentially a population strategy-focused discipline rather than treatment-based.

The essential components of the dual medical categorisation of the opiates in the twentieth century were therefore absent. Tobacco was not a medicine which could be prescribed. Nor was it prescribable in maintenance form for the treatment of continued use. The 'treatment' model was in fact weakly established. A number of anti-smoking clinics were set up in the wake of the Doll–Hill research reports and the RCP publication, but medical involvement was limited. Martin Raw, a psychologist, noted in a article published in the 1970s, how most clinic treatment was psychologically oriented, with walk in clinics and group therapy.[27] Therapy was based on psychological theories of learned behaviour. Hypnosis, aversion therapy, rapid smoking and 'satiation' all had their advocates. But their was little medical involvement. Psychologists were using the theory of dependence – which neatly allied psychological with biomedical theories – but psychiatry established little of a foothold in this area. Nor was the idea of treatment acceptable to all who worked in the smoking arena. The public health activist Simon Chapman attacked the concept because of the need to involve a wider range of health professionals. The concept of treatment was also less welcomed by an anti-tobacco movement which, at least from the 1970s, saw abstinence through self control as the answer.[28]

The rise of the primary health care model and the rehabilitation of the General Practitioner (GP) led to advocacy of his/her potential role in treatment of alcoholism and tobacco smoking. Michael Russell's article of the late-1970s showed the value of 'brief intervention' by a GP in securing a greater degree of smoking cessation (paralleling similar research on alcohol advice through GPs).[29] But, at this stage, primary care had no medical 'treatment' to offer. Prescribing did not enter the discussion; this was simply advice and the image of the authority of the 'family doctor'. The treatment focused medical ownership which had played such an important role in the policy struggles of the 1920s and the 1960s so far as drugs were concerned was only weakly established for smoking, and was operated by psychologists rather than by doctors at the specialist clinic level.

## Policy strategies, the market and medicine

The policy struggles over how this 'substance' was to be defined and regulated therefore took a different form. They operated within the 'drug safety' area of health policy rather than that of medical treatment. This is a crucial defining difference in the history of smoking policy. The policy model considered appropriate in the 1970s was akin to the model of voluntary cooperation used for government and pharmaceutical industry relationships. It was a model of industrial cooperation, rather than the 'medical model' with no industrial involvement that had been put in place for the opiates. The difference in approach is illustrated by the work of the Independent Scientific Committee on Smoking and Health (ISCSH) in the 1970s. The committee was set up in the wake of the government response to the second Royal College of Physicians Report in 1971, after Sir Keith Joseph had signed the first of the voluntary agreements with the industry about the labelling of cigarette packets and the warning notices on advertisements. The Committee's role was to advise both government and the tobacco companies on science; its membership came from a variety of medical specialities. Sir Peter Froggatt, chairman of the Committee in the 1980s, recognised the basic irony: it was tar in cigarettes that did the damage, but most smokers smoked to obtain the nicotine, which so many argued, conferred benefit. Why not remove the tar, or just have nicotine? The objective here, as applied to smoked tobacco, was called 'product modification'.[30] For much of the 1970s, the Committee was preoccupied with an ambitious product-modification project – the launch of alternative tobacco products (New Smoking Material and Cytrel) which were aimed to take over the smoking market. The failure of these products when they were launched in the late-1970s led the Committee to concentrate on modification of existing cigarettes.[31] In doing this, it fell foul of other researchers in the tobacco field. Its second report, issued in 1979, was criticised for its advocacy of low tar-low nicotine cigarettes; critical researchers argued that this could lead to the phenomenon of 'compensatory smoking' which would lead to more harm rather than less.

This 'product modification' line within policy was allied to political moves of relevance to the reconceptualization of the 'substance' of tobacco. In the mid-1970s, David Owen, the new Labour Minister of Health, as part of general moves against smoking, proposed to place all tobacco products, consisting of, or containing, a substitute for tobacco or an additive to tobacco, under the provisions of the 1968 Medicines Act.[32] These products would need a product licence from government. The licence would be granted on advice received from a statutory committee on the safety of the product; the committee was to be based on the existing ISCSH. In the event, this legal redefinition did not occur; Owen moved on and succeeding Ministers were less effective in pushing the strategy forward.

But it is worth reflecting on this period of attempted

renegotiation of boundaries. Much existing commentary is framed in the 'heroes and villains' style, in which events are ascribed to 'industry influence'. Certainly relationships with the industry were close, and both Hunter and the secretary of the committee subsequently moved over to work for the tobacco industry. But there are other, less polemical, perspectives on this sequence of events. At one level, the objective of these policy moves was similar to the 'harm reduction' objectives of the drug policy debates of the 1920s. 'Fundamentally', said Hunter in a article presented to the Royal College of Physicians in Edinburgh in 1976, 'it is accepted that some people will go on smoking'.[33] Given that, the objective was to ensure that smoking was as risk-free as possible, and that it was less addictive, so that fewer people would indulge excessively in the habit. But the arena in which the committee operated was quite different to Rolleston or Brain. This was the drug safety area of regulation, both conceptually and institutionally. A senior civil servant, who had been medical assessor for the Committee on Safety of Medicines, commented,

> Godber wanted food, the environment and chemicals under one man – I moved and smoking was added in. They were similar issues to the CSM (Committee on Safety of Medicines) - it was the dose-response relationship for tar and nicotine...[34]

Hunter, Chairman of ISCSH, also chaired the clinical trials subcommittee of the CSM. The relationships were determined by this conceptual location within a complex that included similar links with the pharmaceutical industry. With both, it was accepted that there was an ultimate difference in objective. Both industries wanted safe products, in order to increase sales, whereas the government regulatory committees sought improvements in health as a primary aim. But both sides accepted relationships with industry as the means of achieving these aims.[35]

The events of the 1970s are significant from the point of view of changing places, in that they marked an attempt, through drug safety, to move tobacco more closely within the boundaries that applied to regulated medicines. We can relate this to a more general redrawing of the boundaries around drugs and medicines in the late 1960s and early 1970s, expressed through the 1968 Medicines Act and through the new Misuse of Drugs Act in 1971, events that are more usually considered in isolation. The boundaries between (illicit) drugs and (licit) medicines were being redrawn and tobacco was potentially being drawn into the regulated medicines camp.

The membership of the ISCSH was medically dominated, but there were also, by the 1970s, strong interests in the field arguing, not for risk reduction, but for the elimination of smoking. Action on Smoking and Health (ASH), founded in 1971 in the wake of the second RCP Report, was the vehicle for these aims. There is no time in this article to dwell on ASH in detail; I have argued elsewhere that, in its formation and operation, it represented a new style of medico-consumerist alliance with a strong emphasis on media publicity to influence policy.[36] Two of its directors, Mike Daube (in the 1970s) and David Simpson (in the 1980s), with their roots in organisations like Shelter and Amnesty, epitomized the change. But the alliance with medicine and the medical case was central. The involvement with the emergent public health agenda for policy was crucial. ASH argued for higher tobacco duty, for advertising controls, for media publicity, rather than for a 'medical model' of treatment or for risk reduction.

## Medicalisation, nicotine and addiction

The sustained push for medicalisation came from a different direction – through the rise of the concept of addiction from the 1970s; through related work on the role of nicotine; and through the debates on the appropriate policy towards this active principle. Should it be maintenance treatment – or prohibited drug? The notion of addiction had been around in various forms in the smoking area for some while, but had never been as strongly established for tobacco as for opium or for alcohol. The concept of inebriety which united those two substances in a late-nineteenth-century medical paradigm, was rarely applied to tobacco. Both the 1962 and the 1971 RCP Reports discussed this aspect of the desire to smoke.[37] The 1961 report noted that there were few occasional tobacco smokers - smoking was more habit forming than drinking. It also noted that it was reported that injections of nicotine could relieve the desire for a cigarette – 'this may be due to nicotine addiction.' The 1971 Report's section on the 'smoking habit' contained discussions of motivation and psychology, including Freudian explanations and the role of personality and inheritance. But it also noted that some craved for nicotine, and that 'dependent smokers' needed special clinics.[38] Psychology was influential in smoking in the early-1970s and 'dependence' was the leading theoretical concept – a construct that was also influential within the alcohol and drugs fields at the same period and which had the authority of WHO behind it. 'Dependence' epitomised an alliance between the older theory of addiction, with its biomedical overtones, and newer personality oriented approaches. It was the 'modernising' approach to addiction, supported by psychology, the lead discipline, with a treatment focus.

At the same time, work on nicotine was more clearly identifying its role in this process. A leading smoking researcher – also medically qualified – pointed out in an interview that knowledge of neurotransmitters and the brain had been underway since the 1950s and 1960s and had included work on nicotine. But this work took place in a different scientific arena to that on smoking. 'Pharmacology talked about nicotine, but the conferences on smoking didn't.'[39] Again technology played a role in developing awareness. Michael Russell and Colin Feyerabend's development of the blood nicotine assay in the early-1970s enabled more precise estimation of blood nicotine concentrations in smokers and led to an expansion of work at the newly established Addiction Research Unit at the Institute of Psychiatry and to significant moves to bring tobacco, alcohol and illicit drugs together under the same conceptual banner.[40, 41] Even earlier work on nicotine had taken place at the Tobacco Research Council's Harrogate laboratories and had been published in *Nature* in 1968.[42] The Harrogate labs pioneered the nicotine work and the use of smoking machines. A scientist there remembered,

> We were free to publish, although that wasn't the case for the skin painting work ...The team was productive and there was a stream of papers. This was the best part of my career ...we were the leading team in the field and at every key symposium....[43]

I cannot give here a detailed 'scientific history' of the emergence of the role of nicotine. Russell's work was taken further in the US in the early 1980s; and in the UK the work of the Tobacco Products Research Trust, funded through a tobacco industry levy as part of the voluntary agreements in the 1980s, and supervised by the ISCSH, saw a programme of research that took in the role of nicotine.[44] This research was published at the end of the decade in a book edited by Nicholas Wald and Sir Peter Froggatt, *Nicotine, Smoking and the Low Tar Programme* (1989).[45] Discussion focused on three areas: the supposed benefits of nicotine; its role in the process of 'compensatory smoking' – the process by which smoke from a cigarette with a high nicotine yield and a given tar yield is inhaled to a lesser extent than smoke from a cigarette yielding less nicotine but the same tar yield (higher nicotine therefore giving less inhalation); and the extent to which nicotine is a co-carcinogen and its maintenance in cigarettes therefore ill-advised.

Manipulation of the tar and nicotine content of cigarettes had been one continuing arm of the ISCSH's 'risk reduction' strategy after the failure of tobacco substitutes. New technology opened up another avenue. The development of nicotine replacement therapy (NRT) through the Swedish pharmaceutical industry and its association with researchers at the Institute of Psychiatry offered a further route to medicalisation and treatment.[46] Here was the 'medicine' which smoking had lacked. But the equivocal status of tobacco again made matters more complex. The CSM licensed nicotine chewing gum in 1980 for general use as an anti-smoking aid, a decision based on the usual grounds of safety and efficacy. But another committee in the regulatory structure, the significantly titled Advisory Committee on Borderline Substances, ruled out its use in NHS prescriptions because of doubts about efficacy. NRT was therefore in the odd position of being the only prescription-based medicine which was not available on the NHS. A doctor who did write such a prescription was brought before an NHS tribunal – an interesting and significant contrast to the policing of heroin prescribing in the 1920s. In the 1990s came further change as some nicotine products moved into the over the counter (OTC) category, meaning that they could be sold under pharmaceutical supervision. But there were still grey areas. In 1995, for example, nicotine nasal spray was prescribable, but the prescription had to be approved by the Family Health Services Authority (FHSA), the GPs local supervisory body.[47] With the election of the Labour government in 1997 and a greater emphasis on anti-smoking policies, doctors were again pushing for NRT to be available on prescription; it was seen both as an aid to stopping smoking, but also as a form of maintenance treatment. There were obvious parallels here with the role of methadone for opiate addiction.

The interplay of addiction with nicotine and the debates it occasioned is an interesting one. At one level, reverting to the 'heroes and villains' mode of much smoking policy analysis, it can be portrayed as a story of 'discovery' and 'concealment', with industry knowing about the addictive properties of a 'dangerous drug' well before other researchers were aware. My view is that the picture is a more complex one. Events again need understanding in the context of the time. Dependence, not addiction, was the construct that found support in its associated scientific community in the 1970s; and work on nicotine proceeded in different scientific arenas. It lacked its scientific 'product champions' within smoking. The significance of this story is more that scientific and activist communities began to change strategy and to focus some of their arguments around nicotine and addiction in the 1980s. The interplay of policy agendas, strategies and science was a symbiotic one. For the mainstream public health constituency, addiction was initially an unwelcome concept, because it removed the notion of individual responsibility, which was central to the public health case. But the late-1980s and 1990s have seen a reversal of that stance; addiction has become a means whereby tobacco industry responsibility can be established through a series of legal actions. But – important for our analysis of the medical–non medical boundary – addiction and the role of nicotine has also strengthened the notion of treatment and of maintenance. Wald and Froggatt noted that addiction was a two-edged sword. It was a reason either to maintain nicotine concentrations or to lower them in order to wean people off the habit.[48]

Michael Russell, long a proponent of nicotine, argued in an anonymous *Lancet* editorial in 1991, that the government should be promoting purified nicotine products at the same time as imposing stringent regulation of the constituents of tobacco smoke. People smoked for nicotine – but the cigarette was essentially a dirty drug delivery system. It therefore seemed logical to offer a cleaner product. There was

> no compelling objection to recreational and even addictive use of nicotine provided it was not shown to be harmful to the user and to others.[49]

Mainstream public health researchers have joined this argument. Ann McNeill, of the Health Education Authority, Martin Raw and others have called for a Nicotine Regulatory Authority for all nicotine products and for nicotine maintenance through a variety of technical means.[50] McNeill and others argue in part from the addiction model, recognising that, despite the declining cultural acceptability of smoking, a 'hard core' will not quit and need 'treatment-maintenance'.[51] The increased visibility of 'poor smokers' and current debates round inequalities have added urgency to these arguments.

The future of these debates is not the subject of the article. But it is instructive to note how they differ from the same science in a different policy context. Nicotine and addiction in the US have not led to the route of medicalization and treatment. Nicotine is to be controlled under the FDA as a 'drug' (not a medicine), and one policy conclusion drawn from the nicotine research is that nicotine should be removed from cigarettes. There is no interest in alternative nicotine delivery systems. One can draw parallels with the 1920s policy moves around illicit drugs in both countries and the divergence between the medicalized and non-medicalized systems that were then established. Nicotine, like heroin and the opiates, is being demonised in the US; while in the UK, partial medicalization is on the agenda, even for public health interests.

## Conclusion: why?

Both substances have shown definitional elements in common – the role of technology; industrial involvement, the rise of the concept of addiction – yet the ways in which these elements have interacted over time have differed. Any explanation of this divergence has to include the broad context of commodities, consumption and culture, and the relationship with technology. Opiates were embryo mass market drugs/medicines in the nineteenth century, with a culture of consumption. But they operated increasingly within systems of medico-pharmaceutical regulation. Technology (the syringe) served to amplify medical ownership. Cultural acceptability was declining by the end of the century – a change that can be related to the expansion of other industry products; to changes within medicine; and to greater access to state run systems of health care. The trading and production economy for these drugs supported greater restriction through international regulation (albeit only as a diversionary tactic, and some companies continued to be involved in the illicit traffic in the 1920s). Tobacco, on the other hand, operated differently within the developing mass market. Systems of medico-pharmaceutical regulation were only weakly established. Technology (the cigarette) amplified a mass market rather than restricting it. Cultural acceptability was increasing.

These issues provide the broader context to more specific policy developments in the post-war period. Here the different routes for medicalization and professional control have been significant. For drugs, the role of psychiatry has been of enormous importance and the treatment model central to policy. Even the 'public health model' apparently established as a response to AIDS relied on treatment, and on methadone maintenance as a preventive strategy. This was a strategy acceptable to the wider 'policy community' around drugs that developed in the 1980s. As one policy researcher remarked, it was in no one's interests to argue that treatment did not work. Policy documents, the Crime and Disorder Bill, for example, link treatment more closely to the criminal justice system and hence reinforce the drug policy community's coherence round this medical issue. The duality of medicine and drug remains.

For tobacco, the picture is less clear cut. While psychiatry rediscovered the concept of addiction for alcohol and drugs in the 1950s, epidemiologists were advancing concepts of probability and risk in relation to smoking. Tobacco was a commodity, and the policy debates in the ISCSH were framed in this context, taking on the 'drug safety' issue. The smoking 'policy community', based in public health-community medicine, had little time for treatment, which was in any case associated with the non-medical discipline of psychology. The 'belated medicalization' of the 1980s and 1990s should be located in changing strategies within this public health constituency and its adherence to the nicotine addiction model, allied to the rediscovery of risk reduction through nicotine. Declining cultural acceptability has also given greater prominence to the 'medical model'. In short then, both illicit drugs and tobacco-nicotine demonstrate how complex and symbiotic interrelationships between scientific constructs, policy alliances, culture and consumption, have helped to determine changing places. And of course, they are not the only substances I could have used to demonstrate this point. The current moves to change the boundaries round definitions of cannabis and to establish its medical utility draw on the history of that drug-substance. That, although another story, also illustrates the general theme.

## Acknowledgements

I am grateful to the Wellcome Trust for funding the smoking research represented in part of this article and also for funding the 'Science speaks to Policy Programme' which has enabled cross-substance comparisons to be drawn. I am grateful to participants in the Anglo–Dutch conference and especially to Henk Van der Velden and Marijke Gijswijt-Hofstra for their comments on my presentation. My thanks are due to Ingrid James for secretarial assistance.

## Notes

1. A. Sherratt, 'Introduction; Peculiar substances' in J. Goodman, P. Lovejoy and A. Sherratt (eds), *Consuming Habits: Drugs in history and anthropology* (London: Routledge, 1995).
2. See also J. Parascandola, 'The drug habit: the assocation of the word "drug" with abuse in American history' in R. Porter, M. Teich (eds), *Drugs and Narcotics in History* (Cambridge: Cambridge University

Press, 1995).
3. J. Pereira, *Elements of Materia Medica*, Vol. 2, 1839–40 (London: Longman, Orme, Browne, Green and Longmans), 1301.
4. These developments are discussed in V. Berridge, *Opium and the People: Opiate Use and Drug Control Policy in nineteenth and early twentieth century England* (London: Free Association Books, second edition, 1999).
5. T. Hardy, *The Trumpet Major* (London: Smith, Elder and Co., 1880), 274.
6. These are discussed in V. Berridge, *op.cit.* (note 4).
7. British Parliamentary Papers. (B.P.P.) *Final Report of the Royal Commission on Opium,* XLIII (1895), 133.
8. H. Richard Friman, 'German and the transformation of cocaine, 1880-1920' in P. Gottenberg (ed.) *Cocaine: Global Histories* (London: Routledge, 1999) ascribes these events more to the stance taken by the German government than to pressure from the German cocaine industry.
9. TBA. *Report of the British Delegates to the International Opium Conference,* British Parliamentary Papers, LXVIII (1912–13).
10. V. Berridge, '"Stamping out addiction": The work of the Rolleston Committee, 1924–26' in G. Berrios and H. Freeman (eds), *150 years of British Psychiatry,* Vol. 2 (London: Athlone Press, 1996).
11. Memorandum by Dr E. W. Adams, 1923, in Ministry of Health papers, PRO MH 58/275.
12. S. Anderson and V. Berridge, 'Opium in Twentieth Century Britain: Pharmacists, Regulation and the People', *Addiction,* 95(2000), 23–36.
13. The heroin ban is touched on in P. Bartrip, *Themselves Writ Large: The British Medical Association,* 1832-1966 (London: BMJ Publishing Group, 1996) and in V. Berridge, 'The Society for the Study of Addiction, 1884–1988', *British Journal of Addiction,* special issue, 85 (1990), 983–1087.
14. Interdepartmental Committee on Drug Addiction, *Report* (London: HMSO, 1965), 7.
15. Interview with Max Glatt, in G. Edwards (ed.), *Addictions. Personal Influences and Scientific Movements* (New Brunswick and London: Transaction Publishers, 1991).
16. G. Stimson, E. Oppenheimer, *Heroin Addiction, Treatment and Control in Britain* (London: Tavistock, 1982).
17. R. L. Hartnoll, M. C. Mitcheson, A. Battersby, G. Brown, M. Ellis, P. Fleming, N. Hedley, 'Evaluation of heroin maintenance in controlled trial', *Archives of General Psychiatry,* 37 (1980), 877.

18. Advisory Council on the Misuse of Drugs, *AIDS and Drug Misuse*, part one (London: HMSO, 1988).
19. A. Brandt, 'The Cigarette, Risk and American Culture', *Daedalus*, Fall (1990), 155–76.
20. B. W. C. Alford, *W. D. and H. O. Wills and the Development of the UK Tobacco Industry*, 1786–1965 (London: Methuen and Co., 1973).
21. J. Welshman, ' Images of Youth: The problem of juvenile smoking, 1900–1939', *Addiction*, 91 (1996), 1379–86.
22. M. Hilton, '"Tabs", "Fags" and the "Boy Labour problem" in late-Victorian and Edwardian Britain', *Journal of Social History*, 28 (1995) 587–607.
23. R. Doll and A. Bradford Hill, 'Smoking and Carcinoma of the Lung. Preliminary Report', *British Medical Journal*, ii (30 September 1950), 739–48.
24. Sir John Charles to Percy Stocks, 18 February 1953, in Ministry of Health papers, (PRO MH 55/1011).
25. For discussion of these developments, see V. Berridge, 'Science and Policy: The case of postwar British smoking policy', in S. Lock, L. Reynolds, and E. M. Tansey (eds), *Ashes to Ashes: The History of Smoking and Health* (Amsterdam: Rodopi, 1998), 143–63.
26. J. Lewis, *What Price Community Medicine? The Philosophy, Practice and Politics of Public Health since 1919* (Brighton, Sussex: Wheatsheaf, 1986).
27. M. Raw, 'The Treatment of Cigarette Dependence' in Y. Israel, F. B. Glaser, H. Kalant, R. E. Popham (eds), W. Schmidt and R. G. Smart, *Research Advances in Alcohol and Drug Problems*, vol. 4 (New York: Plenum Publishing Corporation, 1978).
28. S. Chapman, 'The role of doctors in promoting smoking cessation. Doctors can't do much on their own; public policy can', *British Medical Journal*, 307 (1993), 518–19.
29. M. A. H. Russell, *et al.*, 'Effect of general practitioner's advice against smoking', *British Medical Journal*, ii (1979), 231.
30. P. Froggatt, 'Determinants of policy on smoking and health', *International Journal of Epidemiology*, 18 (1) (1989), 1–9.
31. Independent Scientific Committee of [sic] Smoking and Health, *Second report. Developments in Tobacco products and the Possibility of 'Lower-Risk' Cigarette* (London: HMSO, 1979).
32. For a critical view of these moves, from a public health activist, see M. Daube, 'The politics of smoking: thoughts on the Labour record', *Community Medicine*, 1 (1979), 306–14.
33. R. B. Hunter, 'Smoking and Health. The philosophy of the

Committee', paper presented to the Royal College of Physicians, Edinburgh, 21 April 1976 and reprinted as a pamphlet. British Library official publications library.
34. Interview by V. Berridge with civil servant, UK Department of Health, April 1997. Interview conducted on an anonymous basis.
35. For the pharmaceutical industry, see J. Abraham, *Science, Politics and the Pharmaceutical Industry. Controversy and Bias in Drug Regulation* (London: UCL Press, 1995).
36. See V. Berridge, *op. cit.* (note 25).
37. See, for example, Royal College of Physicians, London, *Summary of a Report of the RCP of London on Smoking in Relation to Cancer of the Lung and other Diseases* (London: Pitman Medical Publishing Co. Ltd, 1962).
38. Royal College of Physicians, *Smoking and Health Now. A new report on smoking and its effects on health from the Royal College of Physicians of London* (London: Pitman Medical and Scientific Publishing Co. Ltd, 1971).
39. Interview by V. Berridge with addiction pharmacologist, Institute of Psychiatry, October, 1997. Interview conducted on an anonymous basis.
40. For an example of this cross substance conceptualisation, see G. Edwards, M. A. H. Russell, D. Hawks and M. MacCafferty, *Alcohol Dependence and Smoking Behaviour* (Farnborough: Saxon House and Lexington Books, 1976).
41. M. A. H. Russell, C. Wilson, U. A. Patel, P. V. Cole, C. Feyerabend, 'Comparison of effect on tobacco consumption and carbon monoxide absorption of changing to high and low nicotine cigarettes', *British Medical Journal*, iv (1973), 512–16.
42. A. K. Armitage et al., 'Pharmacological Basis for the Tobacco Smoking Habit', *Nature*, 217 (1968), 331–4.
43. Interview by V. Berridge with industry researcher, January, 1998. Interview conducted on an anonymous basis.
44. C. Swann and P. Froggatt, *The Tobacco Products Research Trust, 1982–1996* (London: RSM Press Ltd, 1996).
45. N. Wald and P. Froggatt (eds), *Nicotine, Smoking and the Low Tar programme* (Oxford: Oxford University Press, 1989).
46. 'Conversation with Ove Ferno', *Addiction*, 89 (1994), 1215–26.
47. These changes can be traced through the relevant issues of the *British National Formulary*. I am also grateful to Stuart Anderson for advice on this point.
48. Wald and Froggatt, *op. cit.* (note 45).
49. Anonymous, 'Nicotine use after the year 2000', *Lancet*, 337 (1991),

1191–2.
50. M. Raw, *Regulating Nicotine Delivery Systems. Harm reduction and the prevention of Smoking related Disease* (London: Health Education Authority, 1997).
51. A. McNeill, 'Harm reduction and tobacco control', paper delivered at the Society for the Study of Addiction annual conference, Bath, November 1997.

# 2

## Pharmacists, druggists and the spirit of Thorbecke: The shaping of Dutch pharmacy, 1865–c.1920

### Frank Huisman

In 1865, the Dutch parliament promulgated four laws concerning the organisation of the medical profession and the national health care system.[1] An important aspect of this legislation, which was to regulate health care in The Netherlands for many decades, was the elevation of pharmacy to academic levels. Henceforth, the only possibility of becoming a pharmacist was to enrol in the pharmaceutical programme at one of the four Dutch universities. Initially, the legislation was welcomed by the Dutch Society for the Advancement of Pharmacy (*Nederlandsche Maatschappij ter bevordering der Pharmacie,* hereafter *Pharmaceutical Society*) and leaders in the pharmaceutical field. Since the druggist exam was abolished at the same time, it was expected that the druggist trade would gradually disappear. Many believed that the laws had granted pharmacists a monopoly in the field of the preparation and delivery of medicines.[2]

This, however, was not the case. Indeed, it had never even been the intention of J. R. Thorbecke (1798–1872), the Minister of Internal Affairs who had drafted the laws.[3] According to this liberal politician, the state should limit itself to supplying pharmaceutical education of academic standard, and to the inspection of the professional conduct of the academic professions. Consumer choice or inter-professional relationships were no concern of the state. The implication of this was that pharmacists had to earn credit and legitimacy with the public on their own. They had to define (and uphold) their academic identity and professional standards, while at the same time fighting a fierce struggle for survival with many competitors in the medical marketplace, among whom were dispensing physicians, druggists, quacks and the emerging pharmaceutical industry. Here I shall chart relationships in Dutch pharmacy until roughly the First World War, beginning with the crucial Medical Laws of 1865 that were to form the legal framework of Dutch pharmacy up to 1958. I shall do so by looking into the legal and rhetorical aspects of intra-professional relationships against the backdrop of a modernising health care system.

### Raising pharmacy to academic levels

Already in the 1840s there had been powerful pleas for the introduction of a pharmaceutical curriculum at university, in order to raise standards of pharmacy and emancipate pharmacists in the process.[4] In fact, this desire led to the foundation of the Dutch Society for the Advancement of Pharmacy in 1842.[5] In those years, academic pharmacy was part of the medical curriculum; the pharmaceutical doctoral degree could only be granted to physicians (*doctores medicinae*). After many years of laborious debate in parliament, the long-awaited legislation finally materialised in the 1860s and 1870s.

In drawing up his bills, Minister Thorbecke had been led by three guiding principles: first, he wanted to separate pharmacy (*artsenijbereidkunde*) from medicine; secondly, he wanted to enhance the position of pharmacists by allowing those who were qualified to study pharmacy at university; and finally, he intended to limit the competence of druggists to the wholesale trade in medicines. Henceforth, whoever wanted to practise pharmacy had to meet stringent requirements; on top of that, there were strict laws regulating pharmaceutical practice. A Medical State Inspection was installed to supervise compliance with the law. Two later laws completed the process that had been initiated by Thorbecke. The Law on Higher Education (1876) stipulated that pharmacy and toxicology were to become academic disciplines. It created an independent Faculty of Science as well as the possibility of obtaining a doctoral degree in pharmacy. Each of the four Dutch universities got its own chair of pharmacy and toxicology, housed in the newly founded Faculties of Science. Finally, the effect of the Law on Physicians (*artsenwet*) of 1878 was that the practical pharmacists' exam could only be taken by those with a specific preliminary qualification (*HBS: Hogere Burger School*, a new type of school, established in 1863), followed by an exam in physics and theoretical pharmacy. Henceforth, the only road to pharmaceutical competence was through university.[6]

By the end of the 1870s, an entirely new infrastructure of medical education and medical supervision had come into being. Expectations were that it would raise pharmacy to academic levels.

However, there was a long way to go before this could be realised: most pharmacists had not (yet) received an academic education and patients were hardly inclined to value the pharmacist more than other medicine vendors. Given this situation, it was crucial to create a public image of pharmacy and pharmacists that fitted in with the high ideals of the pharmaceutical leaders. Professors of pharmacy and executives of the *Pharmaceutical Society* (NMP) devoted themselves to this task. In their inaugural addresses, in a new historiography – devoted to the history of pharmacy – and in deontological publications they created a professional image of the pharmacist as a man of honour and science, who was entitled to a prominent position in the health care system.[7]

As has been stated above, each of the four Dutch universities got its own chair of pharmacy and toxicology in the wake of the Law on Higher Education. In 1877 and 1878 the four new professors took office. With the exception of the Groningen professor Pieter Cornelis Plugge (1847–1897) all were pupils of Gerrit Jan Mulder (1802–1880), the *paterfamilias* of nineteenth century Dutch chemistry and pharmacy.[8] At Leiden university Eduard Alexander Van der Burg (1833–1890) was appointed, in Utrecht Hendrik Wefers Bettink (1839–1921), while Willem Stoeder (1831–1902) saw his efforts for pharmacy rewarded with a chair in Amsterdam. The last was made responsible for the teaching of pharmacy without pharmaceutical chemistry, which had been taught by Jan Willem Gunning (1827–1900) from 1865.

In their inaugural addresses the new professors sketched the profile of the young academic discipline.[9] All showed a great awareness of the historical moment for pharmacy and pharmaceutical chemistry, as can be concluded from the fact that all called attention to the genesis of the discipline, trying to trace the moment 'pharmacy' had emancipated itself from medicine and become an autonomous discipline. A second theme that ran through their arguments related to the scientific character of pharmacy, considered as the crucial trait of modern pharmacy. A decade before Gunning had dwelt on the specific characteristics of modern science. His inaugural address, delivered on the occasion of his appointment as professor of chemistry and pharmacy at the *Atheneum Illustre* in Amsterdam in 1865, was completely devoted to this theme.[10] At the centre of modern scientific research is the physical object, not the researcher. Gunning argued that this was the trait that distinguished it from past, anthropomorphic, science: 'Nature cannot be explained from man, but only from itself'. He made his point clear using the history of the chemical elements. Classical authors had limited themselves to direct and personal perceptions of nature. Their anthropomorphic conception of nature had led them to accept contemplations of the sensations that had been stirred up by natural objects and phenomena as explanations. According to Gunning, chemistry had become an independent science when analogy and metaphor were no longer accepted as scientific argument. Hence, the fundamental turn in the history of science had been of a psychological nature: the modern scientist found himself in a state of self-denial owing to the fact that he renunciated everyday human subjectivity. As a teacher, Gunning considered it his main duty to instruct his students to an 'objective contemplation of nature'.

In very general terms, this characterises the academic, scientific profile of the modern pharmacist that Gunning and his colleagues envisaged. According to them, chemistry and pharmacy had gone through a major transformation in the nineteenth century. In their modern scientific shape they were being taught at the renewed universities. To the new professors, the superiority of the 'new pharmacy' was self-evident. The only thing they had to do was to convey this optimism to society at large. In 1865, Thorbecke had not much liked the suggestion of the *Pharmaceutical Society* (NMP) that the Netherlands should follow the example of Germany, where pharmacies were subject to strict state control. Instead, the Dutch health care system had very much been organised along the lines of his liberal principles. This implied that the state should only have a facilitating role, creating educational and inspecting institutions as preconditions to a national health care system. Its actual *appearance* should be left to pressures within society. This in turn implied that pharmacists had to create a professional image that was appealing to the public. It was the only way to earn credit and legitimacy, considering the fact that therapeutic possibilities remained rather limited until well into the twentieth century. In short: they had to make clear what distinguished them from both physicians and druggists.

### Creating the new pharmacist

Amsterdam-based Professor Willem Stoeder had been among those who had insisted on the emancipation of pharmacy.[11] He advocated the establishment of university chairs for pharmacy, not just because of the stormy developments within chemistry, but as a logical sequel to the legislation of 1865 – which demanded scientific training for pharmacists – as well. His motto *'La médecine et la pharmacie sont soeurs*' (medicine and pharmacy are sisters) is an indication of his perspective on the position of pharmacy.

In *Pharmaceutisch weekblad*, the weekly magazine of the *Pharmaceutical Society (NMP)*, Stoeder published a series of articles that was meant to contribute to a new representation of pharmacy and its practitioners. In this nine-part series, called 'Letters from the capital', Stoeder developed a deontology for the modern pharmacist.[12] The Medical Laws of 1865 had only created the *possibility* for the development of a class of pharmacists with a high sense of their duties. Now it was up to them to use the possibilities, academic training being the key to success. A pharmacist should earn public esteem as well as patient trust. He was no mere shopkeeper but a scientist. He should not tarnish his reputation by selling secret remedies or non-pharmaceutical commodities like paint, perfumes and the like. In this context, Stoeder contrasted the 'fairground attraction' of the shop-windows of Paris pharmacists with the 'tasteful simplicity and dignity' of their German colleagues. In his 'Letters' Stoeder showed himself to be an advocate of a strict separation between medicine and pharmacy. He did not allow pharmacists to give medical advice. In their own interest as well as in that of public health they should concentrate fully on the preparation of medicines according to the prescriptions of physicians, and on the analysis of, and information on, *specialités*. According to Stoeder, social success would be the logical result of scientific education and ethical elevation.

Stoeder has made another important contribution to the elevation of pharmacists. In 1891, he published a book on the history of Dutch pharmacy, which has remained a standard work for decades.[13] It was meant as a defence of pharmacy as a science and of pharmacists as scientists. Stoeder wanted to offer an alternative to the prevailing image, in which the physician was associated with the provision of services and the pharmacist with commerce.[14] His book was organised along chronological lines, divided into three periods: the first ran from the origin of the independent pharmacist (apothecary) in the fourteenth century to the publication of the first Dutch pharmacopoeia in 1636; the second up to the abolishment of the guilds and *collegia medica* in 1798; and the third up to Thorbecke's legislation of 1865.[15] The first witnessed the emergence of the trade of apothecaries, while medicine disposed of tradesmanlike pharmacy; during the second period pharmacy developed into an organised activity (although apothecaries always remained subordinate to physicians, who were their examiners and the inspectors of their shops). During the third period, pharmacy emancipated itself because of major developments in chemistry. According to Stoeder, the history of both science and trade pointed in the same direction, to which they were a prelude: the liberation of pharmacy in the last quarter of the nineteenth century.

To Stoeder, the Laws of 1865 were a culmination of previous developments. The foundation of the *Pharmaceutisch weekblad* in 1864 he considered a way of meeting the growing need for a platform on which scientific problems could be discussed; the annual reports of the *Pharmaceutical Society* (NMP) of 1866 and 1867 breathed 'a lively scientific spirit'; thanks to the new chairs of pharmacy 'the frontiers of knowledge and abilities' could be pushed back constantly.[16] At the end of the nineteenth century, the pharmacist had reached the same level as the physician.[17] In short: Stoeder was very optimistic and had high hopes for the future of pharmacy.

With regard to the creation of a professional identity through history, the creation of a pharmaceutical hall of fame was at least as important as historiography. For the great men of science memorial stones and statues were being erected. Among them were not only pharmacists and chemists, but botanists, zoologists and mineralogists as well. Pharmacists could follow their shining example.[18] During the last quarter of the nineteenth century many pharmaceutical '*lieux de mémoires*' were erected. To name but two examples: in 1892, a statue of Carl Wilhelm Scheele was unveiled in Sweden, while in the Netherlands, a pharmaceutical museum opened its doors in 1906.[19]

## Competence and competition

To what extent did practising pharmacists meet the professional standards their scientific leaders had created? Thorbecke expected that the Medical Laws of 1865 – together with the Law on Higher Education that was to follow – would raise the 'level of study and competence' of pharmacists.[20] The pharmaceutical leaders shared this expectation. They were very happy with the raising of pharmacy to academic levels and with the doctorate of pharmacy, established in 1876. Stoeder considered the doctorate as a 'fine reward for industry and diligence'; he expressed his wish that Dutch pharmacists would prove themselves worthy of that crown.[21] Evidence suggests the 'field' had less elevated thoughts on the subject. In order to become legally competent as a pharmacist, the state pharmacy exam sufficed. The doctorate added nothing but scientific status. Very few pharmacists have actually used the opportunity to take their doctoral degree in pharmacy.[22] In 1887, Gunning established the fact that out of 130 people who had become pharmacists since 1876, only three had valued the doctorate of pharmacy enough to take their degree.[23] He considered this proved that pharmacists did not consider the doctorate as a prerequisite for the practice of pharmacy or, for that matter, as a means of increasing their social prestige. In fact, Gunning twisted things round by arguing that the laws of 1865 and 1876 had seriously *damaged* patients' trust in pharmacists.

Although the Medical Laws of 1865 raised requirements for entering the profession, the material conditions and social prestige of pharmacists had not improved proportionally. Among other things, this was caused by the enormous expansion of the pharmaceutical industry, which led to the replacement of many 'galenic' remedies – the preparation of which was very much the domain of pharmacists – by chemical ones.[24] Patient demand for manually prepared galenic remedies was declining, whereas manufactured synthetic medicines were a booming business. Secret remedies and specialités were introduced to the market in increasing numbers and varieties. When Johan F. Eykman (1851–1915) took office as professor of pharmacy and toxicology at the University of Groningen in 1897, the situation led him to remark: 'In our days, the industry has taken the preparation of medicines out of the hands of pharmacists almost completely'.[25] This situation had major implications for the social position of the pharmacist, as well as for his relationship with his most important competitors, dispensing physicians and druggists.

### The relationship between pharmacists and physicians

The view that was taken in the inaugural addresses by the first Dutch professors of pharmacy, as well as in pharmaceutical literature, was that pharmacists and physicians were academic equals. In medical practice, they were considered complementary to each other: the pharmacist prepared whatever the physician prescribed. But pharmacists had more to offer, and their scientific training could be put to great social effect. Apart from the preparation and delivery of medicines, pharmacists could be active (doing research, informing the public and advising government) in the fields of forensic chemistry, hygiene, toxicology and food. Moreover, pharmacists could analyse industrial preparations for purity. Like Stoeder, who felt that modern pharmacists were 'inclined to goodness, beauty and truth' his colleague Van der Burg was very optimistic about the future, ending his inaugural address: 'the pharmacy of the future has been granted a worthy task; it will perform it to the happiness of mankind'.

Reality was, however, quite different. In 1865, the relationship between medicine and pharmacy had been far from settled partly owing to the fact that the legislators had been equivocal. On the one hand, they wanted to separate pharmacy from medicine while on the other, they wanted to guarantee pharmaceutical care for all inhabitants of the Netherlands. However, there was a great shortage of pharmacists, especially in the countryside, because most of their clientele lived in the bigger towns. With respect to the countryside, Thorbecke included a transitional provision that until the number of pharmacists increased, physicians were allowed to dispense medicines. In places without a pharmacist, physicians could do so without any restrictions; in places with one pharmacist they had to ask permission from the Provincial Executive (*Gedeputeerde Staten*), who decided after consultation with the provincial Medical Council.[26]

This transitional provision (Stb. 60 article 9) considerably complicated the relationship between pharmacists and physicians for a long time. From the first annual report of the Medical State Inspection onwards, reporting on the year 1866, pharmacists complained that physicians intruded into their territory.[27] Their complaints mainly related to physicians in the countryside, who claimed the right to dispense medicines. From other sources it becomes clear that the law was indeed violated in a number of ways. The *Weekblad van het regt*, a judicial weekly magazine that published jurisprudence, tried to clarify matters when the laws had been unclear or ambivalent. A certain J. Th. A., a physician in Rosmalen, had dispensed medicines to patients in Utrecht, where many pharmacists were based.[28] This was a very clear violation of the letter of the law, and the defendent appealed in vain against the verdict by the district court of Den Bosch that he should pay a fine of 200 guilders. In addition to this, the spirit of the law was being violated many times. Some physicians set up practice just outside the local authority boundary, in order to become dispensing physicians in accordance with the law. Others tried to have the word 'place' in the law refer to a very limited area. In the province of Groningen, a physician claimed the right to dispense medicines, because in Uiterburen – a hamlet in the local authority of Zuidbroek – there was no pharmacist. The district court of Winschoten, considering that Uiterburen did not have its own church (and was therefore not a place, but more like a neighbourhood of Zuidbroek), decided not to honour this kind of linguistic cleverness and made him pay a fine.[29] Still other physicians made an appeal to article 9 directly after the death of a local pharmacist. When they succeeded in getting a dispensing licence, it remained valid for the rest of their professional career.

In practice, article 9 was very much to the disadvantage of pharmacists. Owing to the ingenuity of dispensing physicians and the interpretation judges gave of the law, it proved very difficult for them to build up a clientele in the countryside. The Medical Council of the province of Zuid-Holland took the view that article 9 was meant to promote the supply of medicines in an extensive district; the economic interests of medical practitioners were of minor importance. The most important ground for granting a dispensing licence were the health interests of the population.[30] In spite of all this, Willem Stoeder and Leopold Van Itallie (1866–1952), editor in chief of the *Pharmaceutisch weekblad*, argued that the principle of separation of pharmacy from medicine was never brought to a conclusion.[31]

But how did pharmacists behave themselves? Were they willing to break with their habit of giving medical treatment and medical advice to patients? Before 1865 it had been very common for them to administer enemas and apply leeches. According to the Utrecht professor Wefers Bettink, this was part and parcel of pharmacists' practice.[32] Directly after the Medical Laws had come into effect, the Medical Council for the provinces of Gelderland and Utrecht took the official view that the administering of enemas and leeches included 'a service that was strange to the profession of pharmacy'. Likewise, the Medical Council of the province of Noord-Holland declared that similar treatments should be given up by pharmacists and be left to physicians.[33] However, considering that this was only advice, it is unlikely that this pronouncement had much practical effect.

## The supervision of pharmacists' trade

The laws of 1865 created medical inspectors and medical councils. Neither had administrative powers; they were expected to apply their expertise to investigations in health care matters, in order to be able to advise government. It was their task to collect evidence and report offences. It was up to the public prosecutor to act as he thought fit. Thorbecke had anticipated loyal cooperation from the officials of the Medical State Inspection.

Again, matters proved to be more complicated than the legislators had envisaged. The Medical Laws did not provide definitions of 'medicine' or 'medical advice'. When his Bill was being debated in parliament, Thorbecke had remarked: 'In order to determine whether a substance is a medicine, it is not the nature of the substance that matters, but its purpose and intended use'.[34] It was left to the judge to determine, in each individual case, the legal nature of a substance, taking the spirit of Thorbecke's laws as his point of departure. It will be clear this has led to much legal hairsplitting, misunderstanding and abuse of the law. It is striking that nearly everybody who commented on relationships in health care – whether it be Medical State Inspection, the Society Against Quackery (founded in 1880) or the judge – began with an exegesis of the parliamentary debates of Thorbecke.

The ambiguities of the law had important implications for the behaviour of pharmacists. Indications are that they were less worried about their scientific reputation than about their commercial interests. Many of them appealed to be allowed to deviate from the shop fittings that were prescribed by law. They appealed for permission to sell draperies, liquor, paint, druggist's wares and secret remedies.[35] The last had not been prepared by the pharmacist himself, but had been directly bought by him from the factory. Although the law did not allow pharmacists to sell medicines when they were ignorant of the ingredients, they proved ingenious in sidestepping the law, as can be seen from the following examples. In 1868, a pharmacist stood trial before the Supreme Court of the Netherlands because his wife had sold secret remedies in his house, with his foreknowledge. However, the Supreme Court did not hold the pharmacist responsible for the activities of his wife, who was considered to be an independent merchant.[36] Other pharmacists equipped so-called auxiliary pharmacies or stores for medicines.[37] They tried to use these as sales outlets for secret remedies. In this case, however, the judge took the view that these remedies were part of his stock. In consequence, the pharmacist was liable to punishment unless – as in the above-mentioned case – his wife had acted independently.[38] Another pharmacist tried to justify the sale of secret remedies by appealing to Stb. 61 article 4, which stipulated that pharmacists' stocks should hold all medicines recorded in the Dutch pharmacopoeia. He argued that this applied to the minimum stock; hence, the sale of secret remedies was justified as long as the prescribed number of medicines was in store. The Supreme Court rejected this plea with reference to Stb. 61 article 6, which demanded that the labels of medicines that were not recorded in the pharmacopoeia should explain the nature of their contents. Keeping unlabelled medicines in stock was considered to be a violation of the law.[39] To some pharmacists the trade in secret remedies had become so attractive that they gave up their profession altogether in order to devote themselves to it completely.[40] The attitude of the Society Against Quackery (of which the *Pharmaceutical Society* (NMP) had been an official member since 1888) towards these pharmacists was particularly severe. Attracted by money, they were willing to sell any panacea, even when the *Pharmaceutisch weekblad* had advised against it.[41] Many pharmacists ignored these and similar calls and were repeatedly found guilty of the lucrative sale of laxatives like Holloway pills, Urbanus pills, Mucus pills and Swiss pills.

During the first decades of the twentieth century, these kinds of violations of the law were very common. In 1919, Herman Van Gelder (1848–1933), the former editor in chief of the *Pharmaceutisch weekblad*, complained that many of his colleagues were guilty of the sale of quack remedies; and he added that some departments of the *Pharmaceutical Society* (NMP) even published price lists. This he considered 'a most regrettable phenomenon'. The telling retort of two of his colleagues, who pleaded guilty, was as follows:

> Who does not wish, like our colleague Van Gelder, quack remedies to be non-existent; who does not wish that everything called a medicine is a substance that really heals. However, a price list has nothing to do with idealism; it owes its origin to reality.[42]

Long after the Medical Laws of Thorbecke had come into force in 1865, pharmacists were still being cautioned and warned by the Medical State Inspection (or fined by judges) for dispensing medicines without prescription, for the sale of secret remedies, for the unauthorised practice of medicine, for not complying with the provisions regarding stocks, pharmaceutical weights and scales, for having unauthorised locums in case of absence, or for giving the key to the poison cabinet to unauthorised persons. These examples show that pharmaceutical practice was much less rosy than Thorbecke or the pharmaceutical leaders had had in mind. Although it is very difficult to establish the scale on which these violations took place or, for that matter, the number of pharmacists who followed the book and others who did not, it can be established that the professional consciousness of the pharmacists in the field had not developed as their leaders would have wished. In this context, it is revealing that after their initial prime the number of members and departments of the *Pharmaceutical Society* (NMP) stagnated and even fell.[43]

## Competition with druggists

The Medical Laws of 1865 had aimed at raising scientific standards of pharmacists and at the same time increasing their professional distance from druggists. Since the druggist exam had been abolished, some people expected that the druggist trade would gradually become 'extinct'. However, the opposite happened, since druggists had retained the right of freedom of trade.[44] With regard to the provision of medicines, Thorbecke had tried to steer a middle course between scientific expertise and social freedom, the former being embodied by pharmacists, the latter by druggists. Druggists did not have to take an exam, nor were their shops subject to inspection. The pharmacists, on the other hand, were very much restricted. They were expected to follow rigorous academic studies for many years and after having taken their exam were subject to strict visitations by the Medical State Inspection. The other side of the coin was that pharmacists enjoyed a privileged social position. Formally, they had been the only ones who were authorised to the retail trade of medicines. Druggists were only allowed to deal with the wholesale trade.

The Medical Laws had left much freedom to druggists. Thorbecke had been very much aware of the different positions of druggists and pharmacists; more than that, he had foreseen it and wanted it. During the debates on his bills he asked the following rhetorical question of members of parliament:

> Is there reason to doubt our goal will be attained when by regular inspection we are opening the sources of knowledge and instruction and showing the way, first in some places, then in more and gradually in all?[45]

Thorbecke turned down those who reproached him for damaging the interests of pharmacists. With his laws, he intended quite the contrary. Through pharmacists, the state guaranteed the quality of certain medicines, thereby creating favourable preconditions in health care.[46] However, whereas the quality of certain medicines was safeguarded by the academic training of pharmacists and Medical State Inspection, freedom of choice of the patient had to remain unaffected. By giving in to his critics and treating pharmacists and druggists as equals, the advantages of both principles would be eliminated, and there would be no reason to maintain the differences between them. Thorbecke wanted to limit competition only so far as was required by the public interest.[47]

The situation that had been created by Thorbecke's laws proved especially favourable for the druggists.[48] Contrary to what had been expected, the number of druggists increased dramatically in the decades following the 1865 legislation; their business was thriving, owing to the sale of secret remedies, new synthetic medicines and other remedies that were popular with the public. Stb. 61 article 30 especially was to their advantage. This article held out the prospect of a list of all medicines the sale of which below a fixed weight was forbidden. In 1872, this so-called 'C list' was published.[49] Assuming that the sale of medicines below a certain weight implied sale for medical use – to which only pharmacists were authorised – Thorbecke expected that the introduction of the C list would make druggists wholesale traders and pharmacists retail traders in medicines.

However, the C list was to become the main *causa belli* between pharmacists and druggists. In 1873, the Medical State Inspection established the fact that legal provisions regarding the C list were 'being violated more often than could have been expected, and that secret and other remedies are being sold by unauthorised persons almost everywhere'.[50] For the time being, the inspectors were prepared to believe that most offenders were unaware of the order concerning the C list. For that reason, they limited themselves to warnings to take the law to heart. Later on, however, offenders did not escape prosecution. In 1900, the magistrates' court (*kantongerecht*) in The Hague sentenced 39 druggists at the same time for selling medicines below the weight that had been stipulated in the C list.[51]

Druggists were not the only threat to pharmacists. Apart from them, there were many others who tried to make a living by selling medicines. In the annual reports of the Medical State Inspection, mention was made of the sale of a whole range of medicines by pharmacists' assistants, veterinarians, merchants, housewives, a clergyman, a photographic dealer, a saddler, and an innkeeper.

According to Van Itallie, the problems could be reduced to the definition of the concept of 'pharmacy' in Stb. 61 article 1.[52] To be able to sentence a person for the unauthorised practice of pharmacy, proof had to be delivered that the suspect had both prepared *and* dispensed medicines. It was almost impossible to deliver proof of both facts, even after plain-clothes policemen had been mobilised to buy medicines from unauthorised persons in order to expose them.[53] Therefore, Van Itallie concluded that article 30 had had 'little preventive force'. The law led to more absurd situations: it was possible, for example, that a forbidden secret remedy resulted from the mixing of substances that individually did not occur on the C list. Forensic chemists did not always succeed in providing definite answers to these problems.[54] 'Quack remedies' not containing any substances from the C list could be sold legally. Hence, the medical inspector of Groningen had to admit the legal sale of 'stomach herbs' and a 'corn balm'.[55] Time and again, the definition of 'medicines' caused great legal difficulties; for that reason, the Supreme Court passed a judgment on the matter once more in 1888.[56] It turned out that many judges took the view that only those substances mentioned either in the Dutch pharmacopoeia or on the C list should be considered as medicines in the legal sense. All other remedies they considered as quack remedies. The Supreme Court ruled that a formal distinction was untenable: the category of medicines in the legal sense was not limited to those remedies authorised experts prescribed or dispensed. In each lawsuit the judge was expected to establish the legal status of the substance that had been brought to court.

Already in 1866, the Medical State Inspection had commented that the law on pharmaceutical practice was unclear in many respects. For that reason, the judiciary had little chance of success in the prosecution of unauthorised medical practice. It was considered advisable to proceed to the prosecution of quacks only after thorough consultation with lawyers.[57] In 1886, the Society Against Quackery submitted a request to parliament to amend the laws of 1865 with regard to the paragraph on quackery. It was especially aimed at the retail trade of medicines by unauthorised persons. The Society asked all medical councils for a declaration of support, but in vain. It turned out that the spirit of Thorbecke had taken possession of the councils as well: they refused to give this declaration because they took the view that government only ensured the availability of pharmacists and (dispensing) physicians, so that 'anybody who wants to buy good, sound and well-prepared medicines has the opportunity to do so. In this respect, everybody is perfectly capable of guarding himself from damage'. Of course unauthorised persons should be prosecuted, but that was as far as the state should go.[58]

### Pharmacy between science and trade

In 1877 the new professors had tried to remove current prejudice about pharmacists by creating a new professional image. The traditional pharmacist was a mere shopkeeper, who was subordinate to physicians because he acted on their instructions, written down in prescriptions. He was seen as a medicine mixer, as someone who merely puts together active substances. The modern pharmacist, on the other hand, was a man of science; he was a man with independent views and the equal of physicians. However, the support of the patient was not won by this *image* of the pharmacist as a man of science and high virtue. It turned out that many patients preferred, for whatever reasons, the remedies of druggists and other unauthorised medicine peddlers.

In the liberal political climate of the late nineteenth century, pharmacists had to steer a middle course between the demands of science and those of the public. In his inaugural address, Gunning pointed out that an epistemological gap between layman and scientific expert had come into being in the course of the nineteenth century. In the early modern era, science had still been part of the public domain to a certain extent. In Gunning's own days, it had become the exclusive domain of trained scientists. In early modern times scientific concepts and representations had been comprehensible to everybody. During the second half of the nineteenth century, however, they gradually became estranged from common experience and everyday life. According to Gunning, a student went through a similar process. In order to become initiated into science, it was a prerequisite that he distanced himself from subjective, everyday knowledge. The epistemological gap that was the result of this learning process was deemed to be responsible for the problems pharmacy had in legitimising itself as a public discipline. Whereas science was held in high esteem at modern universities, the public had other standards. This made the legislation of the years 1865 and 1876 Janus-faced: on the one hand, the discipline of pharmacy had become a scientific discipline, whereas on the other hand, the profession of pharmacist had lost its credibility and social cachet.

In an address at the General Assembly of the *Pharmaceutical Society* (NMP) in 1887, Gunning plainly stated that he was pessimistic about the future of pharmacy and pharmacists.[59] In his opinion, the scientific character of pharmacy had been overstated in previous years. At the same time, the social position of pharmacists was worse than ever. Since manually prepared galenic remedies were gradually being replaced by industrial mass-produced chemical substances, pharmacists suffered competition from druggists, dispensing physicians and pharmaceutical companies. Moreover, he thought that the emphasis in health care was shifting from individual curative care to collective preventive care.[60] As a result, 'current pharmacists are hardly more than suppliers of medicines' said Gunning, who saw that their work was simplifying and decreasing. Gunning made a plea for pharmacy as an academic discipline; however, its employment should be adjusted to the changing (hygienic) demands of the time. He thought pharmacists could make an important contribution to society, analysing the quality of the air, the soil, housing, foodstuffs, lifestyles; in short, their field of research was almost infinite.

More than 25 years later, in 1914, Jan Hofman (1866–1942) looked at the matter from a completely different perspective. On the occasion of the 50th anniversary of the *Pharmaceutisch weekblad*, he discussed the development of the social position of pharmacists since Thorbecke's legislation.[61] Hofman blamed people like Gunning and Stoeder for insisting on the scientific and ethical calibre of the pharmacist, neglecting other interests. However, the spirit of enterprise of pharmacists had awakened just in time. He had become aware of the possibilities of new medicines and therapies, as well as of the commercial potential of mineral waters, bandages and *specialités*.[62] Contrary to Gunning, Hofman was very optimistic about the scientific and commercial future for pharmacists. In the same jubilee issue of the *Pharmaceutisch weekblad*, Van Itallie sang the praise of Thorbecke, whose Medical Laws had eliminated many abuses that had been endemic to pharmacy before 1865.[63] At the time, Thorbecke had rightly recognised that the key to the emancipation of pharmacists lay in offering academic training, not in imposing strict legislation. The choice of healers and remedies should always be left to the patient. According to Thorbecke, the only role that fitted the state was a facilitating one; the actual design of the health care system should be left to forces in society.

Late nineteenth century health care has been qualified as a domain full of absurdities, paradoxes and frictions. The medical profession was divided, while quackery was blooming as never before. In this context, medicine has even been called a metaphor for the process of modernisation.[64] At the beginning of the twentieth century however, pharmacists looking back on the preceding decades realised that the problems of their late nineteenth century colleagues were not a sign of a failing discipline. Rather, they appreciated them as one of the most important developmental stages of modern pharmacy.

## Acknowledgements

This research was supported by the Foundation for History,

Archeology and Art History (SHW), which is subsidised by the Netherlands Organisation for Scientific Research (NWO).

**Notes**

1. On nineteenth century Dutch medical legislation, see D. Cannegieter, *150 jaar gezondheidswet* (Assen: Van Gorcum en Comp., 1954).
2. See also: L. Ali Cohen, *Handboek der openbare gezondheidsregeling en der geneeskundige politie, met het oog op de behoeften en de wetgeving van Nederland*, 2 vols (Groningen: Wolters, 1869–1872), Vol. 2, 625.
3. G. G. Van der Hoeven (ed.), *De onuitgegeven parlementaire redevoeringen van mr. J. R. Thorbecke.*, 6 vols (Groningen: Wolters, 1900–1910); see also J. R. Thorbecke, *Parlementaire redevoeringen*, 6 vols (Deventer: n.n., 1856–1870).
4. G. J. Mulder, 'Apothekersstand', *Bijdragen tot geneeskundige staatsregeling*, 1 (1842), 74–8 and 128–33; Idem, 'Over de opvoeding van den apotheker', *ibid.*, 188–202.
5. D. A. Wittop Koning, *De Nederlandsche Maatschappij ter bevordering der Pharmacie 1842–1942* (Amsterdam: Centen Uitgevers Maatschappij, 1948).
6. M. Groen, *Het wetenschappelijk onderwijs in Nederland van 1815 to 1980*, 9 vols (Eindhoven: University of Technology, 1983–1987) Vol. 1, 132–4; Vol. 2, 54–6 and Vol. 7, 65–8.
7. This image is still very much alive today. See, for example, A. I. Bierman, *Van artsenijmengkunde naar artsenijbereidkunde. Ontwikkelingen van de Nederlandse farmacie in de negentiende eeuw* (Amsterdam: Rodopi, 1988).
8. H. A. M. Snelders, *De geschiedenis van de scheikunde in Nederland. Van alchemie tot chemie en chemische industrie rond 1900* (Delft: Delftse Universitaire Pers, 1993). See also H. A. M. Snelders (ed.) *The letters from Gerrit Jan Mulder to Justus Liebig* (1838–1846) (Amsterdam: Rodopi, 1986).
9. E. A. Van der Burg, *Het verleden en het heden der pharmacie* (Leiden: Brill, 1877); H. Wefers Bettink, *Het verleden, het heden en de toekomst der pharmacie* (Utrecht: n.n., 1877); P. C. Plugge, *Eenige beschouwingen omtrent de ontwikkeling en het tegenwoordig standpunt der toxicologie* (Groningen: Schierbeek, 1878); W. Stoeder, *De Nederlandsche pharmacie in hare wording, haar zijn en haar streven* (Amsterdam: Petit, 1878). See also: Groen, *op. cit.* (note 6) Vol. 2, 54–5.
10. J. W. Gunning, *Een eisch van het natuuronderzoek toegelicht uit de*

*geschiedenis der scheikunde* (Utrecht: C. Van der Post, 1865). On Gunning, see J. H. Van 't Hoff, 'In memoriam. Jan Willem Gunning', *Amsterdamsche studentenalmanak voor 1901*, 43–52; *Gedenkboek van het Atheneum en de Universiteit van Amsterdam 1632-1932* (Amsterdam: Stadsdrukkerij, 1932) 592.

11. W. Stoeder, 'Een leerstoel voor de pharmacie in het programma van ons hooger onderwijs', *Nederlandsch Tijdschrift voor Geneeskunde*, 19 (1875) I, 145-7. On Stoeder, see Gedenkboek, *op. cit.* (note 10), 680–1; P. Van der Wielen, 'Bij het afscheid van professor W. Stoeder, op 8 juni 1901', *Pharmaceutisch weekblad*, 38 (1901), 8 June 1901 (supplement).

12. W. Stoeder, 'Brieven uit de hoofdstad', *Pharmaceutisch weekblad*, (11 December 1870); (15 January, 19 February and 19 March 1871); (19 and 26 November, 10 and 24 December 1871 and 14 January 1872).

13. W. Stoeder, *Geschiedenis der pharmacie in Nederland* (Amsterdam: Centen, 1891).

14. In this context, his German colleague Julius Berendes spoke of a 'gewisser Interessenkampf zwischen dem materiellen Gewinn und dem idealen wissenschaftlichen Streben': J. Berendes, *Geschichte der Pharmazie* (Leipzig, 1898), 4.

15. On the problem of periodisation in the history of pharmacy, see Wolfgang Schneider (ed.), *Probleme der Periodisierung in der Pharmaziegeschichte* (Stuttgart: Wissenschaftliche Verlagsgesellschaft, 1962).

16. Stoeder, *op. cit.* (note 13), 420–1, 424 and 432.

17. *ibid.*, 433.

18. K. Van Berkel, 'Natuurwetenschap en cultureel nationalisme in negentiende-eeuws Nederland', *Tijdschrift voor geschiedenis*, 104 (1991), 574–89.

19. W. Stoeder, 'Een standbeeld voor Scheele', *Pharmaceutisch weekblad*, 7 January 1893; P. Van der Wielen, 'Het medisch pharmaceutisch museum', ibid., 39 (1902), 764–71. See also: Carl Frederking, *Grundzüge der Geschichte der Pharmacie und derjenigen Zweige der Naturwissenschaft, aufwelchen sie basirt* (Göttingen, 1874), 5n.

20. G. G. Van der Hoeven (ed.), *op. cit.* (note 3) Vol. 6, 336 (16 June 1871).

21. Stoeder, *op. cit.* (note 9), 26.

22. M.J. Van Lieburg, 'De medische promoties aan de Nederlandse universiteiten (1815–1899)', *Batavia academica*, 5 (1987), 1–17 especially Table 2; see also J. P. Fockema Andreae e.a., *De Utrechtsche universiteit 1815–1936*, 2 vols (Utrecht: Oosthoek, 1936) Vol. 2, 344.

23. J. W. Gunning, *Een blik op de toekomst der pharmacie in Nederland* ('s-Gravenhage: De Gebroeders Van Cleef, 1887), 3.
24. On repercussions this trend had for Dutch pharmacists, see Thijs Rinsema, 'Brocades & Stheeman. Van apotheker-fabrikant tot farmaceutische industrie' in Frank Huisman and Rein Vos (eds), *Farmacie: wetenschap, industrie en markt. De Nederlandse farmaceutische industrie in de negentiende en twintgste eeuw*. Special issue of *Gewina*, 22 (1999), 23–33. On the early history of the pharmaceutical industry in the Netherlands, see Frank Huisman, 'Van bedreiging tot bondgenoot. De transformatie van de farmaceutische industrie in Nederland, 1880–1940' in Willem de Blécourt, Frank Huisman and Henk Van der Velden (eds), *De medische markt in Nederland, 1950–1950*. Special issue of *Tidschrift voor sociale gesciedenis*, 25 (1999), 443–78.
25. J. F. Eykman, *De roeping der pharmacie* (Amsterdam: n.n., 1897), 29.
26. See also G. G. Van der Hoeven (ed.), *op. cit.* (note 3) Vol. 6, 336–7 (16 June 1871: about the countryside) and 375–7 (24 November 1871: about the smaller towns).
27. *Verslag aan den koning van de bevindingen en handelingen van het Geneeskundig Staatstoezigt in het jaar 1866* ('s-Gravenhage: Van Weelden en Mingelen, 1867), 134 and 137–8.
28. *Weekblad van het Regt*, 48 (1886), no. 5358.1.
29. *Weekblad van het Regt*, 42 (1880), no. 4493.3; see also R. J. Opwyrda (ed.), *Geneeskundige wetten van den 1. junij 1865 (Staatsbladen no. 58–61) met de daarover vooral in de Tweede Kamer der Staten-Generaal gewisselde stukken en gehouden beraadslagingen* (Nijmegen: Thieme, 1866), 494–561; *Weekblad van het Regt*, 44 (1882), nos. 4732.1 and 4756.3.
30. *Verslag 1884*, *op. cit.* (note 27), 18 and *ibid.* 1886, 19–20. See also *ibid.*, 59; Th.B. Pleyte, *Verkoop van geneesmiddelen* (Leiden: E. J. Brill, 1891).
31. Stoeder, *op. cit.* (note 13), 418; L. Van Itallie, 'De wetgeving sedert 1864', *Pharmaceutisch weekblad*, 51 (1914), 307–25, especially 312. See also the debate in *Vragen des tijds* (Haarlem 1887) Vol. 1, 347–78; Vol. 2, 169–93 and 309–18.
32. H. Wefers Bettink, 'Voor 60 jaar. Herinnering', *Pharmaceutisch weekblad*, 56 (1919), 913–24, especially 917.
33. *Verzameling van stukken betreffende het Geneeskundig Staatstoezigt in Nederland 1865 en 1866* ('s-Gravenhage, 1870), 70 and 100.
34. *Geneeskundige wetten*, *op. cit.* (note 29), 627.
35. *Verslag 1866*, *op. cit.* (note 27), 177–80.
36. *Weekblad van het Regt* 31 (1869), no. 3078.1.

37. *Verslag 1873, op. cit.* (note 27), 13.
38. *Weekblad van het Regt,* 30 (1868), no. 2975.1 and *ibid.,* 31 (1869), no. 3078.1.
39. *Weekblad van het Regt,* 30 (1868), nos. 2975.1 and 3062.2.
40. J. J. Hofman, 'De maatschappelijke positie der apothekers voor 50 jaar en thans', *Pharmaceutisch weekblad,* 51 (1914), 325–35 especially 331.
41. See, for example, *Maandblad tegen de kwakzalverij* 1 (1881) nos. 1 and 12; 21 (1901) no. 3 and 26 (1906) no. 1. See also Gerrit Van Vegchel, *Medici contra kwakzalvers. De strijd tegen niet-orthodoxe geneeswijzen in Nederland in de 19e en 20e eeuw (Amsterdam: Het Spinhuis,* 1991).
42. *Pharmaceutisch weekblad* 56 (1919), 309-10 (Herman Van Gelder) and 337–8 (retort by J. J. Hofman and W.D. Valkis).
43. Wittop Koning, *op. cit.* (note 5), 26–8.
44. The number of druggists increased from 233 in 1865 to 2000 in 1908 and 6000 in 1942: Wittop Koning, *op. cit.* (note 5), 114.
45. *Geneeskundige wetten, op. cit.* (note 29), 60.
46. *Ibid.,* 624–5.
47. *Ibid.,* 617–18, esp. 618.
48. B. Kruithof, *Het conflict tussen apothekers en drogisten. De professionalisering van twee beroepsgroepen tussen 1865 en 1932* (Houten: Bohn Stafleu Van Loghum, 1995).
49. *Nederlandsche Staatscourant,* 31 July 1872. See also: Weekblad van het regt 49 (1887), no. 5412.3 (G. W. Bruinsma).
50. *Verslag 1873, op. cit.* (note 27), 23.
51. *Verslag 1900, op. cit.* (note 27), 61.
52. Van Itallie, *op. cit.* (note 31), 317.
53. *Verslag 1883, op. cit.* (note 27), 15.
54. *Verslag 1882, op. cit.* (note 27), 16 and *ibid.* 1886, 346.
55. *Verslag 1885, op. cit.* (note 27), 341.
56. *Weekblad van het Regt,* 50 (1888), no. 5518.3.
57. *Verslag 1866, op. cit.* (note 27), 183.
58. See, for example, *Verslag 1886, op. cit.* (note 27), 16–7, 19, 22, 23 and 25.
59. Gunning, *op. cit.* (note 23).
60. See also E. S. Houwaart, *De hygiënisten. Artsen, staat & volksgezondheid in Nederland 1840–1890* (Groningen: Historische Uitgeverij, 1991).
61. Hofman, *op. cit.* (note 40).
62. See also B. Kruithof, 'Wetgeving of marktordening?' Apothekers en drogisten in het Interbellum', Huisman and Vos, *op. cit.* (note 24),

34–45, and Huisman, *op. cit.* (note 24).
63. Van Itallie, *op. cit.* (note 31).
64. John S. Haller Jr, *American medicine in transition 1840–1910* (Urbana, IL: University of Illinois Press, 1981). See also Frank Huisman, 'Shaping the medical market. On the construction of quackery and folk medicine in Dutch historiography', *Medical History*, 43 (1999), 359–75.

# 3

### The 'Dutch drugstore' as an attempt to reshape pharmaceutical practice: The conflict between ethical and commercial pharmacy in Dutch cultures of medicines

## Rein Vos

Since the Second World War the Dutch cultures of medicine have undergone remarkable changes. The pharmaceutical system was shaped by various macrosocial and economic factors, such as the expansion of industrial labour and production, economic scale enlargement, the rapid growth of cities and regional centres, communication and transport, and the increasing roles of science and technology. Cultural factors have been important as well. The role and function of medicines themselves were discussed, for example, in debates about medicalisation and the axiom of medical activism in prescribing medicines, or about medicines as marketing tools and as market products. The development of the medical and pharmaceutical professions has been significantly influenced by these discussions. In the past, political and professional discussions in the Netherlands have emphasised the 'unique' character of the Dutch system, both with regard to the broader aspects of Dutch health care and the specific features of the delivery of pharmaceuticals. The uniqueness of the Dutch healthcare system has often been argued by referring to the strong professional position of midwives and general practitioners, the success of the Dutch Sickness Funds System, the low infant mortality and high life expectancy both for women and men, the fair percentage of national income spent on health care, and the fact that the percentages of prescriptions of drugs by doctors to patients and those of self medication are the lowest in Western Europe.[1]

As for the pharmaceutical profession, the positive character of the system of delivery of medicines is demonstrated by the scientific and professional training of pharmacists who were counterbalanced by a large network of thousands of druggists who mainly provided over-the-counter medicines. However, the scientific and professional character of the pharmacy profession has been continuously discussed and contested, both within the profession and in government and public debate.²

## Donkers' 1955 proposal for the Dutch drugstore

In 1955, at the Annual Meeting of the Foundation of United Dutch Pharmacies, Donkers, put forward his proposal for a 'Dutch drugstore' in a speech entitled 'Flutter the Dovecotes'.³ His conception of the Dutch drugstore consisted of a mixture of ethical, scientific, commercial and economic undertakings:

1. to enlarge the range of articles and goods dispensed by pharmacies;

2. to display articles in the shop window of the pharmacy;

3. to take charge of giving advice to the public;

4. to join with fellow pharmacists to acquire and make use of modern equipment, and to develop collective arrangements;

5. to adapt the academic education of the pharmacist to the needs of society.

Donkers' proposal provoked heated reactions, not only because of its contents, which deviated from common Dutch pharmaceutical practice, but also because of its highly normative tone. According to Donkers, it was necessary to enlarge the range of articles and goods on offer; and there was nothing reprehensible about displaying available articles. It would show that the pharmacist took his role in society seriously. The pharmacist would meet the needs of the public, even when this meant providing articles and goods from abroad. The demands of the public ought to be the pharmacist's guide.

His argumentative strategy was exemplified by the polemical nature of his proposal's title. The Foundation was created in 1930 as a limited liability company, the Dutch Society for the Advancement of Pharmacy being its sole shareholder. The Dutch Society for the Advancement of Pharmacy strove for the establishment of new so-called 'penetration pharmacies' in areas where no pharmacies existed. The aggressive term of 'penetration pharmacies' denotes the competitive spirit of the Dutch pharmaceutical profession, with its concern about 'unqualified' pharmacists, druggists and dispensing physicians. The activities of the Foundation proved to be successful. The number of pharmacists in the Netherlands fell from 639 in 1910 to 614 in 1920, but rose again to 690 in 1934, 708 in 1947, and 816 in 1955.⁴ The Foundation increasingly took measures to bring about a rational distribution of pharmacies in the Netherlands. One objective was to manage and take over pharmacies for which no qualified proprietor was (yet) available. The Foundation became the mediator between pharmacy owners who had no heirs to take over their pharmacy and young pharmacists without adequate financial resources. It mediated between the established members of the pharmaceutical profession and the new generation of pharmacists striving to find a position. This was the context within which Donkers presented his plea to reshape the Dutch pharmaceutical profession.

## Heated responses to Donkers' proposal of the Dutch drugstore

Dutch pharmacists rejected the essential points of Donkers' proposal.[5] What they especially criticised was the overly commercial basis of his proposal. One critic, Van Nunen, responded:

> I get the impression that these views of Donkers are too much based on the commercial attitude which the pharmacists possess due to the nature of their profession.... In the interest of public health the use of medicines should be inhibited rather than encouraged.[6]

The pharmacist Motké reacted:

> Why, colleague Donkers, should we engage in advertising, and drugstore ideas: these will not benefit the sick human being.[7]

In another comment it was stressed that the public should be defended from increasing numbers of medicines aggressively advertised by pharmaceutical companies:

> Medicine is for the benefit of the sick human being... to promote the use of medicines amongst a healthy audience is irresponsible.[8]

Although the arguments in Donkers' proposal were already familiar to Dutch pharmacists, the issue was now coming to a head. Dutch pharmacists were in a certain sense happy with Donkers' extreme formulation. One of them said:

> In any case, by strongly wording this question, he [Donkers] has forced every pharmacist to answer a number of questions, which his suggestions raise. To what purpose have I studied? What is the proper practice of my pharmacy profession? What is outside my authority? Is it my primary task to offer the public everything it asks for? Do I in fact want to enlarge the 'range' of my 'stocked' articles, and why? What is a drugstore cast in the Dutch mould, and what will it become in the future? These are questions the editorial board of the *Pharmaceutical Weekly Journal* cannot ignore.[9]

Many considered Donkers' vision of a Dutch drugstore a nightmare. Business counted less than the integrity of the profession. Their wish was to serve physicians rather than the public at large, and their objective should be the protection of the public from an increasing number of medicines, aggressively marketed by the pharmaceutical industry. Medicines, not goods and articles, should dominate the pharmacist's practice. Nor was there any need to reform academic education. 'Are there any other academic, retail trade, business men?'[10]

The frightening view of foreign drugstores entered the debate:

> Should the pharmacist carry photographic materials, beauty creams, wines and liqueurs, toilet requisites, beach bags, amulets, etc., etc., all goods which one can see displayed in pharmacies in foreign countries?[11]

Motké stated the negative view of Dutch pharmacists regarding their colleagues in foreign countries as follows:

> Most of us have seen pharmacies abroad, and we know what most of them look like. In a single word: insignificant. I wonder how it is possible that our colleague Donkers, as an academically trained person, is impressed by these tiny shops.[12]

These emotional responses were based on the specific way the professional identity of the Dutch pharmacist had developed during the first half of the twentieth century.

### The evolution of the professional identity of the Dutch pharmacist from 1865 to 1950

The four Medical Laws of Thorbecke regulated the medical professions and the healthcare system in the Netherlands from 1865, and significantly improved the position of the pharmacist.[13] The second law provided requirements for the education and examination of medical professionals, including the pharmacist. The fourth law regulated the practice of preparing and dispensing medicines, and defined the basic task of the pharmacist as dispensing medicines prescribed by a physician. It also prohibited pharmacists from supplying medicines whose composition and method of preparation were unknown and uncontrollable. These so-called 'secret medicines' were very popular with the public and were in the forefront of profitable trade. In addition, the new chemical medicines produced by the German, French, British and American pharmaceutical companies – which rapidly developed from the late nineteenth century onwards – were marketed in increasingly large quantities. These medicines were ready-made products, hence not liable to the control of the pharmacist, as stipulated in the fourth Medical Law. These products formed a threat to the professional identity of the Dutch pharmacist.[14]

The Dutch pharmacists attempted to uphold their position by preparing their own products. If, for example, a physician prescribed 'Salipyrin Riedel' (an antipyretic drug made by the German pharmaceutical and chemical company Riedel), then a pharmacist might prepare his 'own' salipyrin. The distinction between 'chemical' name, 'generic' name and 'brand-trade' name was not made in the Netherlands. To protect their products the pharmaceutical companies engaged in many lawsuits in the Netherlands up to the 1920s. Apart from eroding his sense of professional identity, the pharmacist felt threatened with the loss of an important source of income – reward for the skillful preparation of medicines (the *taxa laborum*).

Major pharmaceutical companies started to introduce many specialities at the end of the nineteenth century and during the early part of the twentieth century. The provision of self-medication medicines, commercial specialities, and secret medicines was left to the druggists. In 1865 there were only 133 druggists in the Netherlands, of whom 95 were in Amsterdam. The situation changed dramatically after the Medical Acts in 1865 and changes in the Education Law in 1878, which regulated, among other things, the admission of female students to assistant and apprentice pharmacist training, as well as the general training of pharmacy assistants. Unexpected consequences were the increase in the number of female assistants and pharmacists, whose salaries were less, while male pharmacy assistants started drugstores. At the turn of the century there were already 2000 druggists; in 1940 this number had increased to between 6000 and 7000.[15]

This development has been neither clear cut nor unidirectional. Much confusion reigned in the pharmaceutical profession and in the market for medicines. Druggists very often prepared medicines themselves, although this was forbidden by law. Pharmacists were also involved in druggist activities. In practice, professional pharmacists competed with commercial pharmacies and many pharmacists fulfilled several roles at the same time: the preparation of medicines, large-scale production of mixtures or other pharmaceutical products, wholesale trading, and the delivery of specialities and preparations for general practitioners in rural areas.

Some pharmacies were just like drugstores or they combined different roles, pharmacist–druggist, pharmacist–chemist, pharmacist–public health professional. However, during the twentieth century the Dutch pharmaceutical profession focussed more and more on the preparation of prescription medicines or cheap chemical substitutes.

Dutch pharmacists were mainly located in the cities, leaving the rural areas to dispensing physicians and druggists, a situation little changed during the twentieth century. When sickness funds were introduced, initially in the cities, pharmacists and sickness funds became mutually interdependent. In 1900 about 10 per cent of the Dutch population was insured through sickness funds. This had increased to 31 per cent by 1926, to 48 per cent by 1941, and to 72 per cent by 1963 (51 per cent of the population insured compulsorily, 15 per cent voluntarily, and 6 per cent as pensioners).[16] The Dutch sickness funds are exceptional because they insured to cover the cost of provision of medicines and medical care and not to protect against the economic consequences of disease. Sickness funds and pharmacists negotiated the prices of medicines and the fees for preparing medicines. Likewise, physicians were urged to prescribe cheap medicines, to substitute specialities for cheap medicines prepared by pharmacists, and to keep prescriptions as simple as possible. Dutch pharmacists became the mediators between the physicians, the patients and the sickness funds.

Other European countries, such as France, Germany and the United Kingdom, have evolved different systems of delivery. Outside the Netherlands a large number of pharmacies developed in such a way that each community possessed its own pharmacy.[17] Many pharmacists outside the Netherlands performed a mediating role in healthcare consultations. In the Netherlands, a dual system of delivery of medicines developed in which a limited number of pharmacists cherished their specific professional role, yet also had to compete with dispensary physicians and druggists.

Throughout the twentieth century the tension between 'ethical' and 'commercial' pharmacy influenced the pharmacy profession.[18] It was this tension that underlay the comments on Donkers' proposal for the Dutch drugstore in 1955.

### The political nature of the debate: the society's fear of emerging commercialism

Many pharmacies already practised what Donkers proposed as the official philosophy of the Dutch pharmaceutical profession. In subsequent addresses by the president of the Dutch Society for the Advancement of Pharmacy during the 1950s, fellow pharmacists were warned not to expand into commercial ventures, nor to encourage the advertising and selling of specialities and packaged medicines. The Dutch Society was very sensitive to these developments, particularly because at the time the Society was engaged in the enactment of a new medicines law meant to replace Thorbecke's laws regulating the supply and delivery of medicines.

In 1952 a new Bill for a Medicines Act was submitted – based on a Bill from 1938, which left the position of the pharmacist open, much as the 1865 Law had. However, the Bill contained a number of significant changes to the architecture and arrangement of the pharmacy, apparatus and equipment, and quality control of medicines. Further extensions and specifications of these requirements continued from the 1960s onwards.

Similarly, the Bill regulated the establishment of pharmacies with relation to dispensing physicians. A system of licensing was proposed for the establishment of pharmacists in areas in which no pharmacies existed, through national (central) and provincial committees 'for area indication'. These committees consisted of pharmacists, dispensing physicians, pharmaceutical and medical sanitary inspectors, and a neutral chairperson. Furthermore, the Bill regulated the licensing and quality control of novel medicines. The principle of 'exclusive pharmacy medicines', a category of medicines that could only be prescribed and delivered by pharmacists, in addition to prescription and self medication medicines, was incorporated into the Bill. These included medicines with a more potent pharmacological action, such as analgesics or sedatives in higher doses or those with potentially serious adverse effects, but which involved no intricate diagnosis and therapy on the part of the physician. This principle was based on a private agreement among a broad alliance of druggists, pharmacists, pharmaceutical wholesalers, and companies in the 1930s.[19] The three-fold division in pharmaceuticals established the unique professional position of the pharmacist in the Netherlands.

More important from the perspective of the pharmacist, however, was Article 15, which declared that a pharmacist was forbidden to practise his profession in the service of non-pharmacists. Some exceptions were allowed, such as pharmacists working in the military, hospitals, or the pharmacies of sickness funds, and pharmacist heirs.

The Bill was finally accepted in 1958, although it was another five years before the law came into effect. The process was eventually speeded up by the thalidomide disaster. The delay caused a fierce political debate during the 1950s concerning the roles of druggists and grocers.

There was a broad political consensus that the delivery of prescription medicines should be the business of physicians, pharmacists and the sickness funds. Yet the role of druggists and grocers in supplying self medication medicines was indisputable. The motives of pharmaceutical companies were held in some suspicion, although they had launched a myriad of new branded medicines on to the market, some of great value, but many with dubious effects. The druggists and grocers were the supply channel of branded self medication medicines to the public. The government, the sickness funds, and the medical and pharmaceutical professions, all firmly agreed that prescription medicines, as well as medicines with potent pharmacological effects (the Pharmacy Exclusive medicines) were a matter of health care. The supply and delivery of self-medication medicines was a matter of economics and business. The need for strict separation between health care and economic interests dominated the debate.[20]

There were those who even pushed this separation one step further. The renowned physician, Heyermans, made the following point:

> We hope that the druggist will be forbidden to sell medicines, because this is the profession of the pharmacist. The pharmacist is the only specialist who is capable of ensuring that the patient will be given the correct medicine of good quality.[21]

In the 1950s several cases of the incorrect supply of medicines of great potency or causing harmful effects became the focus of public debate. Dutch pharmacists responded in unison:

> Here lies the essential difference between the pharmacist and the druggist. The former will take responsibility for health care and hence will minimise the use of medicines. The latter considers medicines as a profit item.[22]

The government slowed down the acceptance of the Medicines Supply Act until the legislation licensing new businesses was in place, regulating the position of druggists and grocers. The pharmaceutical profession reacted cynically to the government's position:

> We await, and look forward with interest, to the debate in the Second Chamber on the question of delaying the enactment of the

healthcare law concerning the settlement of establishment regulations for druggists, the foodstuff industry, grocery shops and hairdressers' shops.[23]

The druggists were the stumbling block in the development of the Medicines Supply Act and the further professionalisation of pharmacy, according to the pharmacists. The druggists advertised medicines, displayed articles and medicines in shop windows, and promoted the use of medicines during consultations with consumers.[24] In fact, druggists did precisely what Donkers wanted, and what the pharmacists despised. This commercialisation of drug use was, in the eyes of the pharmacists, the result of the partnership between the public, with its need for self medication, pharmaceutical companies, with their need for high profit, and the druggists, with their desire to establish their position as suppliers of branded medicines. In particular, pharmacists pointed to reprehensible practices in foreign countries, especially in the United States, presenting several examples of unqualified advertising in foreign medical journals, such as the ad in the *Journal of the American Medical Association* in 1950 for a new cold medicine:

> New antihistamine. Safe even for children. Kills Colds Fast. Can Stop Cold Symptoms In A Single Day. Helps prevent bad colds and their complications – also prevents passing colds on to others.[25]

The desire of the American public for this type of medicine was truly great, since sales by druggists were estimated at US$72 million, and sales by prescription at US$28 million: 'Indeed, for drugstores, eager for an extensive sale of medicines, it was a tempting business.'[26]

Serious adverse effects, such as sleeplessness, nervousness, lack of concentration, disturbance of balance, were the concern of the medical and pharmaceutical communities. The Board of Directors of the Royal Dutch Society for the Advancement of Pharmacy warned Dutch pharmacists to refrain from supplying this type of medicine 'in the interest of pharmaceutical–scientific standing, as well as of health care'.[27] Clearly, many pharmacists had started to engage in activities similar to those practised by druggists. This growing practice among pharmacists was viewed as a serious threat. When Donkers appeared on the scene declaring this form of practice as an official policy for professional pharmacy, the stakes were already high.

Moreover, psychological motives played a part. In 1951 the Annual Meeting had formulated and accepted the general guidelines for professional ethics and the conduct of pharmacists. In 1953 these guidelines were summarised in the *Honorary Code for Pharmacists* which contained rules of professional conduct regarding propaganda and advertising, dispensing of medicines without prescriptions, agreements with physicians, dentists, veterinary surgeons, and other healthcare workers, relations with the sickness funds, and price calculations.

The Medicines Supply Act was accepted in 1958, incorporating many of the views put forward in the pharmacists' *Honorary Code* by law. Donkers chose a critical moment to propose his idea of a Dutch drugstore. He was the spokesman of an emerging practice which the professional societies of the pharmacists tried to suppress. In 1953 the General Dutch Pharmaceutical Students' Society accepted the following resolution:

> Dutch pharmaceutical students, assembled at the general meeting in Amsterdam, voice the wish that, in the interest of health care, the supply of medicines to the Dutch population be legally and exclusively assigned to the Dutch pharmacist, and that the pharmacist for his part impose restraints on himself regarding whatever is, directly or indirectly, connected with the supply of medicines.

The positive editorial comment in the *Pharmaceutical Weekly Journal*, the official journal of the Royal Dutch Society for the Advancement of Pharmacy, reads:

> It is gratifying to note that the prospective generation dissociates itself in such a clear cut way from the tendency to commercialisation observable here and there within the profession of the pharmacist.[28]

### The pharmacist as contributor to the welfare service: his position within the sickness fund system

Another issue that came to the fore at this time, and which was also framed in terms of professionalism versus commercialisation in the Dutch pharmacy profession, concerned the role and function of the pharmacist within the Dutch sickness fund system. During the 1950s the Royal Dutch Society for the Advancement of Pharmacy undertook serious negotiations with the sickness funds, both at the national and regional levels, to ensure the position of the pharmacist. At the time pharmacists played an important public health role as producers of cheap medicines of high quality, a counterbalance to the expensive new medicines produced by pharmaceutical companies.

The importance of the sickness funds to Dutch pharmacists is

## Table 3.1
### The distribution of pharmacies supported by sickness funds (n=776) in May 1953.[29]

| Number of insured patients per pharmacy | Number of pharmacies | Percentage of total number of pharmacies |
|---|---|---|
| less than 1000 | 39 | 5.0 |
| 1,000-1,999 | 61 | 7.9 |
| 2,000-2,999 | 65 | 8.4 |
| 3,000-3,999 | 86 | 11.1 |
| 4,000-4,999 | 94 | 12.1 |
| 5,000-5,999 | 100 | 12.8 |
| 6,000-6,999 | 75 | 9.7 |
| 7,000-7,999 | 63 | 8.1 |
| 8,000-8,999 | 47 | 6.0 |
| 9,000-9,999 | 38 | 4.9 |
| 10,000-10,999 | 35 | 4.5 |
| 11,000-11,999 | 17 | 2.2 |
| 12,000-12,999 | 13 | 1.7 |
| 13,000-13,999 | 17 | 2.2 |
| 14,000-14,999 | 9 | 1.2 |
| 15,000 or more | 17 | 2.2 |

shown in Table 3.1. For many decades most pharmacies depended on sickness fund patients for their sales. In 1939 two-thirds of all sales came from the sickness funds.[30] In the 1940s and 1950s this must have been the case as well, although relevant data are lacking. Rijpkema found in his study of 18,111 prescriptions in one month from 24 pharmacies in 1951 that 12 per cent were for branded medicines, whereas more than 80 per cent were for pharmaceutical preparations.[31] By the first quarter of 1964, only 31 per cent of the 3952 prescriptions of one pharmacy were for specialities.[32] Go estimates the percentage of specialities in 1964 to be between 35 and 40 per cent.[33] In January 1967, 49 per cent of the 12,250 deliveries to the account of the Hertogenbosch and Surroundings General Sickness Fund' were for specialities.

In the pharmacies supported by sickness funds, the percentage of specialities was much lower. Only 24 per cent of the 2,193,769 prescriptions of the Municipal Pharmacy of the Hague in 1966 – which also supplied about 20 hospitals in the region – were specialities. In practice, however, there was diversity among pharmacists depending on the individual pharmacist's entrepreneurship, organisation, and technical and economic perspectives, and, last but not least, on the scale of the pharmacy and the nature of the prescriptions of the physician involved.[34]

The Dutch percentages of prescribed specialities are very low compared with other countries in the two decades after the Second World War.[35] In France more than 90 per cent of the prescribed medicines were for specialities. In the United States the percentage were even higher. Various factors kept the Dutch pharmacist in his role of producer of pharmaceutical preparations much longer, and to a much greater extent, than his foreign colleagues.

During the 1950s tough negotiations took place between the sickness funds and pharmacists, precipitated by a crisis in 1954, which resulted in arrangements that lasted for many years. Did pharmacists working for the sickness funds have independent professional status? To what extent were procedures and the organisation of labour in the pharmacy under the control of the sickness funds? The sickness funds proposed that efficiency experts visit pharmacies to check whether medicines were being prepared in the most efficient and economic way (including audits of time, order and the division of labour within the pharmacy). The Royal Dutch Society for the Advancement of Pharmacy tried to separate the professional and financial aspects of the issue. Thus, the pharmacist was both a professional with loyal ties to the sickness funds and an independent professional who was master of his own pharmacy and who had control over the allocation of his time for other activities. This was a delicate position, which left no space for commercial entrepreneurship within the pharmaceutical profession. The Dutch Society for the Advancement of Pharmacy stated:

> As we request that certain principles affecting the pharmacist as an independent agent be acknowledged, so too it is the right of the sickness funds that the pharmacist should continuously participate in the important social development which is firmly rooted in the Dutch Sickness Funds System.[36]

The Chairman of the Royal Dutch Society for the Advancement of Pharmacy had serious reservations:

> Alas, honesty forces us to admit that not all members individually weigh their duties as much as their rights. Without going into details, I feel obliged to voice a serious warning, that some egoistical

individuals can destroy what your representatives have built up with so much patience, tact and hard work.[37]

This warning note was accompanied by a strong plea:

> I have to make a serious appeal to you all for your full participation in accomplishing our task, which is the responsible and adequate supply of medicines to sickness fund patients, so that the patients are reassured that their care is sound in all respects.[38]

The Dutch pharmacists were aware of their unique position in the world, and the announcement continued:

> It is through the efforts and labour of the pharmacist that those who are insured in the Netherlands receive complete and cost-effective pharmaceutical provision which the surrounding European countries can only envy.[39]

Against this background, Donkers' attempt to elevate the emerging practice of commercial pharmacists to official policy of the Dutch pharmaceutical profession was doomed to failure. Two years later, the new president of the Royal Dutch Society for the Advancement of Pharmacy, the pharmacist, H. A. A. J. Martens, again boasted of the unique position of the Dutch sickness fund system and the special role of the pharmacist:

> Our sickness fund system is completely different from that of surrounding countries. Both the way in which remuneration is set at fixed rates, and discussions about what can be prescribed have resulted in the situation that the use of medicines per head per year in the sickness funds sector is considerably lower than in the surrounding countries. I believe that this is principally due to the system of subscription here, and also to the calm and sober attitude of the average Dutch physician and the Dutch pharmacist.[40]

### Some further considerations and concluding remarks

The practice of Dutch pharmacists in the 1950s focussed on the preparation of medicines and the specific role the pharmacist played in the welfare system of the Netherlands.[41] The organisation, labour, formal and informal procedures for controlling and instructing personnel were all accommodated by the lay-out of the pharmacy. The central task of Dutch pharmacists was the preparation of medicines, their proper professional business, which distinguished them from druggists and commercial suppliers of medicine. Many in the Netherlands considered the Dutch pharmacy to be truly unique.

The public, on the other hand, played no direct role in the triangular relationship between physician, pharmacist and sickness funds. This structure was based on a mixture of healthcare ideals, professional motives and economic considerations, and was supported by a broad political and social consensus. It was counterbalanced by the market for branded medicines, and self-medication products in which pharmaceutical companies, drugstores and the public all played a part. The Dutch system of supplying pharmaceuticals was seen as the cheapest system in the world and one that met the highest standards of professional quality.

This system was radically transformed during the 1970s. A myriad of developments contributed to the changes: the close relations that developed between the pharmaceutical companies and physicians and pharmacists; the process of re-urbanisation, a process that was accompanied by shifts of pharmacies from the centre to newly founded suburbs; the sudden rise in the prices of bulk materials for pharmaceuticals; the rising costs of labour and medicines; the elimination of the pharmaceutical cartel; the increasing roles of science and technology, automation and computerisation. Last but not least, the paternalistic organisation of the healthcare system was finally eliminated through a process of individualisation and emancipation.

Healthcare came to cater for the patient, and the pharmaceutical market was transformed into a consumer-oriented business. As a result of these developments the specific role of the pharmacist in health care was eliminated. The delicate balance between the pharmacist's position as healthcare worker and as an 'element' in the pharmaceutical business chain was disturbed. The pharmacists developed from independent professionals into powerful players in the market. Attempts were made to counterbalance this tendency by formulating 'New Tasks' for the pharmacist – medication surveillance, patient education and physician advice – and more recently 'pharmaceutical care' as the pharmacist's primary activity.

Throughout this process of transformation, various parties continued to stress the unique character of the Dutch system. They referred, however, to a reality, in which prices of Dutch medicines appeared to be the highest in Europe, with pharmacists who appeared to be monopolistic and to be operating as powerful market players. Other European countries such as France, the United Kingdom, Germany and Scandinavia, were held up as shining examples of how to frame Dutch policy on medicines.

Most of the requirements of the Dutch Medicines Supply Act of 1958 have now been abolished, and an attempt is being made to create a new counterbalance to the pharmaceutical companies and wholesale trading companies, and to re-establish the pharmacist in his professional role as a healthcare worker.

I have shown the specific way in which the Dutch pharmacy profession developed during the 1950s, both with regard to its internal operation and its relation to the sickness funds, physicians, and the public. Commerce has always shaped the organisation of drug delivery within the Dutch healthcare system. Donkers' specific approach of matching professional and economic considerations and combining the emerging roles of the pharmacist as a contributor to the welfare service and as an entrepreneur, provoked much debate. At a deeper level this debate exposed the profound tension that exists between the market and the ideals of health care, between economic interests and ethics. This tension still underlies the current reform of the healthcare system and the role of various parties in the Dutch cultures of medicine, particularly the pharmacy profession.

## Acknowledgement

The author wishes to thank Edwin Schothorst (MPharm) for his help with collecting materials for an analysis of developments in the Dutch pharmaceutical profession during the 1950s.

## Notes

1. This is not to deny that the various parties have referred to common themes and parallel developments in Western countries in these discussions. Furthermore, the supposed 'positive' unique features have been accompanied by a perception of negative characteristics as well, e.g. the notorious patchwork structure or 'spaghetti' model of the Dutch health-care system and the delivery of medicines. The issue is not so much to describe the unique character of the Dutch system – that question can only be answered on the basis of a comparative analysis of developments in different countries. The issue is how this supposedly unique character of the Dutch system has influenced perceptions, attitudes and the collective activities of the participant groups in Dutch cultures of medicines, in particular the Dutch pharmacy profession
2. J. J. Van der Werf, 'Openbare apotheker op een kruispunt – marktwerking in een gepolitiseerde branche', *Pharmaceutisch Weekblad*, 131 (1996), 160–4; Rein Vos, 'Spanning tussen markt en zorg. De Pharmaceutische Vereniging Kampen, 1862–1889',

*Pharmaceutisch Weekblad*, 131 (1996), 1390–7; Frank Huisman and Rein Vos, 'Farmacie: wetenschap, industrie en markt', *Gewina* [special issue], 22 (1999), 5–11.
3. The full title was 'Flutter the dovecotes: A few ideas on the practice of the pharmacist occupation in the future', Report of the General Meeting of the Foundation of United Dutch Pharmacies, 29 April 1955 in *Pharmaceutisch Weekblad*, 90 (1955), 437.
4. W. R. Siegmann-Slingerland, *De apotheker en de geneesmiddelenvoorziening* [dissertation Universiteit van Amsterdam] (Nijmegen: Thoben Offset Nijmegen Drukkerij – Uitgeverij, 1968), 81.
5. These comments have been translated by the present author.
6. J.A.J. Van Nunen, 'Comment', *Pharmaceutisch Weekblad*, 90 (1955), 535.
7. H. P .Motké, 'Comment', *Pharmaceutisch Weekblad*, 90 (1955), 536.
8. Anonymous, 'Comment', *Pharmaceutisch Weekblad*, 90 (1955), 499.
9. *Ibid.*, 498.
10. *Ibid.*, 500.
11. *Ibid.*, 499.
12. Motké, *op. cit.* (note 7), 536.
13. Frank Huisman, 'Pharmacists, druggists and the spirit of Thorbecke: The shaping of Dutch pharmacy', in this volume.
14. Rein Vos, *Met de rug naar de toekomst - leren in en van de geschiedenis van de farmacie*, [Inaugural Speech, 26 November 1996], (Groningen; Stichting Drukkerij Regenboog, 1996). With regards to how such products influenced the development of the Dutch pharmaceutical firm Gist-Brocades: Thijs Rinsema, 'Brocades & Stheeman. Van apotheker fabrikant tot farmaceutische industrie', in: Frank Huisman and Rein Vos, *op. cit.* (note 2), 23–33.
15. B. Kruithof, *The Conflict between Pharmacists and Druggists*, (Houten/Diegem: Bohn Stafleu van Loghum, 1996), 231.
16. Siegmann-Slingerland, *op. cit.* (note 4). See also Rein Vos, Job Wolters en Willy Van der Schuit, *OPG 100 jaar. De geschiedenis van een bijzondere apothekers cooperatie*, (Utrecht: OPG, 1999).
17. This is not the present author's view of the pharmacy system in other countries.
18. Van der Werf, *op. cit.* (note 2); Vos, *op. cit.* (note 2); Vos, Wolters, Van der Schuit, *op. cit.* (note 16).
19. B. Kruithof, 'Wetgeving of marktordening? Apothekers en drogisten in het interbellum' in Huisman and Vos, *op. cit.* (note 2), 34–45. See also Vos, Wolters en Van der Schuit, *op. cit.* (note 16).
20. Vos, Wolters and Van der Schuit, (1999), *op. cit.* (note 16).

21. Editorial comment, 'Professional Interests', *Pharmaceutisch Weekblad*, 89 (1954), 857–8.
22. *Ibid.*, 857.
23. Anonymous, 'Comment', *Pharmaceutisch Weekblad*, 92 (1957), 344. Increasingly, however, the position of the druggists and the grocers became less dependent on medicines. New markets opened up for them: cosmetics, bath products, insecticides, plastics, etc.
24. Quote taken from *De Drogist*, (1951), 24 October, 144, by the author of: Anonymous, 'Comment', *Pharmaceutisch Weekblad*, 92 (1957), 344.
25. Anonymous, 'Comment', *Pharmaceutisch Weekblad*, 85 (1950), 334, for reference to and quotation from the *Journal of the American Medical Association*, (1950), February 25.
26. *Ibid.*
27. *Ibid.*
28. Anonymous, 'Editorial comment', *Pharmaceutisch Weekblad*, 88 (1953), 406.
29. J. Winters, 'Comment', *Pharmaceutisch Weekblad*, 88 (1953), 204.
30. Anonymous, 'Editorial comment', *Pharmaceutisch Weekblad*, 76 (1939), 372.
31. B. H. Rijpkema, *Een onderzoek naar het geneesmiddelengebruik in Nederland* (Dissertatie, Amsterdam, 1954). See also: K.J. Van Deen, *Arbeidsanalyse in een plattelandspraktijk* (Dissertatie, Groningen, 1952).
32. Siegmann-Slingerland, *op. cit.* (note 4).
33. *Ibid.* with reference to L. S. Go, 'Comment', *Pharmaceutisch Weekblad*, 99 (1964), 967.
34. Siegmann-Slingerland, *op. cit.* (note 4).
35. *Ibid.*
36. H. A. A. J. Martens, 'Presidential address 102nd General Meeting KNMP' (Tuesday, 4 June 1957 in Enschede), *Pharmaceutisch Weekblad*, 94 (1959), 424–33.
37. *Ibid.*, 425.
38. *Ibid.*, 425–6.
39. *Ibid.*, 426.
40. H. A. A. J. Martens, 'Presidential address 104th General Meeting KNMP' (Tuesday, 2 June 1959 in Amsterdam), *Pharmaceutisch Weekblad*, 94 (1959), 393–402, especially page 399.
41. Oral history interviews with Dutch pharmacists on their practical work in the 1950s indicate as much. See project on Oral Histories and the History of Pharmacy in the Netherlands in the Twentieth

*Rein Vos*

Century, Rein Vos, Elles Bulder and Edwin Schothorst, History of Pharmacy, University of Groningen, Health Ethics and Philosophy, University of Maastricht.

# 4

## Community pharmacy in Great Britain: Mediation at the boundary between professional and lay care, 1920 to 1995

*Stuart Anderson*

Throughout the twentieth century, community pharmacists in Great Britain have had strong links to the traditions of lay care and to popular medicine. For most of this period they were usually referred to as 'chemists', by both the public and themselves, as a shortened version of 'pharmaceutical chemist'. In this chapter the word 'pharmacist' will be used except where 'chemist' appears in an official title or quotation. Community pharmacists have been a readily accessible and unpaid source of health information, advice and support, available in most communities in Britain over extended hours and without appointment. Yet they have long occupied an indeterminate terrain, spanning the boundaries between business and profession, between orthodox and non-orthodox medicine, and between professional and lay care. These are tensions that remain largely unresolved today. This chapter is concerned with how these boundary issues were managed during the twentieth century.

### The training of the pharmacist

In Great Britain, unlike the Netherlands, there is only one category of qualification as a pharmacist, namely Membership of the Pharmaceutical Society, or MPS (the Society became Royal in 1988, and the qualification became MRPharmS). For most of the century, training was by means of an apprenticeship of between three and five years duration, followed by one or two years at college. The one-year course led to the award of the Chemist and Druggist Certificate; whilst the two-year course, taken by the minority who could afford an extra year at college, led to the Pharmaceutical Chemist (PhC) Diploma. Both qualifications allowed holders to have their names included on the Register of Pharmaceutical Chemists, and hence call themselves pharmacists. No legal distinction was made between the two groups as to what they could or could not do. The PhC Diploma was seen as a higher level qualification needed for careers in industry or academia. Although the first degree course in pharmacy was offered in the 1920s, pharmacy in Great Britain only became a degree entry profession in 1967. Since 1970 all entrants to the profession have had to hold a degree, and undertake a one-year period of pre-registration training. The duration of the degree course became four years in 1997.

### The practice of pharmacy in the community

Throughout the century pharmacists who worked in shops have been helped by assistants. In many cases the principal source of assistance was provided by apprentices, who were paid very little, but who could themselves expect to qualify in due course. However, some of the apprentices did not go on to college to complete their training, usually for financial reasons, and stayed on as qualified assistants or 'improvers'. Training courses were provided for dispensing assistants, most notably by the Society of Apothecaries, but none of these groups received a university education, and all worked under the supervision of a pharmacist. In Great Britain, therefore, unlike the Netherlands, there has only ever been one type of community pharmacy (or chemist's shop), which has to be under the supervision of a registered pharmacist. In this chapter the word 'pharmacies' will be used to describe these shops.

There was, however, great diversity amongst these pharmacies, not least in their ownership. A number of multiples developed following a legal case in 1880, and today two multiples, Boots and Lloyds, each own over 1000 of the 12,000 registered pharmacies in Great Britain. There are, in addition, several hundred other chains with varying numbers of branches, but even in 1998 just over half of community pharmacies were still owned by individual proprietors. Premises vary in size, location and client base, in the range of merchandise sold, and in their financial dependence on the dispensing of prescriptions, although for many smaller pharmacies this now accounts for over 70 per cent of income. Community pharmacy is highly regulated in relation to the supply of medicines, and regional differences in practices are minor.

In the early part of the century, pharmacists were mainly white and male. In 1920 women represented only seven per cent of the names on the register of pharmaceutical chemists; by 1941 this figure had risen to over 15 per cent, and by 1953 to 18 per cent. The proportion of women on the register continued to rise in the post-war period, from 26 per cent in 1964 to 36 per cent in 1984; by

1995 women represented over 40 per cent of a total register exceeding 40 000. Their customers, however, were largely female, as women generally took responsibility for treating the ailments of the whole family.

### Scope of the chapter

In this chapter I shall explore the boundary between medical and pharmaceutical practitioners in the community, examine why patients decided to visit one rather than the other, and consider how this balance has changed over time. Many factors influenced this decision, but crucial amongst them was the cost and accessibility of the doctor relative to the pharmacist. Four time frames can be identified; an early period up to the introduction of the National Health Service (NHS) in 1948, during which access to the doctor was limited largely by cost, and access to the pharmacist was very easy; a middle period starting in 1948 and continuing until 1982, during which access to the doctor was easy whilst at the same time the pharmacist became less accessible; a period of transition commencing in 1982, during which the pharmacist began to become more visible again; and a final period, commencing in 1989 and continuing to the present, during which the pharmacist has taken on a variety of so-called 'extended' roles, whilst at the same time access to the doctor has become more difficult for many people.

These changes will be considered in relation to the key relationships involved; between the patient and the pharmacist, between the patient and the doctor, and between the doctor and the pharmacist. The history of pharmacy in Great Britain during the twentieth century in relation to these issues is under-researched, although some studies relating to the nineteenth century have been reported.[1] One rich source of evidence is interviews with pharmacists themselves, and the changes discussed here are illustrated with material from an oral history of community pharmacy, in which the life stories of fifty retired community pharmacists were recorded.[2] This chapter provides a preliminary analysis of the evidence available from this source.

### The 'traditional' pharmacist: 1920 to 1948

The early period of the 'traditional' pharmacist was characterised by the pharmacist's ready accessibility, availability and low cost, during a time when access to the doctor was restricted, largely on the grounds of cost. Before the advent of the NHS in 1948, only a minority of the population had free access to a doctor. The national scheme of insurance against sickness and disability provided under the National Health Insurance Act of 1911 applied only to wage-earners over the age of 16 with an annual income of less than £160, which was the limit for exemption from income tax. In the first 13 years of the service, medical benefit was provided to 15 million people each year. National Insurance was never extended to cover dependents, but the income limit was progressively raised, partly because of inflation, from £160 to £250 in 1920, and again to £420 in 1942. By 1938 over 20 million workers (representing 43 per cent of the population) were covered by the scheme. By 1946 the number had risen to 24 million, about half the British population. It was not until the National Health Service was established in 1948 that free health services became available to all.[3]

## Barriers to the doctor

For at least half of the population a visit to the doctor was not to be considered lightly, because they would have to pay. For many women and children, for the elderly and the unemployed, a visit to the doctor was justified only for life-threatening conditions, or for mental conditions. Elizabeth Roberts, in her study of the management of diseases by the Lancashire working class between 1890 and 1939, found that:

> until the advent of the National Health Service, the majority of working-class people treated themselves and their families for all but nervous illnesses; seeking outside advice, if at all, only from the chemist, much more rarely the doctor.[4]

In some areas a number of lay practitioners were available, including local wise women, charmers and travelling salesmen, but many of these operated mainly in the countryside. If people did go to the doctor, they would as likely as not be given a prescription, which they would then have to pay for at the pharmacy. So for many people pharmacists were the first port of call on health matters. They were readily available, they could offer advice over a wide range of problems, and they could make up an appropriate remedy for a few pence.

Elizabeth Roberts found that pharmacists at that time 'frequently provided free diagnosis, free advice and cheaper medicine than the doctor'. As part of her study she interviewed two retired pharmacists. According to one of them:

We were the first filter as it were. The trouble was that we had to do things that are not really proper for a chemist. We had to do a bit of diagnosing in our own way and be responsible for it.

*Would they for example bring children in and say 'what is the matter?'*
Oh my goodness, yes.
*What sort of things would be the matter with them?*
It might just be nettle rash, it might be measles and teething trouble, a little feverishness, constipation, or something like that. The usual childish ailments, but we had to be very, very careful in case there were little yellow spots behind the throat, and then right to the doctor.
*You didn't charge for this advice?*
Oh dear, no. Anything had to be inexpensive. It had to be inexpensive or away it went to the doctor.[5]

## The ready availability of the pharmacist

At the beginning of the century the dispensing of prescriptions was a rare event in most pharmacies.[6] Even when numbers began to increase once the National Health Insurance Act was implemented in 1913, most of the dispensing was done by the apprentice (where there was one). This left the pharmacist free to greet and assist customers in the front of the shop, and to make up medicines and sell ingredients for home remedies. Ronald Benz, during his apprenticeship in a small pharmacy in Eastbourne, East Sussex, in 1926, recalls that:

> At the end of the counter there was a gap, and then another small counter where the boss used to stand. He would interview chosen customers. He would make notes and keep his eye on the business generally. No one else was allowed to stand there. There was a fireplace behind so that he could keep himself warm in the winter. The spot was 12 to 15 feet away from the shop door. He was there to greet the more affluent customers and doctors who came in.[7]

One of the main reasons for this attitude was the ready accessibility of the pharmacist. The shop was usually readily identifiable as a pharmacy, and was often in a prominent position. It was common practice for the shop door to be kept permanently open. Alan Kendall remembers the shop on the High Street in Shipley, North Yorkshire, where he was undertaking his apprenticeship in 1936.

The door to the shop had to be kept open winter and summer. A closed door was a barrier to the customer. There was no minimum temperature for inside the shop. We used to see how cold it was using a bottle of glacial acetic acid. On a very cold day it would go like ice in seconds when you took the stopper out and blew on it!

In the 1930s and 1940s the pharmacist was generally held in high regard by the public. Alan Kendall remembers that, in the 1930s

> Patients looked upon the chemist with respect. They would always do as he recommended. I can't remember anyone asking for something different from what was recommended. But it was an age of discipline. People took note of what those in authority suggested.[9]

Joyce Gilbert undertook her apprenticeship in a small shop in Leicester in the early 1940s. She remembers that the public's attitude to the pharmacist at that time was

> fairly deferential. My father used to have one older assistant who had been there a long time, and the people often used to come in and ask for 'Dr Raymond'. We thought that was quite funny. But whether they really thought he was a doctor, or whether it was simply because of his age, I'm not sure.[10]

Reliance on the pharmacist, particularly by the poor, continued at least until introduction of the NHS in 1948. Grace Goodman undertook her apprenticeship in a privately owned pharmacy in a poor area of Bedford in the early 1940s.

> Poor people relied quite heavily on the chemist, because they could not afford the doctor.[11]

People with fairly minor complaints would go to the pharmacy in the hope of getting relief for a few pence. Jack Maskew undertook his apprenticeship with Banners Pure Drug Company in Liverpool in 1943.

> They'd come in and say 'I've got a bad cough. Can you give me something for it?' I would ask what type of cough it was. Was it tight or loose, that sort of thing. You'd say 'Just hang on a minute'. Then I'd make something up for them. We didn't keep proprietary cough mixtures. We would supply our own from a stock bottle. We had our own standard bottle for coughs. It was called 'Black Magic'. There were also other house nostrums with names like 'Black Lightning', 'Banners Tonic' and 'Strawson's Tonic Mixture'.[12]

Such nostrums continued well into the 1960s, and only finally disappeared with the implementation in 1973 of regulations under the Medicines Act of 1968, which effectively prevented small-scale manufacture in community pharmacies.

## The relationship between the pharmacist and the patient

But the role of the pharmacist was more than just that of supplier of medicines. In many communities the pharmacist was one of the few people who had received much of an education. The public would come to the pharmacist as a source of general advice and wisdom, and to have important documents read. Wilfred Ayres had his own shop in Nottingham in the 1930s.

> You didn't go to the lawyer if you could possibly help it, and the teacher vanished after school. You had to pay to see the doctor, so the only person left was the pharmacist, with the shop and the ever-open door. You knew him, standing there, you saw him every day. We became father confessors, giving advice on all sorts of subjects.[13]

The public felt less inhibited about telling the pharmacist things that they would not be prepared to say to the doctor.

> There was for us the constant listening to troubles and the giving of advice. I seem to remember most often I would ask the patient 'and have you told the doctor all that you have told me?' and usually the answer was 'no'. The public expected a great deal from myself and my contemporaries.[14]

Most of these conversations took place in the open shop. There was never a separate area set aside for consultations, and patients were not invited into the dispensary for more private discussion. Privacy was virtually non-existent, and the best that could be hoped for was that voices would be kept down and that there would be few other customers about. Very few could afford the greater privacy offered by the doctor's surgery, and in any case for many patients such a visit was filled with fear and trepidation. They answered the doctor's questions, but received no information about either the diagnosis or the treatment. Pharmacists themselves were not allowed to tell patients anything about the medicine, such as what it contained or what it was for. Jack Bearman undertook his apprenticeship in a pharmacy in Rickmansworth, Middlesex, in 1933.

The doctor issued the prescription and the chemist dispensed it. You were not supposed, or even allowed, to discuss the prescription with the patient. Nowadays, of course, it's entirely different. But in those days, to reveal to the patient what was in the prescription was considered wrong. It was written in bush Latin, and they probably couldn't read it at all. And you weren't allowed to tell them what it was at all, and you certainly weren't allowed to suggest to a patient that they should be on such-and-such. The doctor was God Almighty, and what he said went.[15]

## The relationship between the doctor and the pharmacist

At the beginning of the century the pharmacist was essentially subservient to the doctor, although contact between them was at best infrequent and at worst non-existent. But the doctor's patients were the pharmacist's customers, and the pharmacist was keen to keep the doctor happy. Often, when doctors came into the shop a great fuss would be made of them. Ronald Benz began his apprenticeship in a small pharmacy in the seaside resort of Eastbourne in 1926. He recalls that

> doctors used to come in quite frequently. They would leave prescriptions for dispensing. The chemists were somewhat subservient to the doctors. [When a doctor came in] the boss would lean forward and half bow, and say, 'Good morning, doctor, and how may I help you?' Doctors were a class apart.[16]

Many pharmacists went out of their way to avoid having to contact the doctor. Joyce Gilbert remembers from early 1940s Leicester that you only contacted the doctor as a very last resort.

> Of course, it was considered to be a great art NOT to have to ring anyone up. You deciphered what they wanted.[17]

Even when pharmacists did contact the doctor their intervention was not always welcome. During his apprenticeship in Rickmansworth, Middlesex, in the early 1930s, Jack Bearman recalls having to contact doctors with queries about prescriptions.

> If it was a dose which was well over the limit you were expected to phone the doctor and tell him. You weren't supposed to dispense it just like that. I can remember about half a dozen cases like that, and generally speaking they just said 'well just reduce it to so-and-so'. But some of them could be quite awkward. They would take the view

that 'you're interfering with my prescribing, aren't you? If that's what I've written, that's what I meant.[18]

But not all doctors were so defensive, and some were positively friendly. Alan Dickman took over his father's shop in Berkhampsted in the 1930s, and always had good working relationships with the doctors.

> There was a nice arrangement in those days that if a doctor brought in a new partner he would bring him in here and introduce him to us. It doesn't go on now.[19]

### The 'invisible' pharmacist: 1948 to 1982

The introduction of the NHS in 1948 brought with it an enormous increase in the number of prescriptions requiring dispensing. Numbers almost quadrupled, from about 71 million in 1947 to over 241 million in 1949.[20] The numbers of state prescriptions written by doctors and dispensed by pharmacists are shown in Figure 4.1.

*Figure 4.1*
*The numbers of state prescriptions written by doctors and dispensed by pharmacists, 1905–1995*

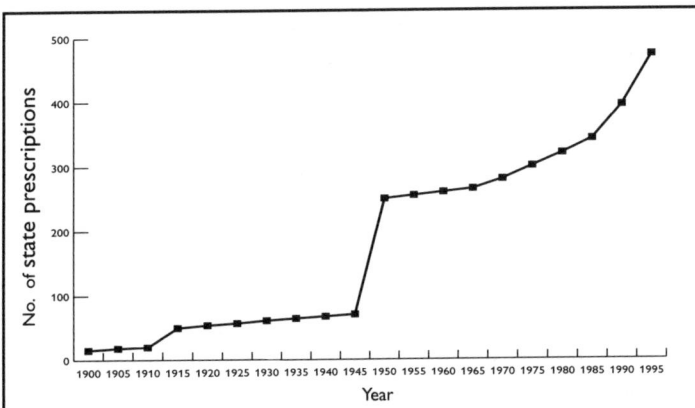

Sources: Jones, I. F. (1998), *Supplement to the Pharmaceutical Journal*, July 4, NHS 23: Department of Health Statistical Bulletin, 15 July 1997; Office of Health Economics, 1995, Compendium of Statistics, Ninth Edition, Table 4.26: Loudon, I., Horder. J. and Webster, C., *General Practice Under the National Health Service 1948 to 1997* (London: Clarendon Press, 1998), 305; Holloway, S. W. F. (1991), *op cit.* (note 6), 341–5: Anderson-Stewart, J., *op. cit.* (note 3), 33–35.

The impact of the NHS on the practice of pharmacy in Great Britain was dramatic. Access to doctors became freely available to all, and any medicines prescribed would also be without charge. The public could and did visit the doctor for advice about the most trivial of complaints.

So visits to the pharmacist for advice on even the most trivial of complaints diminished substantially. The increase in prescription numbers meant that pharmacists now had to spend a significant part of their day at the back of the shop in the dispensary, since most of the prescriptions prescribed in the early days of the NHS still needed to be made up individually. The consequence of these developments was a dramatic shift in the balance between the use by the public of the pharmacist rather than the doctor for less serious conditions.

### The changing relationship between the patient and the pharmacist

Many pharmacists thus began to spend most of their working days out of sight of the public in the dispensary. Over a period of years this came to be accepted as normal practice, such that by the 1960s the role of the pharmacist was perceived by new recruits to the profession as a backroom person dispensing prescriptions, rather than as a readily-available health professional in the front of the shop eager to dispense advice. Slowly, the traditional role of the pharmacist changed to a less visible one. Grace Goodman worked as a locum pharmacist in Lowestoft, Suffolk, in the early 1960s, and she witnessed this transition at first hand.

> I think with this particular pharmacist he had always been a 'doctor' to his customers. He had been there a long time. He was of the old school, and the customers came to him for help and advice because that is what they had always done. But I think in other pharmacies I went to the reverse was happening. The pharmacist tended to be in the dispensary, and there was very little advice offered or help given unless someone specifically asked for it. They [the pharmacists] would give the prescription to the assistant to give out, and there was, I think, very little contact between the pharmacist and the patient.[21]

The public quickly began to see the pharmacy, not as a place to obtain advice on a wide range of health issues, but as the place where they got their prescriptions dispensed. Following the introduction of the NHS Mr Gorman recalled that:

> it was nice to be able to go to the chemist with your prescription, and you got the thing for nothing. It was nice particularly for people who had two or three children. Oh yes, it was a marvellous thing, that you could have a doctor at any time. And you didn't have to think, 'oh, I'll have to pay'.[22]

But even during this period the community pharmacist was a respected member of the community. Geoffrey Knowles ran a small pharmacy in a tough area of Ellesmere Port on Merseyside during the 1950s.

> People round there were very respectful to the pharmacist. I remember one evening, just before closing around 5.55 pm, two youngsters aged 14 or 15 came onto the doorstep. One said to the other, 'Are you going in there?' The other boy replied, 'Yes, I'm going for me mum', or something like that. 'Well then', said the other one, 'Don't forget you have to say "please" in there!'[23]

### The impact of prescriptions written by doctors

For pharmacists there was little incentive to spend more time in the front of their shops building relationships with their customers. Income from the dispensing of prescriptions transformed many of their businesses. Pharmacy owners who contracted to provide services under the NHS at its inception received a generous remuneration package. This included an on-cost allowance of over 33 per cent, to cover all overhead expenses and to provide a modest profit margin, and a container allowance of tuppence ha'penny per prescription.[24] As a result most pharmacy owners made a comfortable living and many became rich, particularly those who had invested in a number of pharmacies.

As financial dependence on the dispensing of NHS prescriptions grew, the key incentive for the pharmacist was to build up this side of the business as much as possible. The change in the training of the pharmacist, from an apprenticeship-based system to one based on university education, meant that the traditional source of cheap labour (the apprentice) was no longer available. Although many pharmacists did train assistants as dispensers, most chose to continue with the dispensing themselves.

The supply of medicines under the NHS free of all charges was not to remain for long. In 1951 prescription charges were introduced for the first time, initially at one shilling per prescription.[25] This fairly quickly became one shilling per item, as doctors increased the number of items per prescription. Prescription charges undoubtedly represented a barrier to adequate health care for the poorest patients, and some no doubt opted to return to the local pharmacist to buy a trusted remedy for a few pence.

Many doctors went out of their way to help their patients, even helping them financially out of their own pockets. Christine Homan worked in a shop in Lambeth, South London, in the mid-1950s.

> We were in regular contact with one of the local doctors. He had the poorest patients. He would write [NHS] prescriptions, and quite frequently would pay the prescription charge himself, at one shilling per item. The charges had started at one shilling per form, but later became one shilling per item. He was an Irish doctor.[26]

### Building bridges to the doctors

Relationships between doctors and pharmacists took a turn for the better with the introduction of the NHS. Indeed, the Secretary and Registrar of the Pharmaceutical Society of Great Britain at the time, Sir Hugh Linstead, went so far as to describe them as 'cordial'.[27] Improved relations nationally were mirrored in the situation locally. Ronald Crisp was running his own pharmacy in Wipton, Exeter, at the time the NHS was introduced.

> There seemed to be a better relationship with the doctors following implementation of the NHS, in the early 1950s. It was only with the younger doctors; you had got older and you knew a lot of older doctors. They saw you as an ally, as a conscientious pharmacist; someone who would do their best for the patient. You were the link between the doctor and the patient.[28]

There were other opportunities to build bridges to the local doctors. Amongst these were several changes in prescribing practices that were introduced in the 1960s and 1970s. These included a switch to the English language from Latin, the use of proper names on medicines, and metrication. John Savage ran his own pharmacy business in York in the 1960s.

> Metrication was implemented reasonably smoothly. It gave me (I don't know about other pharmacists) a nice point of contact with the doctors; because there were plenty of doctors who had their own little nostrums, and they wanted their nostrums converted into metric quantities. If you were very nice to them and did the conversions, you built a bridge. Local doctors would come into the

shop and talk about the impending metrication; they were unhappy about being unable to prescribe half pints any more. They wanted to know what the quantities they could prescribe looked like physically. A lot of doctors had no more idea than the man in the moon what 200ml [millilitres] looked like. They knew what eight ounces looked like. But 200ml was a foreign thing. Other doctors you might have to phone up [to find out] what quantities they wanted dispensing, if they'd written their nostrum in apothecaries measures. I always offered to re-formulate them in metric measures, and to send them a copy of the formula. I made a lot of contacts, and built a lot of bridges in that way.[29]

Clive Murray had his own pharmacy business in Tipton, West Midlands, during the 1960s. He recalls that:

Sometimes doctors took exception to the chemist using his initiative, and saw it as an attack on their professional autonomy.[30]

Such contacts occasionally soured the relationships between doctors and pharmacists, often lasting for many years. Clive Murray remembers that:

There was a GP in Tipton who prescribed Mysteclin Paediatric Drops. When he prescribed them they were no longer available; they had been discontinued by the manufacturer. I tried to ring him but he wasn't in. The woman customer was desperate to give these drops to the child. I don't just remember the drug in Mysteclin [tetracycline with nystatin] but some sort of antibiotic. I had Ledermycin Drops in, and I made the decision to supply the woman Ledermycin Drops and then to let the doctor know what I had done as soon as possible, which I did. The man went through the roof faster than any rocket. It [the animosity] lasted 25 years.[31]

By the end of the 1970s there was a recognition that all was not well within the pharmaceutical profession. Despite the steadily increasing numbers of prescriptions, the government was gradually cutting back on the profit margins of pharmacy contractors, and some of them were beginning to feel the financial pinch. Many of the pharmacist's traditional areas of business were under attack. Over-the-counter medicines appeared on the shelves of grocers, specialist photographic shops took much of the developing and printing trade, and health food shops took much of the vitamin trade. The list seemed endless. To make matters worse, the public esteem of the pharmacist was at an all time low, and there was a feeling that there was a need to promote the role of the pharmacist directly to the public.

### The re-emergence of the pharmacist: 1982 to 1995

The initiative was eventually taken in 1982 by the body that represents the independent proprietor pharmacists, the National Pharmaceutical Association. It decided to begin a press campaign designed to persuade the public of the benefits of seeking advice from the pharmacist. So began a long-running campaign to 'ask your pharmacist', which appeared in newspapers and magazines.[32] The campaign slowly changed public attitudes, as increasing numbers of them took up the advice. But not all people were equally keen to take up the advice offered; social class distinctions still remain. David Barbanel runs his own pharmacy in the East End of London.

> People would ask to see the pharmacist. Working class people are more likely to ask. Middle class people tend to say 'I want some of that Tagamet'. Then they get upset if you ask them lots of questions. Working class people want to know, they ask for your advice, and they value your input more. Less educated people see the pharmacist as someone they can trust, and who is knowledgeable about the situation.[33]

### 'Can I speak to the pharmacist?'

The impact of the 'ask your pharmacist' campaign was to draw the pharmacist out of the dispensary at the back of the shop to talk face to face once again with the public. Peter Homan was a manager with Boots during this period in Surrey.

> Due to the campaign brought about by the National Pharmaceutical Association and the Pharmaceutical Society, people gradually became a lot more aware of what the pharmacist can do, and in the early days of the campaign [during the early 1980s] there was a lot more of 'can I speak to the pharmacist?' and I think certainly the role of the pharmacist has increased.[34]

Even in the 1980s symbols of authority and professional status remained important. Jerzy Naks worked as a pharmacy manager for Boots in North London during this period.

> When I wore a white coat I felt like an ice-cream salesman or a greengrocer. But people do relate to you straight away if you are wearing a white coat.[35]

But by the mid-1980s the importance of building up personal relationships with customers was again at the top of the priority list when establishing a new business. Pharmacy received a new lease of life from the Report of the Nuffield Inquiry into pharmacy.[36] When Jennifer Andrews took over a business in 1987 she concentrated on building up good customer relations.

> I offered a very personal service. I wanted to give my customers access to me at all times. The public now views me as an accessible professional, someone who is available at all times. It is one of the major bases of the business.[37]

### 'Go to your chemist – he'll tell you'

However, ready accessibility to the pharmacist was only one part of the challenge. For pharmacists to regain the lost role of mediator at the professional-lay care boundary they also needed to regain the trust and respect of those members of the public in whom it had been lost. It was something that the pharmacists had neglected in their daily battle with the dispensing of prescriptions. Yet trust was something that the public generally seemed willing to give, and pharmacists were generally good at responding to confidences. Geoffrey Knowles retired from his shop in Hoylake on the Wirral in 1989. Reflecting on his career in 1995 he says:

> I think that chemists, then and now, are held in good esteem by the public, more so than most pharmacists realise. I've noticed it more since I retired. They are quite definitely the first line when there is illness. Therefore, there must be respect for people to do that, mustn't there? Because confiding is a difficult thing. But pharmacy seems to be able to cope with confiding. By back reflection that means that they are held in high esteem by the public.[38]

Although doctors now rarely conceal any information about either the diagnosis or the treatment from the patient, sometimes they do not have the technical knowledge necessary to answer all the patients' queries, and they will advise patients to obtain this from the pharmacist. John Herman still manages a pharmacy in Olympia, London.

> A lot of customers treat us as the people who know about the drugs. But the doctors can't explain to them some of the things [they ask about]. They say 'go to your chemist – he'll tell you'. Doctors are now advising the patients to ask the pharmacist. We had a customer

only yesterday who wanted blood pressure tablets, Tenormin. But one of the ingredients there is maize starch, and they said 'we can't take starch in any form'. We had to phone the manufacturers and find out if any of them make atenolol [generic name] tablets without maize starch.[39]

### 'Thank you for bringing this to my attention'

With the increasing complexity of the therapeutic armamentarium and the greater the consequences of any error, doctors began to see the pharmacist as an ally rather than as a threat to their professional autonomy. Computers, too, had a major impact on the relationship between the doctor and the pharmacist. Peter Homan was a manager for Boots in Surrey during the 1980s.

> By the early-1980s computers had begun to be introduced into many pharmacies. The doctors don't use their computers as well as we do. There is no adverse drug reaction section on the surgery computer. The computer will throw up any reaction. Whether it's one that's of concern you would have to use your judgement, and you would have to phone the doctor. Many's the time I have phoned the doctor, with the result that the medicament has been changed, or that the doctor has confirmed that he would actually want this. And the way things are with doctors these days he would actually say, 'Thank you for bringing this to my attention', which is an aspect which wouldn't have happened in the earlier days of my career [in the early-1960s]. We are all aware of the great advances in therapeutics there have been in recent years and of the caution with which they have to be used now.[40]

Jennifer Andrews took over a pharmacy business near Peterborough in 1987, and made a point of introducing herself to the local doctors.

> I then built up regular contact with the doctor's surgery. And I found that eventually they were contacting me. It was some of the younger women doctors in practice, and their trainees, who rang most often for advice. They began to see me as a fellow professional.[41]

### The less accessible doctor: 1989 to 1995

The public's increased willingness to 'ask the pharmacist' was reinforced, at least in part, by a decrease in public perceptions about the accessibility of the doctor, through appointment systems and high prescription charges. Combined with this was the fact that people in the 1980s were living a much busier life than in earlier decades, and their better education meant that they had more realistic expectations of what the doctor might be able to do for them.

### 'I haven't got time to visit the doctor'

Jerzy Naks came across these attitudes repeatedly during the late 1980s.

> People are now more willing to go to the pharmacist. They'll come in and say, 'I've got a cold. What would you recommend? I haven't got time to visit the doctor, and probably the doctor won't be able to help me anyway'. There has been a major shift. A lot more advice is now sought from pharmacists.[42]

Clive Murray recalls working in his pharmacy in Tipton in the West Midlands during the 1980s.

> Everywhere you go you see 'ask your pharmacist'. [advertisements] Patients will come in and say, 'I've come to see you. I don't think I need to bother the doctor. What do you think?' Well, you listen to what they say, and most of the time you don't think they do need to, but there are the occasional times when you think it would be better if they went. And I do make that decision too, not often, but I do make it.[43]

The continuing rise in the cost of prescription charges has also been a key factor in the public's decision to visit the pharmacist rather than the doctor during the 1990s. Manjula Patel, who manages her own shop in North London, reports that:

> The public now see the chemist as an important person to talk to before they go to see the doctor, because they don't want to pay £5.25 per item in prescription charges; and they don't want to spend a lot of time at the doctors, only to be fobbed off with the same medication [as they could buy for themselves at the chemist's]. I have a lot of people who come in saying, 'I only came to you because I don't want to go to my doctor. I know you will give me as good advice as a doctor would give me'. It makes you feel good.[44]

### 'We know all about that'

But not all patients appreciated the detailed questioning by the pharmacist that by this stage often accompanied a visit to the pharmacy. Some just wanted to collect their medicines and depart.

John Cave managed his own pharmacy in Harlow, Essex, until 1988.

> I know that it is advocated that the pharmacist should always give out the prescription and discuss it with the patient, but this doesn't really work out in practice; and if you do start discussing it with some people it will put them off; because they say, 'We know all about that'. So you have to be very diplomatic in what you say to people.[45]

Geoffrey Knowles reported the same experience in his pharmacy in Hoylake on the Wirral in the late 1980s.

> There are some people who don't want to see the pharmacist. They just want their prescription, or to buy a proprietary medicine. 'If I can't buy my Nurofen without being asked a lot of questions, I'll buy it somewhere else'.[46]

### 'Second line of defence'

A great deal depended on the personal relationship between the pharmacist and the doctor. Sometimes they became firm friends, or at least close colleagues working together over a period of years. Edith Spivack continued to run her pharmacy in Kingsbury, North London, until the 1980s, and got to know many of her local doctors well.

> The chap round the corner, he had his practice not far from here. I rang him up one day. 'Hello Alan!' 'Oh, I know', he said, 'You can't read my writing'. I didn't even have to ask! He was proud of himself.
> *How did you get to know the doctor?*
> He came into the shop. We became great personal friends. We retired at the same time.[47]

So the attitude of the doctor to the pharmacist has undergone a considerable transformation since the introduction of the NHS. The doctor has come to recognise the value of the pharmacist checking his prescribing. As Peter Homan says:

> I think that doctors now look upon the pharmacist as a second line of defence, that they will be grateful that the pharmacist picks up on any errors they might make. They realise that the pressures they are under are far greater than they used to be, and I think that they are comforted by the fact that there is somebody there to help. You still

get the doctor who says, 'Don't bother me. If that's what I wrote then that's what I want!' But these are fast becoming a minority now, and most doctors will say, 'Thank you for phoning.'[48]

Doctors today are on the whole only too aware of just how easy it is to make a prescribing error. David Barbanel established a successful pharmacy in the East End of London during the 1970s, and has established close working relationships with his local doctors. He had computerised medication records for many of their patients in his pharmacy. He recalled that:

> Only yesterday a doctor had returned from holiday. He had done four repeat items by hand for his patients. The last item he had written amiodarone [for heart irregularities]. I looked at the patient's medication record. She was on amlodipine [for hypertension]. There was nothing wrong with the amiodarone prescription. Now if she hadn't come into me, maybe the pharmacist [she had taken it to] would have said, 'Does he want the 100mg or the 200mg tablets? I'll phone him up to confirm'. And then the doctor would have said, as he said to me, 'Oh my God, I've made a mistake! I meant amlodipine.'[49]

So changes in the relationship between the doctor and the pharmacist, and between the pharmacist and the patient, and also in the nature of the medicines available, meant that by the end of the twentieth century the transition of the pharmacist from 'poor man's doctor' to 'doctor's safeguard' was all but complete.

## Conclusions

Evidence considered in this chapter, obtained from oral history, can often be corroborated by information published elsewhere, and whenever possible this has been done. However, caution is needed in the interpretations, since only pharmacists' perspectives are presented here, and those selected may themselves not be representative of the many thousands of pharmacists who practised in the community during the course of the twentieth century. Significant differences may be apparent in terms of space, time and gender. Nevertheless, a number of general conclusions can be drawn. Throughout the twentieth century the community pharmacist in Great Britain has acted as mediator between professional and lay care, and specifically as mediator between the doctor and the patient. Before the introduction of the National Health Service in 1948, a visit to the pharmacist was a cheaper, and often the only, alternative to visiting the doctor. But the decision was not necessarily straightforward. The decision to seek help outside of the family depended on how illness was defined, and the threshold of severity that would trigger such action. The medical market was also far less clear. Whose help was sought depended as much on local tradition and family circumstances as on judgements about the competence of the individual concerned. Clearly, many people did make use of local untrained women practitioners and other lay sources. But the pharmacist was generally there as an option for sound advice and low cost remedies. The pharmacist supported lay care by making available ingredients for home remedies, selling medicines over the counter, and providing a variety of welfare services, such as weighing babies and offering first aid.[50] This mediating role has fluctuated over time, according to the relative ease of access to the pharmacist and the extent of the barriers placed in the way of access to the doctor. Initial barriers to access to the doctor, principally cost, were removed with the introduction of the NHS in 1948. However, new barriers emerged in the 1980s in the form of prescription charges, appointment systems and time spent on the visit. Conversely, access to the pharmacist diminished dramatically with the introduction of the NHS as a result of the quadrupling of prescription numbers, and the migration of the pharmacist from the front to the back of the shop. This was accompanied by a substantial loss in many areas of the pharmacist's traditional business, such as photographic developing and printing, health foods, and toiletries.[51] Initiatives such as the 'ask your pharmacist' campaign started in the early 1980s sought to remind the public of the availability of pharmacists, of their training and expertise, and emphasised the diversity of services provided by them. Such activities can be seen as an attempt by the profession to regain the historic role of the pharmacist as mediator between professional and lay care.

## Acknowledgements

The research on which this chapter is based was funded by the Wellcome Trust, through a project grant for an oral history of community pharmacy practice in Great Britain, awarded to Professor Klim McPherson and Professor Virginia Berridge at the London School of Hygiene and Tropical Medicine. The assistance of Miss Helga Mangion in the compilation of Figure 4.1 is gratefully acknowledged.

## Notes

1. H. Marland, 'The medical activities of mid-nineteenth century chemists and druggists, with special reference to Wakefield and Huddersfield', *Medical History*, 31 (1987), 415–39.
2. The oral history study involved recorded life story interviews with 50 retired community pharmacists. These represented a variety of locations (inner city, suburban, rural), of ownership (independent proprietors to large chains), and of customers (from the very rich to the very poor). Eleven of the participants were women, and the sample included representatives of the Jewish, Polish and Asian communities. Participants practised in England, Scotland and Wales, during the period 1911 to 1995. The questionnaire schedule included items such as reasons for entering pharmacy, education and training, the range of activities undertaken and of products sold, and relationships with doctors and patients. Participants were also asked how, why and when changes in practice occurred. Quotations are taken from interviews recorded by Stuart Anderson during 1995. They are used, and interviewees are identified, with permission. The Pharmacy in Practice (PIP) series of tapes are lodged with the National Life Stories Collection of the National Sound Archive at the British Library in London as C816, Oral History of Community Pharmacy.
3. S. W. F. Holloway, *Royal Pharmaceutical Society of Great Britain 1841(1991: A Political and Social History* (London: The Pharmaceutical Press, 1991).
4. E. Roberts, 'Oral History Investigations of Disease and Its Management by the Lancashire Working Class 1890 to 1939', in J. V. Pickstone (ed.) *Health, Disease and Medicine in Lancashire 1750 to 1950: Four papers on Sources, Problems and Methods* (Manchester: Department of History of Science and Technology, UMIST, 1980), 44–5.
5. Mr C6L, born 1896 and Mr H10L, born 1915, *op. cit.* (note 4).
6. J. Anderson-Stewart, 'Jubilee of the National Insurance Act', *Pharmaceutical Journal*, 189 (1962), 33–5.
7. Ronald Benz, retired pharmacist, born 1910, PIP/18.
8. Alan Kendall, retired pharmacist, born 1920, PIP/48.
9. Alan Kendall, *ibid.*
10. Joyce Gilbert, retired pharmacist, born 1923, PIP/47.
11. Grace Goodman, retired pharmacist, born 1925, PIP/33.
12. Jack Maskew, retired pharmacist, born 1926, PIP/39.
13. Wilfred Ayres, retired pharmacist, registered 1930, recorded in 1990,

Pharmacy in Nottingham Collection, Nottinghamshire County Library, Nottingham.
14. Wilfred Ayres, retired pharmacist, registered 1930, contribution to *Dusting and Dispensing: A Collection of Memories and Anecdotes by Nottingham Pharmacists to mark the 150th Anniversary of the Royal Pharmaceutical Society of Great Britain* (Nottingham: Splendid Productions, 1992).
15. Jack Bearman, retired pharmacist, born 1917, PIP/02.
16. Ronald Benz, retired pharmacist, born 1910, PIP/18.
17. Joyce Gilbert, retired pharmacist, born 1923, PIP/47.
18. Jack Bearman, *op. cit.*(note 15).
19. Alan Dickman, retired pharmacist, born 1915, PIP/34.
20. S.W.F. Holloway, *op. cit.* (note 3).
21. Grace Goodman, retired pharmacist, born 1925, PIP/33.
22. Mr Gorman, reported in *Can We Afford The Doctor?* (London: Age Exchange, 1985).
23. Geoffrey Knowles, retired pharmacist, born 1919, PIP/36.
24. S. W. F. Holloway, *op. cit.* (note 3).
25. I. F. Jones, 'The History and Development of NHS Prescription Charges', *Supplement to the Pharmaceutical Journal*, 261 (1998), NHS22–23.
26. Christine Homan, retired pharmacist, born 1938, PIP/46.
27. *The Times*, (7 July 1958).
28. Ronald Crisp, retired pharmacist, born 1914, PIP/19.
29. John Savage, retired pharmacist, born 1934, PIP/27.
30. Clive Murray, retired pharmacist, born 1933, PIP/30.
31. Clive Murray, *ibid.*
32. Anonymous, '75 Years of the National Pharmaceutical Association', *Supplement to the Pharmaceutical Journal*, 256 (1996), NPA2–8.
33. David Barbanel, practising pharmacist, born 1946, PIP/28.
34. Peter Homan, retired pharmacist, born 1938, PIP/08.
35. Jerzy Naks, practising pharmacist, born 1962, PIP/41.
36. *Pharmacy : A Report of an Enquiry* (London: Nuffield Foundation, 1986).
37. Jennifer Andrews, practising pharmacist, born 1947, PIP/25.
38. Geoffrey Knowles, retired pharmacist, born 1919, PIP/36.
39. John Herman, retired pharmacist, born 1922, PIP/14.
40. Peter Homan, *op. cit.* (note 34).
41. Jennifer Andrews, *op. cit.* (note 37).
42. Jerzy Naks, *op. cit.* (note 35).
43. Clive Murray, *op. cit.* (note 30).
44. Manjula Patel, practising pharmacist, born 1953, PIP/44.

45. John Cave, retired pharmacist, born 1919, PIP/10.
46. Geoffrey Knowles, *op. cit.* (note 38).
47. Edith Spivack, retired pharmacist, born 1911, PIP/22.
48. Peter Homan, *op. cit.* (note 34).
49. David Barbanel, practising pharmacist, born 1946, PIP/28.
50. S. C. Anderson, V. S. Berridge, 'The Role of the Community Pharmacist in Health and Welfare, 1911 to 1986', in J. Bornat, R. B. Perks, P. Thompson, J. Wamsley (eds), *Oral History, Health and Welfare* (London: Routledge, 2000), 48–74.
51. S. C. Anderson, V. S. Berridge, 'L'Heritage Perdu du Pharmacien: Professionalisation, Specialisation et Accroissement de la Protection Sociale', en O. Faure et A. Opinel (eds), *Les Thérapeutiques: Savoirs et Usages* (St Julien en Beaujolais, France: Fondation Marcel Merieux, 1999), 317–37.

# 5

## Homoeopathy and its concern for purity: The Dutch case in the early-twentieth century

*Marijke Gijswijt-Hofstra*

The history of homoeopathy can be partly written as a history of disputes over the definition and the preservation of purity. It all began with homoeopathy's founder, Samuel Hahnemann (1755–1843) of Saxony. In his *Organon*, first published in 1810, he qualified his new therapeutic system as gentle, prompt, certain and lasting.[1] However, if these promises were to come true, he warned, his therapy should be strictly applied. Hahnemann kept stressing this. As he said in German: 'macht's nach, aber macht's genau nach'; which means: imitate it, but imitate it accurately. Deviation from his principles was not to be tolerated.

It would soon become clear that Hahnemann's followers were not all as true to him as he wished. This resulted, from the 1830s onwards, in conflicts and splits within homoeopathy. In fact, since that time there was no longer one homoeopathy, but several. This is still the case today, two centuries later. The question as to what homoeopathy is, is therefore incorrectly formulated, at least from the historian's point of view. One should rather ask what those who claimed or claim to practise homoeopathy understand by homoeopathy, what they actually have in common, and where their paths part. Most homoeopathic practitioners would agree that homoeopathy should be qualified as a distinct type of drug therapy, the common denominator being the *similia similibus curentur* principle: like can be cured by like. Even so, this still leaves room for different emphases and interpretations, including those that move towards a decidedly spiritualised approach to homoeopathic drugs.

Given these internal differences within homoeopathy, and Hahnemann's intolerant attitude towards deviance, it is hardly surprising that the definition and preservation of purity was to become an issue from an early stage. However, the extent to which it became an issue, and its outcome, varied significantly in different countries and over time. In this contribution, special attention will be paid to developments in the Netherlands in the early twentieth century. I shall argue that the production of a homoeopathic supplement to the Dutch pharmacopoeia brought to light serious differences of opinion amongst university-educated homoeopathic practitioners, which until then had been suppressed or had perhaps even been non-existent. Whereas the late nineteenth century could be characterised as a period of 'compromise, not conflict'[2] on the part of Dutch homoeopathic practitioners, this was no longer the case from 1910 onwards. By then the issue of homoeopathic purity was being brought into the open, even in the Netherlands. How and why this happened, and what the consequences were, will be the central concern in my paper.

### Hahnemann's homoeopathy and conflicts over purity

What was homoeopathy, or what should it be, according to Hahnemann? In 1796 he formulated the basic principle of his therapy, the *similia similibus curentur*. By this he meant that patients can be cured by drugs that would produce the symptoms of the disease in a healthy person. Drugs were to be tested on healthy persons. Once their effects were known, they could be prescribed in a (much) lower dosage to patients with similar symptoms. In 1807 Hahnemann named his therapy homoeopathy, as opposed to 'allopathy', Hahnemann's label for orthodox medicine, which, so he said, prescribed 'allopathically', according to principles *other* than symptom similarity. In 1810 Hahnemann expounded his theory for the first time in a more systematic way in his *Organon*.

But that was not all. Through the years Hahnemann kept adding new elements to his theory or elaborating old elements. The five later editions of the *Organon* (the last was published posthumously in 1921), as well as his other publications, bear witness to this. The assumption of a vital force played an especially prominent role in his later work. According to Hahnemann, externally perceptible symptoms point to the derangement of the vital force, and medicines affect the deranged vital force in a dynamic way. In this context Hahnemann developed a preference for the so-called high potencies: highly diluted and shaken or triturated medicines. The higher the dilution and therefore the smaller the substance of the drug, the more powerful and potent would be the stimulation of the vital force.

From 1828 onwards Hahnemann also developed a theory of chronic diseases, in particular the *psora* (scabies) theory. Chronic diseases were traced back by him to three miasmatic (contagious) diseases: syphilis, sycosis (Hahnemann apparently meant gonorrhoea) and *psora*. By far the most chronic diseases were caused by *psora*. Among later generations of homoeopaths *psora* has been regarded as a constitutional factor.

Problems over homoeopathic purity started with Hahnemann himself. According to Hahnemann, only one, and moreover, only a simple (as opposed to a compound) medicine, was to be used at one time. He strongly objected to deviation from this norm. He likewise condemned those who were not prepared to follow his example, by using increasingly smaller doses. But in his opinion it was worst of all, indeed downright apostasy, when his followers also prescribed allopathic medicines.

This is exactly what happened already in the early 1830s in Germany: a schism occurred between 'pure' and 'free' (or bastard) homoeopaths.[3] Later on the terminology would switch to terms like classical (instead of pure) and (scientific) critical (instead of free). Similar conflicts and schisms occurred sooner or later in other countries, for example in England and France in the 1840s, in the United States in the 1870s, and again in Germany in 1914.[4] In these latter schisms Hahnemann's metaphysical turn also had an impact: for to what extent should the idea of a vital force and the highly diluted medicines be considered as an essential part of homoeopathy? And what about the *psora* theory? For many of his followers the master had obviously gone too far.

### Homoeopathy and the Dutch in the nineteenth century

In the Netherlands the situation stayed much quieter, at least until the early twentieth century. This is hardly surprising, given the weak position of homoeopathy in the country during most of the nineteenth century. The Netherlands proved much less receptive to homoeopathy than the United States, which attracted most converts, or countries like England, France, Belgium, Italy, and Germany itself. Although Hahnemann's *Organon* was translated into Dutch as early as 1827, and several Dutch physicians in those days published on the pros and cons of homoeopathy – most reactions were fairly negative – it was not until 1886 that Dutch homoeopaths organised themselves nationally, much later than elsewhere. Even then homoeopathy's share in the Dutch 'medical market' remained modest, at least if the number of homoeopathic practitioners with a medical doctor's degree is taken as a measure. In 1887 there were still only four of them. Although it can be taken for granted that the Dutch demand for homoeopathic treatment was larger than the number of homoeopathic practitioners suggests – Dutch patients also consulted foreign homoeopathic practitioners – the image still holds that homoeopathy did not gain much popularity amongst the Dutch in the nineteenth century.

Elsewhere I have offered some tentative answers to the question as to why homoeopathy did not meet with a warmer welcome in the Netherlands in the nineteenth century.[5] Initially it was not as though the lack of enthusiasm on the part of Dutch medical practitioners was due to the Medical Act of 1818, for qualified practitioners were free to choose the therapy they deemed best, and to make and sell their own medicines. However, the intellectual climate at the universities was less favourable to homoeopathy, and practitioners who wanted to find out about the new therapy had to rely on their own initiatives and maybe get in touch with German colleagues. The presumed surplus of qualified practitioners from the 1830s onwards may have deterred practitioners from striking out along new paths. It could equally well have provided the very stimulus to do that, especially if they anticipated a demand for homoeopathic treatment.

However, the main problem at this early stage was that the backing of a leading doctor and the example of upper-class support were lacking – the Dutch nobility was a relatively small group anyway. In other European countries, homoeopathy initially thrived on the example of the upper classes. Insofar as members of the Dutch upper classes felt themselves attracted to Hahnemann's therapy, they would have consulted German or Belgian homoeopathic practitioners. Other conditions for a successful introduction of homoeopathy in the medical market, such as the poor state of orthodox medicine and dislike of 'heroic therapy' on the part of upper- and middle-class patients, and possibly also a tradition of self-help, seem to have been amply met in the Netherlands.[6]

Only much later, in the 1850s, are there signs of both upper- and middle-class support. Thus it was reported that the German homoeopathic practitioner C. G. Kallenbach had set up practice in Utrecht at the request of 'many highly placed people'. But it was Rotterdam that in those years became the centre of Dutch support for homoeopathy. The Dutch-speaking Münster homoeopathic practitioner Baron Clemens Maria Franz von Bönninghausen (1785–1864) attracted a fairly large Rotterdam clientele from the early 1850s onwards.[7] This favourite disciple of Hahnemann was highly instrumental in furthering the homoeopathic cause, especially in Rotterdam. Here a Society of Champions of Homoeopathy (*Vereeniging van Voorstanders der Homoeopathie*) was founded in 1857. The Society succeeded in attracting three homoeopathic practitioners to Rotterdam: in 1857 the Germans F. W. O. Kallenbach (1829–1917), a son of the Kallenbach in Utrecht, and A. J. Gruber (1820–1896) set up practice there. In 1859 they were joined by the Dutch homoeopath and doctor of medicine S. J. Van Roijen (1828–1909). Both Kallenbach and Van Roijen, who had to leave Rotterdam after only two years for lack of paying patients, would become prominent promoters of the Dutch homoeopathic cause.

Although the demand for homoeopathic therapy was growing at that time, very few Dutch practitioners had been converted to homoeopathy, and this would continue to be the case until the very end of the nineteenth century. An explanation for this should be sought in the predominantly scientific orientation of the Dutch medical faculties and the absence of homoeopathic training in the Netherlands. There was no chair at a Dutch university, and the first Dutch homoeopathic hospital was only opened in 1914. The standard route to homoeopathic practice was to take first a medical degree at a Dutch university, and then receive homoeopathic training in Germany or Prague, or, from the 1870s onwards, in Budapest with Professor Theodor von Bakody. The Medical Act of 1865 presented a kind of barrier, not so much to becoming a homoeopathic practitioner but to practising as one, since medicines could no longer be freely distributed. A way out of this problem was to interest pharmacists in selling homoeopathic medicines which had been purchased in Germany.

This was the setting in which the Society for the Advancement of Homoeopathy in the Netherlands (*Vereeniging tot Bevordering van de Homoeopathie in Nederland*) was finally founded in 1886, with, from 1890 onwards, its own publication, the *Homoeopathisch maandblad*. The young doctor of medicine and homoeopathic practitioner N. A. J. Voorhoeve (1855–1922) of The Hague became chairman of the Society, in which both laymen and doctors participated. From the 1890s onwards the homoeopathic practitioners were on the increase: their numbers rose from four in 1887 to 14 in 1900, and 31 in 1914. For a long time it would remain an all-male business. Only in 1938, when there were about forty homoeopathic practitioners, would the first female homoeopathic practitioner join them. Just before the turn of the century, in 1898, the Society of Homoeopathic Practitioners in the Netherlands (*Vereeniging van Homoeopathische Geneesheeren in Nederland*) was founded, its chairman being S. J. Van Roijen, the former Rotterdam homoeopath, but by then practising in Utrecht. Two years later the Society of Homoeopathic Practitioners started to publish its proceedings (*Handelingen*).

The Society for the Advancement of Homoeopathy in the Netherlands was active on many fronts, raising funds for homoeopathic training abroad, for a homoeopathic hospital, and, at local level, for a homoeopathic practitioner's salary, persuading pharmacists to sell homoeopathic medicines, and publishing on homoeopathy. However, they failed to have a homoeopathic chair instituted, something opposed by both parliament and the medical faculties. As support for homoeopathy grew, and as the homoeopaths became organised and let their voices be heard and above all began to request scientific and official recognition, criticism from the 'allopaths' became in turn more severe. The homoeopathic practitioners believed they had a monopoly of the truth, and said so frequently. This caused irritation on the part of their non-homoeopathic colleagues, who were often no less convinced of their rightness, supported by what they regarded as scientific truth. Some attempts were made at conciliation by both groups, but more often homoeopathic practitioners were treated as outsiders.

### Dutch homoeopaths and the problem of internal purity in the early-twentieth century

To what extent was homoeopathic purity an issue, or did it become so, once the Dutch homoeopathic practitioners had become organised? There certainly was some discussion over the question as to what homoeopathy was, or should be. Dutch homoeopaths were indeed concerned about the purity of homoeopathy, and they also used this term, *zuiverheid* in Dutch. But it appears that their interpretation of homoeopathic purity tended to be somewhat broader than the one that Hahnemann himself had chosen.

What Dutch homoeopathic practitioners considered to be pure homoeopathy, and to what extent they tolerated impurity can, to begin with, be deduced from their publications. Most of these have appeared in the monthly journal of the Society for the Advancement of Homoeopathy in the Netherlands, the *Homoeopathisch maandblad*, in the *Handelingen* of the Society of Homoeopathic Practitioners in the Netherlands, the *Homoeopathisch tijdschrift* (a Dutch edition of the *Leipziger Populäre Zeitschrift für Homöopathie* of Willmar Schwabe, appearing from 1911 to 1914) and in a limited number of books or brochures by Dutch homoeopaths. These are the main sources on which the following sections are based. Thereafter special attention will be paid to the vicissitudes of the homoeopathic supplement to the Dutch pharmacopoeia between 1902 and 1913. For this subject the archives of the *Centrale Gezondheidsraad* (Central

Health Council) have also been consulted.

Some preliminary ordering seems to be called for. The discussion over homoeopathic purity covered three different, but partly overlapping issues. First of all it was an internal discussion with respect to Hahnemann's therapy, namely over the question what homoeopathy is or should be. Secondly it was again an internal discussion, but this time over the question of who should be allowed to practise homoeopathy: were lay homoeopathic healers to be trusted, and what about self-medication? Thirdly, homoeopathic purity was discussed in terms of external relations, namely those between homoeopathy and 'allopathy'. One of the questions in this context was whether homoeopathic practitioners should also be allowed to use 'allopathic' methods and prescribe 'allopathic' medicines. The problems around the homoeopathic supplement to the Dutch pharmacopoeia related to both the internal issue about the essence of homoeopathy and the external issue about the relationship between homoeopathy and orthodox or regular medicine.

To start with the first issue, the question as to what homoeopathy is or should be. This issue was a relatively popular one. It was regularly and more or less extensively discussed in the *Homoeopathisch maandblad* (from 1890 onwards) and in various brochures. This was by way of information for the readers who, in the case of the *Homoeopathisch maandblad*, were mostly laymen. As could be expected with this type of source there was no proper debate, but one does find information about what was considered to be essential in homoeopathy.[8] In the *Handelingen* of the homoeopathic practitioners (from 1900 onwards) there are some signs of a debate, but on the whole they appear to have agreed with each other. However, this source can misrepresent what went on among them: not all of them became or stayed members of the Society of Homoeopathic Practitioners in the Netherlands (in 1916 only 25 of the 32 homoeopathic practitioners were members).

It would lead too far afield to present the relevant items in the *Homoeopathisch maandblad* and the various brochures extensively. Generally speaking, it comes down to the following. The basic principles and the results of homoeopathy were stated with a great deal of verve and with a variety of rhetorical means, such as an explanation of the principles, a defence against criticism, narrative rhetoric, stories about conversions of allopaths to homoeopathy, and statistics proving homoeopathy's superiority. The aim was to convince and impress the reader of homoeopathy's value. Not surprisingly 'allopathy' was often given the blame. Initially in the 1890s this was done more firmly than later on.

Still, it appears that Hahnemann was not followed in every respect. In the *Homoeopathisch maandblad* of August 1900 it was stated by Johannes Voorhoeve, homoeopathic practitioner in Dillenburg, that:

> we cannot accept all of Hahnemann's publications as the expression of the present-day position of homoeopathy. Our sincere striving has as its aim: the fundamental principle of homoeopathy: 'similia similibus', of which truth we are convinced, and the truly scientific elements of homoeopathy: the employment of a single medicine and research into the effects of medicines by testing them on healthy people.[9]

Voorhoeve further remarked that the doses of the drugs still formed a bone of contention amongst homoeopathic practitioners, but that most of them agreed that certain drugs had more effect in low dilutions, and that the homoeopathic practitioner had the right and the freedom to use the whole range of potencies. One year earlier a similar position had been formulated by his uncle N. A. J. Voorhoeve, the chief editor of the *Homoeopathisch maandblad* and chairman of the Society for the Advancement of Homoeopathy in the Netherlands, namely that:

> the present homoeopathic practitioners by no means agree to everything that Hahnemann has said and taught, for example about the psora theory, about the way in which the weaker, natural disease is removed by a stronger, artificial disease, about the vital force, about potentisation, etc. As far as the inessentials are concerned, there is no doubt that hardly any scientifically educated homoeopath will take sides with Hahnemann; but with respect to the essentials all those who can claim the name of homoeopath agree with Hahnemann.[10]

Similar views were offered in the following years.[11]

The *Homoeopathisch maandblad* does not make mention of internal disputes amongst Dutch homoeopathic practitioners. As F. W. O. Kallenbach, the Rotterdam homoeopath but by then retired for three years, formulated it in 1902: 'Union is strength', and to this adage the Dutch homoeopathic society had successfully adhered.[12] Five years later the editors of this monthly journal commemorated the fiftieth anniversary of Kallenbach's setting up practice in Rotterdam. They called him the Nestor of the Dutch homoeopathic practitioners, an ardent advocate of homoeopathy's basic principle, the *similia similibus*, but also a stern and relentless opponent of everything that bordered on mysticism in Hahnemann's doctrine.[13] If conflicts amongst homoeopaths were mentioned, they were fought out in other countries. In 1914, for example, an article titled 'De potentie-strijd' (The battle over potency) reported that 'the old battle between "Hoch- and Tief-Potenzler" [proponents of high or low potencies] which had already started during Hahnemann's life and has since been raging periodically and in several countries amongst his followers, ...has now broken out once more in Germany.'[14]

In the *Handelingen* of the Society of Homoeopathic Practitioners in the Netherlands the question as to what constitutes homoeopathy, was also considered, and fairly unanimously at that. Already in the first series from 1900 a contribution by N. A. J. Voorhoeve was included on 'What is homoeopathy?' He deemed it useful to establish what according to Dutch homoeopathic practitioners should be understood by homoeopathy, for 'it seems that not all those who call themselves homoeopathic practitioners answer this question in the same way.'[15] According to Voorhoeve one can only speak of a purely homoeopathic treatment if it meets the following four requirements: a correct knowledge of the illness syndrome, including both objectively observable symptoms and subjective complaints; a thorough knowledge of the medicine syndrome via experiments on healthy people or animals; the employment of one drug, after having compared the illness syndrome with the medicine syndrome; and administration of the chosen drug in such a dose, that no deterioration of the existing abnormal state occurs.[16] Voorhoeve moreover fully agreed with the explanation of Hahnemann's method by Theodor von Bakody (1825–1911), the professor in Budapest from whom many Dutch homoeopaths had received their homoeopathic training. 'Anyone who adheres to these principles [as put forward by Bakody] I can recognise as an homoeopathic colleague, even if he is different from me in many respects (for example the size of dosing, alternating medicines etc.).'[17]

The reactions were positive. But that was not all. F. W. O. Kallenbach remarked that these requirements were now and then violated: he warned against dosages that were too small and against stretching the simile-concept.[18] D. K. Munting (1862–1932), homoeopathic practitioner in Amsterdam, took Kallenbach's side.

> The deviations from these basic principles, which are common practice nowadays, are the inevitable consequence of the expansive

tendencies of the homoeopathic school.

New drugs were being insufficiently tested, according to him. And to this he added that it cannot be denied:

> that knowledge of pathological-physiological and histological changes in our time should be considered as absolutely necessary for the complete knowledge of the effects of medicines. Indeed, one can no longer be content with Hahnemann's idea that diseases ...are nothing other than the sum of the externally observable symptoms. We know, that the essence of the matter is more deeply situated, that each externally observable phenomenon, whether objective or subjective, meets the alterations in the normal course of life processes, which have their base in the unity of organic life: the cell.[19]

It hardly needs saying that Munting, who had been Bakody's first Dutch student, was making a truly deep bow to university medicine! Interestingly, Munting puts the cause of homoeopathy in perspective even further, be it with somewhat mixed feelings:

> It is true, that not the principle should be the main point in our therapeutic treatment, but the success. Still, I have to say, that it is a somewhat disappointing thought, that perhaps by us, homoeopaths, homoeopathic treatment should be substituted in many cases by serum therapy.[20]

Although neither the *Homoeopathisch maandblad* nor the *Handelingen* makes explicit mention of disputes over the principles of homoeopathy amongst Dutch homoeopathic practitioners, at least not before 1910 when problems arose over the homoeopathic supplement to the Dutch pharmacopoeia, it was in 1907 hinted at by a critic of homoeopathy, E. A. M. Droog, that Dutch homoeopaths were internally divided over the matter of the very small dosages.[21] J. Mieg (1865–1911), homoeopathic practitioner in Haarlem, thought it wise to minimise these differences by pointing out that they only regarded theoretical explanations of the workings of their drugs, but not the basic principles of homoeopathy.[22]

The second internal issue had a much lower priority on the official homoeopathic agenda: the question as to who should be allowed to practice homoeopathy. The Society of Homoeopathic Practitioners in the Netherlands set the tone in 1898, in the first year of its existence. J. I. A. B. Van Roijen (1870–1925), homoeopathic practitioner in Rotterdam and son of the founder and chairman S.J. Van Roijen, gave a talk on lay practice.[23] He and his audience agreed that professional lay practice should be prevented, but that self-medication still had a reason for existence. It was also stressed that homoeopathy's expansion had been mainly due to laymen.

Only the *Homoeopathisch maandblad* contains notices about specific unqualified homoeopathic healers and unqualified sellers of homoeopathic drugs. But these notices are very scarce indeed. A first notice appeared already in 1893. It was about lawsuits against two unqualified homoeopaths, and the discharge of further prosecution of one of them. The editors greatly rejoiced, because the man had only given free advice on the basis of a homoeopathic 'family doctor', a health-care manual, to an incurably ill person.[24] The only other notice followed in 1906. This time the tone was negative: it concerned a lawsuit in Nijmegen, against an unqualified homoeopathic pharmacist and healer, R. Haverhoek, by then living in The Hague, against whom the readers were warned.[25] Much later, in 1916, the author of an article on quackery even explicitly supported the cause of anti-quackery. He was also quite negative about homoeopathic self-medication by laymen.[26]

Indeed, this last issue was discussed somewhat more frequently, both in the *Homoeopathisch maandblad* and in the *Handelingen*. It is hardly surprising that homoeopathic practitioners had their reserves. Of course it was no problem if people doctored for themselves as long as they had minor affections, and the more so if no homoeopathic practitioner was on hand. In that case a homoeopathic medicine box, as provided by the Leipzig pharmacist Willmar Schwabe, and an edition of a homoeopathic 'family doctor' would certainly come in useful. But people should be careful not to wait too long before consulting a proper doctor, for otherwise things could go irrevocably wrong. What is more, irresponsible self-medication gave homoeopathy a bad name, and that should be avoided at any cost.[27] In 1907 special attention was paid to the *Homoeopathische Bibliotheek* (Homoeopathic Library), a series of publications on homoeopathy for the lay public. It was thought that these publications would damage the prestige of scientists and of practising doctors, and also presented a danger to the patients themselves.[28]

## Dutch homoeopaths and 'allopathy' in the early-twentieth century

Dutch homoeopathy appeared to be on the way up. Since 1898 the university-educated homoeopathic practitioners had their own society, and their numbers were growing. Moreover, the Society for the Advancement of Homoeopathy in the Netherlands was active on many fronts and successful in raising funds, although its membership was falling (from about 400 in 1900 to about 300 in 1910). Thanks to the Society's financial help young doctors were able to receive homoeopathic training abroad, some outpatients' clinics could be instituted, in 1907 a homoeopathic ward for 25 patients in the Utrecht Deaconesses' hospital could be realised, and finally, in 1914, the homoeopathic hospital at Oudenrijn near Utrecht was opened. The Society had also succeeded in persuading a growing number of pharmacists to sell homoeopathic medicines. At the beginning of the twentieth century these were still mostly provided by the Leipzig homoeopathic drugs factory of Willmar Schwabe. In 1895 a Dutch depot for Willmar Schwabe's products had been set up in the international pharmacy at Amsterdam. This depot was replaced in 1902 by nine depots in pharmacies in various parts of the country. The first all-homoeopathic pharmacy in the Netherlands dates from 1909. This pharmacy was run by Carl Theodor Voorhoeve (1883–1969), a son of N. A. J. Voorhoeve, at The Hague. Thereupon Schwabe tried to consolidate his position by establishing a Dutch branch in Zaandam, where pharmacist F. Van Dijk started producing homoeopathic drugs from 1910 onwards.[29]

However, Dutch homoeopaths were less successful in dealing with their 'allopathic' colleagues, much as they tried. At the beginning of the twentieth century the time seemed ripe for another attempt to institute a university homoeopathic chair and for the official registration of homoeopathic medicines. With the Calvinist Abraham Kuyper (1837–1920), an ardent supporter of homoeopathy, as prime minister from 1901 to 1905, the political climate was certainly favourable. But this was hardly the case at the universities. There was much opposition and scepticism towards homoeopathy. Still, in 1903 Kuyper almost managed to have a homoeopath appointed to a vacant pharmaceutical chair at Leiden university. It was for lack of a suitable candidate that the plan failed. The homoeopathic practitioner P.L. Van der Harst (1865–1936) at Leiden is said to have declined an offer for this chair, while attempts to persuade the Parisian homoeopath Dr G. Sieffert failed as well.[30] Embarrassed by the situation the Dutch homoeopathic practitioners postponed their attempts to get a special homoeopathic chair instituted. Instead they organised homoeopathic training at the Utrecht Deaconesses Hospital (1907) and later on at the Homoeopathic Hospital at Oudenrijn (1914). Nor would later attempts to establish a homoeopathic chair be successful. Next best, a *'privaat-docentschap'* (an unsalaried university lecturership) for homoeopathic pharmacology was instituted in 1960 at the Free University at Amsterdam at the request of and funded by the Society for the Advancement of Homoeopathy. The history of the homoeopathic supplement to the Dutch pharmacopoeia, which will be told in the next section, shows a similar pattern: a promising start followed by (partial) failure.

Why these failures? Were they only due to opposition on the side of orthodox medicine and possibly, after Kuyper's term in power, to a lack of political support, or were they also caused by internal dissension amongst the homoeopathic practitioners themselves? As it turns out, there was more dissension than the discussions over the internal aspects of homoeopathic purity have so far revealed. This becomes clear when we take a closer look at how homoeopathic practitioners dealt with 'allopathy' and the issue of what could be called external purity.

Until the end of the nineteenth century homoeopathic authors tended to depict the relationship between homoeopathy and 'allopathy' in strongly antagonistic terms. For homoeopaths, homoeopathy was nothing but the truth, and 'allopathy' an error. Conversely, 'allopaths' were just as quick to condemn homoeopathy. The well-known medical professor in Amsterdam, B.J. Stokvis, had in 1888 by no means been the first opponent to call homoeopathy a scientific error.[31] Both S.J. Van Roijen and F. W. O. Kallenbach felt compelled to react promptly.[32] It is interesting that Kallenbach already at that time made an attempt at conciliation. He agreed with Stokvis that it was no longer correct to call university medicine 'allopathy'. He further claimed that homoeopathy was part of general medicine, and that the new generation of medical practitioners should be acquainted with all forms of therapy, many of which had been recently developed. He even admitted that scientific proof of the *similia* principle was still lacking, something he would repeat in 1910.[33] Van Roijen was not yet prepared to give up the term 'allopathy', nor did he mention the absence of scientific proof of homoeopathy's basic principle. But otherwise his ideas corresponded fairly well with those of Kallenbach.

Once the Society of Homoeopathic Practitioners in the Netherlands had been founded, its members were no longer inclined to voice severe public criticism of university medicine. On the contrary, like their orthodox colleagues they kept stressing that a scientific approach to medicine, homoeopathy included, was absolutely necessary. It is quite obvious that it was scientific respectability that counted. But this was exactly what proved so difficult to obtain for homoeopaths. Even today this is still a serious problem, as was recently noticed at the hundredth anniversary of the Society of Homoeopathic Practitioners in the Netherlands.[34]

Following Kallenbach, and to a lesser extent Van Roijen's position of 1888, N. A. J. Voorhoeve reported a decade later in a fairly tolerant manner on the relationship between homoeopathy and 'allopathy' – he still used this term.

> That we are doctors, and not homoeopathic specialists in the first place, we will all agree about. For in many respects we are not different from our allopathic colleagues. Although in the field of surgery and obstetrics homoeopathic drugs may come in useful, we are still not homoeopathic surgeons or obstetricians. Even in the field of the general therapy of internal diseases we are by no means only homoeopaths, but we act in this extensive field in all sorts of cases in the same way as doctors from the other schools.[35]

Munting would, as has already been shown, vent a similar view.[36]

Much to the regret of Van der Harst and his fellow members of the society not all homoeopaths behaved as moderately as they themselves. In 1907 he criticized in particular Johannes Voorhoeve's black and white representation or rather misrepresentation of 'allopathy' versus homoeopathy in the second edition of his *Homoeopathie in de praktijk*.[37] Dutch homoeopathic practitioners preferred not to be seen any longer as antagonists of university medicine, but as a special branch of medicine. They were conscious of the fact that the new university medicine had much more to offer than the old medicine which had been so severely criticized by Hahnemann and his followers.

But did this more lenient attitude towards university medicine on the part of homoeopathic practitioners also mean that they themselves felt free to prescribe non-homoeopathic drugs? Could they still consider themselves to be homoeopaths if they also used 'allopathic' medicines? Where was the limit? For Hahnemann it had been clear enough: homoeopaths were no longer homoeopaths once they started prescribing 'allopathically'. Kallenbach, no longer that young, but even so impressed by the development of university medicine, was positively inclined to have the best of both worlds, although it would be interesting to find out if his words were also corroborated by his prescriptions.

However, many Dutch homoeopaths were as liberal as he seemed to be. There are several indications that not all of them agreed on this point. When it was discussed in 1903 who could become a member of the Society of Homoeopathic Practitioners and if candidate members should be examined, it was suggested asking them if they put into practice the *similia similibus curantur* [sic] principle and whether they sometimes prescribed a different type of medicine if their patients asked for it.[38] The *Handelingen* do not report the outcome. But so much is clear that at least some members of the society wanted to maintain stricter boundaries than people like Kallenbach. This may also reflect part of the internal problems around the creation and acceptance of the homoeopathic chair.

In 1901, the year in which Abraham Kuyper became prime minister and home secretary, J. Mieg, the homoeopathic practitioner in Haarlem, had pleaded for state inspection of homoeopathic medicines, the compilation of a homoeopathic pharmacopoeia, and the establishment of homoeopathic chairs in the medical faculties, with homoeopathy as a compulsory subject.[39] In early 1903, a few months before Kuyper's attempt to attract an homoeopathic candidate for the pharmacological chair at Leiden university became stranded, N. A. J. Voorhoeve reacted positively to the first part of Mieg's proposal, but he could not agree with the last part. One homoeopathic chair would do, and homoeopathy should not become a compulsory subject. J. T. Wouters (1871–1953) preferred a clinic with an instructor, but without exams. In the line of Wouters it was decided unanimously that the home secretary would be asked to institute a homoeopathic clinic with government funds and totally separate from the university.[40] Obviously, this request was not granted. Instead, as has been shown, the homoeopaths themselves organised homoeopathic training in Utrecht and later in Oudenrijn.

Whereas the discussions over a homoeopathic chair in these early years do not point to internal dissent, this changed after 1910. The subject of the homoeopathic chair was resumed in the wake of the conflict over the homoeopathic supplement to the Dutch pharmacopoeia. Both Kallenbach on the one side and Wouters on the other showed a remarkable consensus on this one point: in view of the lack of unanimity over Hahnemann's doctrine, neither of them deemed it opportune to attempt to have a homoeopathic chair established.[41] It was Wouters who advocated the cause of a 'pure' homoeopathy in the line of admittedly true adherents of Hahnemann's theory, like Skinner in England, or Hering and Kent in America, while homoeopaths like Kallenbach and the editors of the *Homoeopathisch maandblad*, N. A. J. Voorhoeve and Munting, represented a more critical approach, as for example advocated by Theodor von Bakody. According to Wouters this last group adhered to a narrow (*eng* in Dutch) view of Hahnemann's doctrine, whereas the group to which he belonged was devoted to the more comprehensive (*ruimer* in Dutch) and 'purer' conception. It was natural, but nevertheless regrettable, that most Dutch homoeopaths had not yet worked themselves up to the comprehensive conception: this, he added, was a consequence of their training.

### The homoeopathic supplement to the Dutch pharmacopoeia

As it turned out, Wouters had also played a crucial role in blocking the homoeopathic supplement to the Dutch pharmacopoeia in his function as a private member (1902–1925) of the Central Health Council. In 1901 Mieg had not only pleaded for homoeopathic chairs, but also for an official homoeopathic pharmacopoeia. In 1902 the Society of Homoeopathic Practitioners in the Netherlands had presented a petition to Crown and Parliament to introduce official requirements for homoeopathic medicines. After the petition had been granted, a committee was installed in 1904 consisting of S. J. Van Roijen (chairman), P. Van der Wielen (secretary, pharmacist), N. A. J. Voorhoeve, M. L. Van der Stempel (1870–1943), (homoeopathic practitioner at Zaandam) and I. S. Cohen (pharmacist) who was replaced in 1905 by G. H. Van den Wal (pharmacist). Neither of the pharmacists was a homoeopath. When Van Roijen died in 1909, Van der Wielen succeeded him as chairman, while Van der Stempel was appointed secretary.

The committee was charged with the task of making a draft for a supplement to the Dutch pharmacopoeia, containing the processing of homoeopathic medicines, and, as often as this would be necessary, to complement, alter or renew this supplement. In 1905, the first results were put before the Dutch homoeopathic practitioners. The reactions were positive, except for a minor point which the committee changed accordingly. In November 1909 the committee submitted the completed draft of the homoeopathic supplement to a long list of parties concerned.

In July 1910 the committee was ready. The wishes that had been put forward to the committee had been taken into account as much as possible. Medicines of which neither the preparation nor the research could be carried out by the pharmacist had not been described. If these medicines were often used as homoeopathic medicines in the Netherlands, they had been simply mentioned, including the way of preparing the dilutions.[42] The draft supplement was offered for approval to the government. However, because of an unfavourable recommendation by the Central Health Council, the government decided that the time was not yet ripe for official recognition and therefore dissolved the committee.

The Society of Homoeopathic Practitioners in the Netherlands thereupon decided to ask the government permission to publish the supplement themselves. This request was granted, provided that nothing would be altered in it and all relevant documents relating to the work of the committee would be printed as well. So it happened: in 1913 the *Nederlandsch homoeopathisch artsenijboek* was finally published. C.Th. Voorhoeve, the homoeopathic pharmacist at The Hague, gave quite a positive judgement:

> the Dutch Homoeopathic pharmacopoeia strikes the golden mean, for it keeps strictly to Hahnemann's principles and it still brings the preparation of drugs in conformity with science.[43]

Other pharmacopoeias, according to Voorhoeve, either take over Hahnemann's prescriptions including their shortcomings (for example the *Pharmacopoeia Polyglotta*, published by Willmar Schwabe), or they avoid Hahnemann's mistakes wholly or partially, but then also more or less discarded his principles with regard to preparation and potency determination. Voorhoeve concluded that the Dutch homoeopathic pharmacopoeia was far superior.

The archives of the Central Health Council reveal that Wouters had strongly protested against the draft supplement, because prescriptions about high-potency drugs had been excluded. His protest certainly contributed to the negative advice by other members of the advisory committee of the Central Health Council. For, as they realised, homoeopaths were not just internally divided about the extent to which medicines should be diluted, as the committee for the homoeopathic supplement had pretended. Their controversy was a much more fundamental one, for it concerned the question of whether grinding and diluting only resulted in dividing the drugs, or that this processing also gave the drugs a mysterious force. It was concluded that homoeopaths should first agree about this fundamental issue amongst themselves. But the committee members could not refrain from adding that they completely disagreed with Wouters about the supposedly great force of high potencies.[44]

The gap between Wouters and a few other classically oriented homoeopaths on the one hand, and the dominant group of critically oriented homoeopaths on the other, was further revealed in publications from both sides.[45] Wouters was heavily criticized, and he even stopped being a member of the Society of Homoeopathic

Practitioners in the Netherlands. It is not yet clear whether this decision was his own initiative or not. In his turn Wouters vented his critique on the state of Dutch homoeopathy, which had deviated from what he understood to be pure homoeopathy. The *Homoeopathisch tijdschrift*, which published his grievances in 1913 just after this former Leipzig-Schwabe journal had gained independent status and adopted as subtitle 'The most widely distributed organ for homoeopathy in the Netherlands and the colonies' (the September 1914 number would be the last one), reveals still more.

In an editorial, M. L. Van der Stempel, the former member of the committee for the homoeopathic supplement to the Dutch pharmacopoeia, and R. A. B. Oosterhuis, a young homoeopathic practitioner in Amsterdam, wrote that they thoroughly disagreed with the plans to publish the draft homoeopathic supplement as the Dutch homoeopathic pharmacopoeia.[46] They considered this to be 'incorrect and contrary to the interests of homoeopathy, quite apart from the value which should be attached to the draft as such.' As they were fairly positive that the majority of homoeopathic practitioners shared their opinion, they were going to set up a postal survey, since 'the Society of Homoeopathic Practitioners, of which no longer all homoeopathic practitioners are a member, does not represent this opinion correctly.'

Soon after this critical editorial two more substantial critiques were published. Hugo Platz, pharmacist and director of the Homoeopathic Central-Pharmacy of Dr Willmar Schwabe in Leipzig, stated that the Dutch homoeopathic pharmacopoeia was deficient, in that detailed instructions for trituration had been omitted and that the adherents of homoeopathy would therefore have no guarantee that their medicines would be prepared exactly according to Hahnemann's prescriptions.[47] Wouters quite agreed with Platz. Indeed, people would be at the mercy of the pharmacists' discretion.[48]

Notwithstanding (or possibly due to) these negative verdicts, the response to the postal survey was disappointing: only about one third of the Dutch homoeopathic practitioners sent in their answers. The majority of the respondents, some seven of them, were as negative and worried as the editors and Wouters themselves. The editors concluded that there was 'strong opposition' to publication of the Dutch homoeopathic pharmacopoeia (which had by then been published) because its principles were no longer 'purely Hahnemannian' and would therefore only cause confusion.[49]

## Homoeopathy's dilemma: between trust and truth

Once the numbers of Dutch homoeopathic practitioners had started growing and they had to admit what they stood for, as in the case of the homoeopathic pharmacopoeia, homoeopathic purity turned into a real issue, even in the Netherlands. The majority of Dutch homoeopathic practitioners was still in favour of a critical scientific approach. Thus, Kallenbach explicitly stated in 1913 that one group of homoeopaths recognized the thesis fairly generally accepted amongst scientists, that matter and force form an unbreakable unity, from which it follows that drugs should still contain matter to be effective. The other group of homoeopaths was convinced that force could be separated from matter and be passed on to neutral substances, and thus have a healing effect by itself.[50]

Before the first decade of the twentieth century, internal homoeopathic purity had hardly been a matter of concern to Dutch homoeopathic practitioners. Moreover, as orthodox medicine had increasingly more to offer, they aimed at compromise, not conflict. However, when the time seemed ripe to harvest a homoeopathic chair and a homoeopathic supplement to the Dutch pharmacopoeia, this failed to come true. This failure did have the unintended effect of the publication of the non-official Dutch homoeopathic pharmacopoeia. This in turn evoked homoeopathic 'purists' to voice their criticisms even more loudly.

It looks as though two alliances were formed between the central Schwabe firm at Leipzig, including the Dutch branch at Zaandam, and a younger generation of classical homoeopaths like Wouters, Van der Stempel and Oosterhuis on the one hand, and the slightly older group of Voorhoeve's, including the pharmacist at The Hague, the Van Roijen's, and Kallenbach on the other. Homoeopathic theory was one thing, but neither should pharmaceutical and medical interests be downplayed. Homoeopathy represented an interesting, albeit small, part of the pharmaceutical and medical market. Schwabe's firm was by no means happy with the competition on the part of Voorhoeve's homoeopathic pharmacy.

Still, homoeopathy's dilemma was, and is, that scientific proof for both the *similia* principle and the effectivity of highly diluted drugs is hard or maybe even impossible to come by. Homoeopaths have to have trust in Hahnemann's therapy, whatever they understand by it, and whether or not they aspire to scientific status. Their truth is based on trust. And the more they aspire to scientific truth, the less 'pure' their homoeopathy will tend to be.

## Notes

1. In German *sanft, schnell, gewiss und dauerhaft*. Samuel Hahnemann, *Organon der rationellen Heilkunde nach homöopathischen Gesetzen* (Dresden: Arnold, 1810). The later editions, published after 1819, were called *Organon der Heilkunst*.
2. Marijke Gijswijt-Hofstra, 'Compromise, not conflict. The introduction of homoeopathy into the Netherlands in the nineteenth century', *Tractrix*, 5 (1993), 121–38.
3. See Renate Wittern, 'Le développement de l'homéopathie en Allemagne au XIXe siècle', in Olivier Faure (ed.), *Praticiens, patients et militants de l'homéopathie* (Lyon: Boiron, 1992), 33–58; Karl-Heinz Faber, 'Die homöopathische Zeitschrift Hygea als Spiegel einer neuen Heilmethode', in Martin Dinges (ed.), *Homöopathie. Patienten, Heilkundige, Institutionen. Von den Anfängen bis heute* (Heidelberg: Haug, 1996), 255–69.
4. See Phillip A. Nicholls, *Homoeopathy and the Medical Profession* (London: Croom Helm, 1988); Phillip A. Nicholls, Peter Morrell, 'Laienpraktiker und häretische Mediziner: Grossbritannien', in Martin Dinges (ed.), *Weltgeschichte der Homöopathie. Länder, Schulen, Heilkundige* (München: Beck, 1996), 185–213; Olivier Faure, 'Eine zweite Heimat für die Homöopathie: Frankreich', in Dinges (ed.), *ibid.*, 48–73; Harris L. Coulter, *Divided Legacy. The conflict between homoeopathy and the American Medical Association*, second edn (Richmond, VA: North Atlantic Books, 1982); Naomi Rogers, 'Ärzte, Patienten und Homöopathie in den USA', in Dinges (ed.), *ibid.*, 269–300.
5. Marijke Gijswijt-Hofstra, *op. cit.* (note 2).
6. These conditions have been suggested by: Coulter, *op. cit.* (note 4), 101; Olivier Faure, *Le débat autour de l'homéopathie en France 1830–1870. Evidences et arrière-plans* (Lyon: Boiron, 1990), 158–59; Wittern, *op. cit.* (note 3), 38. For the tradition of self-help, see, for example, Melitta Schmideberg, *Geschichte der homöopathischen Bewegung in Ungarn* (Leipzig: Willmar Schwabe, 1929), X; Ursula Miley, John V. Pickstone, 'Medical Botany around 1850: American Medicine in Industrial Britain', in Roger Cooter (ed.), *Studies in the History of Alternative Medicine* (Houndmills and London: Macmillan Press, 1988), 139–54, 148.
7. Marijke Gijswijt-Hofstra, 'Homoeopathy's early Dutch conquests: The Rotterdam clientele of Clemens von Bönninghausen in the 1840s and 1850s', *Journal of the History of Medicine and Allied Sciences*, 51 (1996), 155–83.

8. The *Handelingen*, first series (1900–1904), 24, mention that at the meeting of 15 February 1899 N. A. J. Voorhoeve had explained that the board of the Society for the Advancement of Homoeopathy in the Netherlands had decided not to publish an article in the *Homoeopathisch maandblad* about the risks of self-medication and lay practice. It was written by his colleague, H. Van Roijen, and was to be signed by all homoeopathic practitioners because it was feared that polemical writing would create a wrong impression and disturb the good relationships within the Society.
9. Dr J.V. [J. Voorhoeve], 'De grondbeginselen der homoeopathy', *Homoeopathisch maandblad*, 11 (1900), 154–6. His book, *Homoeopathie in de praktijk*, first published in 1905, was to become very popular.
10. Dr N.A.J.V. [N. A. J. Voorhoeve], 'Voordracht van den Arts van Eden', *Homoeopathisch maandblad*, 10 (1899), 33–5.
11. See, for example, J.M. [J. Mieg], 'Wat is homoeopathie?', *ibid.*, 19 (1908), 153–4; Dr F.W.O.K. [F. W. O. Kallenbach], 'Over de grenzen van de genezing met artsenijen', *ibid.*, 19 (1908), 180–2; Dr F.W.O.K. [F. W. O. Kallenbach], 'Uit het homoeopatisch en allopathisch kamp', *ibid.*, 21 (1910), 105–6.
12. F. W. O. Kallenbach, 'Voordracht van Dr Kallenbach', *ibid.*, 13 (1902), 33–6, 34.
13. Editorial, 'Een jubileum', *ibid.*, 18 (1907), 9.
14. Dr J.N.V. [J. N. Voorhoeve], 'De potentie-strijd', *ibid.*, 25 (1914), 41–3. In 1914 Jacob Nicolaas Voorhoeve, a son of N. A. J. Voorhoeve, had also set up practice in The Hague. In 1915 he was to become the second director of the Homoeopathic Hospital Oudenrijn near Utrecht. Earlier, in 1909, his brother, Carl Theodor, had set up an all-homoeopathic pharmacy in The Hague, the first in The Netherlands.
15. N. A. J. Voorhoeve, 'Wat is homoeopathie?', *Handelingen*, first series (1900–1904), 7–13, 8.
16. Voorhoeve, *op. cit.* (note 15), 12–13.
17. *Ibid.*, 9–10.
18. F. W. O. Kallenbach, 'Wat is homoeopathie?', *Handelingen*, first series (1900–1904), 82–9.
19. D. K. Munting, 'Eenige opmerkingen naar aanleiding van Dr Kallenbach's "qu'est ce que l'homoeopathie?"', *Handelingen*, first series (1900-1904), 90–106, 99.
20. Munting, *op. cit.* (note 19), 100.
21. E. A. M. Droog, *De homoeopathie voorheen en thans voor artsen en ontwikkelde leeken toegelicht* (Haarlem: Erven F. Bohn, 1907), 39–44.

22. J. Mieg, *"Macht's nach!"*. *Eenige opmerkingen naar aanleiding van "De homoeopathie voorheen en thans" van Dr E. A. M. Droog* (Zwolle: La Rivière & Voorhoeve, 1907), 24–5, 35.
23. J. I. A. B. Van Roijen, 'De leekenpraktijk', *Handelingen*, first series (1900–1904), 20–4.
24. *Homoeopathisch maandblad*, 4 (1893), 25, 46.
25. *Ibid.*, 17 (1906), 143.
26. A. D. de Leeuw, 'Kwakzalverij', *ibid.*, 27 (1916), 20–3, 28–32.
27. F. W. O. Kallenbach, 'Similia Similibus Curantur II', *ibid.*, 25 (1914), 33-4. See also Dr N.A.J.V. [N. A. J. Voorhoeve], 'Misbruik van homoeopathische geneesmiddelen', *ibid.*, 19 (1908), 116–17; A. B., 'Leekenpraktijk – een gevaar!', *ibid.*, 21 (1910), 139–40; Dr F.W.O.K. [F. W. O. Kallenbach], 'Over vijanden der Homoeopathie', *ibid.*, 21 (1910), 146–7.
28. H. Van Roijen, 'Het schrijven van geneeskundige werken voor leeken', *Handelingen*, second series, no. 2 (1907), 58–9. The *Homoeopathische Bibliotheek* was published by La Rivière & Voorhoeve in Zwolle. Most of the books were written by Johannes Voorhoeve. In addition to his *Homoeopathie in de praktijk*, which was first published in 1905, books appeared by him on influenza, whooping cough, and neurasthenia in the same year.
29. H. E. M. de Lange, 'De Nederlandse homeopathische tijdschriften sinds 1836', *Similia similibus curentur*, 17 (1987), 125–31, 127–8. See also Schwabe's advertisement in *Homoeopathisch maandblad* 13 (1902), 8.
30. O. E. A. Goetze, 'Geschiedenis van de homeopathie', in H. G. Bodde, O. E. A. Goetze and E. S. M. de Lange-de Klerk (eds.), *Leerboek homeopathie* (Utrecht & Antwerpen: Bohn, Scheltema and Holkema, 1988), 3–28, 26; H. E. M. de Lange, 'Vereniging Homoeopathie Nederland: een eeuw van betrokken zijn bij de opleiding tot homoeopathisch arts', *Similia similibus curentur*, 16 (1986), 92–8, 94.
31. B. J. Stokvis, *Voordrachten over homoeopathie, gehouden aan de Amsterdamsche universiteit* (Haarlem: Erven F. Bohn, 1888).
32. [S. J. Van Roijen], *Professor B. J. Stokvis' voordrachten over homoeopathie beoordeeld* ('s-Gravenhage: C. Blommendaal, 1888); F. W. O. Kallenbach, *De aanval afgeslagen. Antwoord op de door H. H. Prins Wielandt en Dr B. J. Stokvis tegen de homoeopathie gerichte brochures* ('s-Gravenhage: C. Blommendaal, 1888).
33. Kallenbach, *op. cit.* (note 11).
34. *VHAN Nieuwsbrief Homeopathie* (April 1998).
35. Voorhoeve, *op. cit.* (note 15), 7.

36. Munting, *op. cit.* (note 19).
37. P. L. Van der Harst, 'Homoeopathie in de praktijk', *Handelingen*, second series, no. 2 (1907) 72–78, 73. J. Voorhoeve, *Homoeopathie in de praktijk*, second improved edition (Zwolle: La Rivière & Voorhoeve, 1907).
38. H. Van Roijen, 'Examens', *Handelingen*, first series (1900–1904), 195.
39. J. Mieg, 'Ons ideaal', *ibid.*, first series (1900–1904), 77–81.
40. Second appendix, discussion 11 February 1903, *ibid.*, first series (1900–1904), 119–24.
41. J. T. Wouters, 'Homoeopathie en Homoeopathen', *Homoeopathisch tijdschrift*, 3 (1913), 57–9, 73–6; F. W. O. Kallenbach, 'Oprichting van een leerstoel voor Homoeopathie', *Homoeopathisch maandblad*, 24 (1913), 141–2; Editorial [N. A. J. Voorhoeve and D. K. Munting], 'Een Homoeopathische Leerstoel', *ibid.*, 145–6; F. W. O. Kallenbach, 'Nog eens: "Een Homoeopathische Leerstoel."', *ibid.*, 157–8.
42. See the introduction to the *Nederlandsch homeopathisch artsenijboek*. Publication by the Society of Homoeopathic Practitioners in the Netherlands (Amsterdam: J. H. de Bussy, 1913).
43. C.Th. Voorhoeve, *Het Nederlandsche artsenijboek* (Zwolle: La Rivière & Voorhoeve, 1913), 16.
44. ARA, Archive Centrale Gezondheidsraad 378, nr. 48 (1912): Rapport van de Commissie van praeadvies etc., 1 March 1912.
45. Wouters, *op. cit.* (note 41); this same article was also published in *Vox medicorum*, 13 (1913), 75–6, 90–1. It gave rise to a discussion between Wouters and the pharmacist, G. Wieringa, at Arnhem, who considered himself to have been unfairly treated by Wouters. This discussion was published in *Vox medicorum*, 13 (1913), 154, 164–6, 171–2, 181, 186–7; and in *Homoeopathisch maandblad* 24, appendices 8 and 9 (1913). Kallenbach, *op. cit.* (note 41).
46. Editorial, *Homoeopathisch tijdschrift*, 3 (1913), 1–2.
47. Wouters, *op. cit.* (note 41); Hugo Platz, 'Eenige opmerkingen naar aanleiding van de brochure van Dr N. A. J. Voorhoeve', *ibid.*, 21–4.
48. Wouters, *op. cit.* (note 41), 75.
49. Editorial, 'Onze enquête over het concept der Homoeopathische Pharmacopee', *Homoeopathisch tijdschrift*, 3 (1913), 184–6.
50. Kallenbach, *op. cit.* (note 41), 157.

# 6

## Drugs for healthy people:
## The culture of testing hormonal contraceptives for women and men

*Nelly Oudshoorn*

The oral contraceptive is a very special type of drug. In contrast to other pharmaceuticals, contraceptive drugs are used by healthy and fertile adults, rather than by people who suffer from a specific illness. The fact that contraceptives are not curative drugs raises an important question about the nature of the development of these pharmaceuticals. To what extent does the practice of making contraceptives differ from the making of medicines in general? In this paper I shall explore the specificity of the culture of contraceptive development by focusing on the clinical testing of these pharmaceuticals.

The first aspect that needs attention is the way in which clinicians succeed in enrolling volunteers for clinical trials. Since contraceptives are not related to a specific category of patients, scientists need to develop specific procedures for gaining access to people who want to participate in clinical trials. To what extent can clinicians rely on existing routines in the testing of drugs? Do they face specific constraints in recruiting volunteers for the testing of new contraceptives? If so, how do they try to overcome these constraints? A second feature of the testing of contraceptives that differs from the testing of drugs in general involves the procedures for obtaining approval for testing and marketing by regulatory agencies. Since contraceptives are not developed for treating or preventing diseases, the criteria for assessing the safety and acceptability of health risks are likely to be different from those used for the testing of other drugs.

To explore these questions I shall analyse two case studies: the testing of the first oral contraceptive for women in the late 1950s and early 1960s, and the testing of a hormonal contraceptive injection for men in the 1980s and 1990s. I shall use these examples to analyse the procedures to test the first generation of hormonal contraceptives for women and one of the first prototypes of hormonal contraceptives for men as a new type of pharmaceutical. I shall first describe the procedures used to gain access to volunteers for clinical trials, and then proceed to analyse the procedures used for obtaining approval for the testing and marketing of these pharmaceuticals.[1]

## The quest for 'healthy patients'

Although the possibility of using hormones as contraceptives was mentioned as early as 1921, it took three decades before scientists actually began to develop contraceptive hormones. When the pill eventually came into existence, it was greeted with enthusiasm. By the late 1950s and early 1960s, less than a decade after initial testing in animal studies, the pill was being consumed daily by millions of women all over the world. Never before in medical history had a medical technology witnessed such rapid and broad diffusion.[2]

The contraceptive pill was a novelty in the market for contraceptive methods at that time. It was the first physiological means of contraception; that is, it prevented pregnancies by intervening in the internal processes of the body, rather than by means of an extraneous device.[3] All conventional contraceptives depended on setting up a mechanical or chemical barrier to prevent sperm cells from reaching egg cells.[4] Contraception might now be achieved by taking an 'aspirin-like pill that would be unrelated to sexual intercourse.'[5] Moreover, the pill was a novelty since it was one of the first drugs given to healthy people for a social purpose, i.e. to limit population growth.[6] When Gregory Pincus, the American biologist specializing in endocrinology and reproductive functions, who eventually became the 'father' of the pill, began testing hormones as contraceptives in 1951, he could not easily follow the routines of other clinical testing.

The testing of drugs to cure a specific disease relies on patients who can be assessed in clinical settings. For the pill, such patients did not exist. The testing of the pill required 'healthy patients' who did not suffer from any particular disease and consequently did not belong to the clientele of a specific clinic. Moreover, the development of the first oral contraceptive for women took place during a period in which contraceptive research was highly constrained by political and moral taboos against contraception. In the United States, federal and state laws prohibited the dissemination of contraceptive information, including contraceptive devices, until well into the 1960s.[7] Pincus faced the problems of where to find test subjects and a politically feasible test location.

Owing to these constraints, the history of testing the pill reads like a detective story, in which the actors try to conceal their real intentions from anyone who might hinder their endeavours. In this respect, the first trial in which hormones were tested in women speaks volumes: the contraceptive potential of the hormones was tested first among women who were being treated for infertility problems! At a scientific conference in 1952, Pincus happened to meet John Rock, a professor of gynaecology at Harvard, with whom Pincus had collaborated in an earlier research project. Rock, the director of the Free Hospital for Women, one of the busiest infertility clinics in the US, was a major advocate of the application of hormone research to clinical gynaecology.[8] At this conference Pincus learned about Rock's clinical studies, in which he tested progesterone among his women patients for a purpose diametrically opposed to that of Pincus: the treatment of infertility. Rock's studies were based on the hypothesis that infertility might be related to underdevelopment of the fallopian tubes and womb. The administration of progesterone (and estrogens) was expected to stimulate the growth of these organs and thus facilitate fertilization and pregnancy.[9] The Free Hospital appeared to be an ideal test site for Pincus's purposes as well. The hospital attracted many leading gynaecologists and functioned as a private research clinic.[10] Despite their different missions, Rock and Pincus seemed to follow similar approaches. Actually, they were working on different aspects of the same problem - the manipulation of the process of conception - and they shared an interest in the same hormones.[11] Cooperation between the laboratory and the clinic could be of mutual interest: it would provide Pincus with the conditions required for testing progesterone as a contraceptive in women, while Rock might profit from the collaboration, since it promised a much broader investigation into the development of infertility drugs. Rock, who well knew the contraceptive effect of progesterone, accepted Pincus's request to extend his research on progesterone to explore the compound's potential use as a contraceptive.[12] The first testing of oral contraceptives thus took place as a parallel study in the context of Rock's infertility research.

In 1953, Rock began a second series of clinical trials, in which 27 women were enlisted, all patients with infertility complaints drawn from the Free Hospital clinic, this time with the explicit aim of testing the effects of the trial compounds on ovulation.[13] The results of this first trial did not answer the question of whether oral progesterone could be made into an effective contraceptive. The participating women were all suffering from infertility problems, and were not exactly ideal subjects to test contraceptives. Both Rock and

Pincus felt that further clinical trials were needed. A single study of 50 and then of 27 infertile women did not suffice to convince their colleagues. Actually, Pincus met with severe criticism when he first presented their findings in public. At the fifth meeting of the International Planned Parenthood Federation held in Tokyo in 1955, Pincus's presentation was received with yawns and scepticism. The tests used by Rock to check whether women had ovulated were criticized by other scientists as inconclusive.[14] However, large-scale clinical trials for the explicit purpose of developing contraceptives were practically impossible to carry out, since they would have violated the law. Rock and Pincus knew that legally they could not organize such trials at the Free Hospital without risking criminal prosecution.[15] Pincus considered an escape route: Puerto Rico, a location outside the continental US. In Puerto Rico, laws prohibiting contraception did not exist at that time. Laws prohibiting birth control had been repealed as early as 1937, owing to the successful lobbying of the birth control movement in Puerto Rico.

This clinical experiment in Puerto Rico did not last long. The recruitment of volunteers was problematic. Most of the medical students dropped out, owing to graduation and a reluctance to adhere to the troublesome requirements of the study: taking daily temperatures and vaginal smears, collecting urine samples, and submission to an endometrial biopsy. The trial included 23 female medical students, of whom only 13 remained in the project for three months. Disciplining women to the rigorous conditions of the trials was obviously not easy. Garcia, after a vain attempt to recruit new students, then turned to female prisoners as potential subjects. These women, however, expressed objections to participation. The final setback for this Puerto Rican trial came when university officials learned about the contraceptive implications of the study and withdrew their support.[16]

After this debâcle in Puerto Rico, Pincus tried another escape route: a mental hospital. He approached the Worcester State Hospital, a mental institution located near his laboratory, with which he had cooperated in earlier experiments.[17] The hospital's director agreed to the organization of a clinical trial with 15 patients, all classified as psychotics. The group consisted of seven women and eight men, the first (and last) male test subjects in the research project. Despite the fact that the hormone preparations had a definite contraceptive effect in the male patients, men were not included in later trials because of adverse effects. One subject in this trial was found to have smaller testicles after five months of taking progestin tablets. Pincus encountered other constraints as well. The psychotic men did not make easy subjects. The men's mental disturbances made it rather difficult to collect semen samples, one of the requirements for investigating the effects of progestin.[18] The results of this trial, to put it mildly, did not provide a decisive answer to Pincus's quest for the 'universal contraceptive'.

This episode in the making of the pill illustrates that Pincus's quest to find locations to test the contraceptive was not an easy one. Initially, Rock's clinic seemed to offer a perfect solution. The clinic provided Pincus with access to women who could be made into the first test subjects for the contraceptive-in-the-making. Pincus successfully reoriented Rock's research from conception to contraception. Nevertheless, Rock's clinic, and the other settings that Pincus selected, failed to provide the proper conditions for testing the contraceptive activity of hormones. The development of progestins into contraceptives required access to large groups of healthy, fertile women. However, large-scale trials could not be organized in the gynaecological clinics of medical schools, since these trials were even harder to conceal than small-scale trials. Pincus and Rock had to find a test location outside the domain of the established medical institutions. The quest for 'healthy patients' could only be solved by moving the trials to a completely different location: the infrastructure of the family planning organizations, particularly the Family Planning Association in Puerto Rico. Pincus again found refuge in Puerto Rico, where the family planning movement had a wide-spread institutional base in the form of birth control programmes and clinics. The making of the pill thus required the creation of what might best be described as 'a laboratory in the field.' The test location had to provide the same controlled conditions that were present in the clinical setting. It was quite clear that the field location had to meet specific requirements so that these trials would not fail altogether.

The prerequisite was that the location had to guarantee that women would not easily drop out of the project. But where could one find such a "cage of ovulating females", as McCormick bluntly put it?[19] In this respect an island seemed a perfect solution, since its population tended to be stable. The 'miniature world' of Puerto Rico seemed an ideal location for the testing of progestins.[20] In 1956 Pincus and his colleagues selected a location in one of the suburbs of the capital, San Juan, where large slum-clearance operations were being carried out, involving a new housing project. Many of the families who had just moved into these new houses had previously lived in hovels. This situation promised to minimize the risk that women would become lost to the continuous checks and examinations required in the trials. Puerto Rico thus promised to meet one major requirement of the laboratory. But an island in itself is, of course, not enough to make a 'laboratory in the field'. The development and introduction of new technologies requires an organizational infrastructure within which this testing can take place. Puerto Rico also met this requirement in the form of its Family Planning Association. In the early 1950s the family planning movement had a well-established base in Puerto Rico. The Family Planning Association was founded in 1953 as the direct successor to the Population Association and other previous birth control organizations in Puerto Rico, and had inherited a widespread network of family planning workers and clinics. The displacement of the clinical tests from the medical institutions to the clinics of the family planning organizations had enormous consequences in terms of the women who eventually became the major test subjects for the contraceptive pill. Following the trials in Puerto Rico in 1958, clinical trials were organized in the continental US (trials were carried out by Dr Edward Tyler in Los Angeles in 1958)[21] and the UK (preliminary small-scale trials were organized in a private birth control clinic and a hospital in London in 1958 and in Birmingham in 1960),[22] but the first large-scale trials preceding the marketing of the first oral contraceptive for women did not take place among the white majority of Americans or Europeans. It was Caribbean women who entered this history as the guinea pigs of one of the most revolutionary drugs in the history of medicine. A further testing of the pill took place when oral contraceptives were introduced on to the European market. In the UK trials were organized to develop an easier regimen for taking the pill and to adjust the dose of the pill in order to limit adverse effects.[23] In the Netherlands, Organon, currently one of the leading firms in the market of female contraceptive pills, sought to enter the hormonal contraceptive market in the late 1950s by trying to buy a licence from Syntex, but this company had already sold the exclusive rights to the US firm Parke, Davis & Co. Consequently, Organon had to develop their own product, and initiated chemical research to synthesize new steroids with contraceptive activity. In 1957 they received a Dutch patent for lynestrenol, a modified progesterone, which eventually became the major compound of the first Dutch contraceptive pill, Lyndiol. In the early 1960s Organon organized pre-marketing and post-marketing clinical trials of its new product. In 1965 Lyndiol was tested among 200 Dutch women.[24]

Summarizing the pre-marketing testing of the first oral contraceptive for women in the late 1950s, we can conclude that the quest for 'healthy patients' would have been much simpler if contraceptive research had not been constrained by political and moral taboos against birth control. If contraceptive research had not been prohibited, Pincus would not have been forced to find a test location outside the medical institutions. He might well have persuaded other gynaecological clinics to participate in the clinical trials. The major constraint on the testing of the first oral contraceptive for women is thus not specific for the culture of the clinic but imposed by society at large. Contraceptives have become part and parcel of our culture since the 1970s and the testing of contraceptives for women can nowadays easily follow the routines of other clinical testing. Clinical trials for new contraceptives for women usually take place in gynaecological clinics, as happens with other drugs related to reproductive functions.

### News media as tools for gaining access to male volunteers

Given the changed attitudes towards contraceptives, one might expect that the enrolment of people for the testing of new contraceptives would no longer require any specific procedures. However, the testing of new contraceptives for men, shows how the quest for 'healthy patients' – if these 'patients' are male – still cannot follow the routines of other clinical testing.

The development of hormonal contraceptives for men first appeared on the research agenda in the early 1970s. Compared with the testing of the first hormonal contraceptives for women, the testing of hormonal contraceptives for men showed a much wider variety of test locations, both in Northern and Southern countries. The first small-scale clinical trials took place primarily in the US and the UK in the early 1970s. The first large-scale clinical trials included test locations in Europe, the US, Latin America, and Asia.[25] Since the pharmaceutical industry did not show much interest in the development of new male contraceptives, research and development in this new technology was mainly performed by non-profit public sector agencies, most notably the WHO and the Population Council. The testing of male contraceptives thus depended largely on the creation of alliances with the news media. For most clinicians, 'going public' was a completely new role. Paulsen, a professor in reproductive physiology at the Medical School in Seattle, and one of the pioneers in male contraceptive research, recalled his first contacts with the media as follows:

> I never used to call up the television and say 'hey I'm working on such and such' ...You don't hold press conferences every day so it was somewhat foreign to me to go public... But they (the media) have been very useful.[26]

Approaching the media to recruit volunteers was obviously so delicate that it had to take place outside Paulsen's medical centre; Paulsen asked his secretary to contact the media from her own phone number and to answer any phone calls at home.[27] In Britain, male contraceptive researchers had similar experiences. Fred Wu, who participated in the multicentre clinical trials organized by the WHO in 1990, concluded that:

> The media are very important. I don't like doing it though, because I didn't think I'm trained to deal with the media, but I'm forced to do it, because its the only way I can get the recruitment.[28]

Although scientists did not consider themselves experts in approaching the media, British scientists were nevertheless very successful in attracting media attention. In July 1993, Fred Wu and his colleagues at the public relations department of the University of Manchester drafted a press release and organized a special press conference. The trial was described as the most extensive trial of the 'male pill' ever carried out in the UK, launched by the University of Manchester, Department of Medicine, based at Hope Hospital, Salford.

The press release also described the volunteers they were looking for: they needed to have specific qualities such as age (between 21 and 45 years), they should have 'a stable relationship', and they should be 'highly motivated, determined people' with a 'strong commitment' to the trial. Quite remarkably, the press release was addressed not to men but to 'couples'. Men who wanted to participate in the trial should bring their partners with them. The new male contraceptive was presented as a technology particularly suited to 'couples' in 'stable relationships', 'who are not sure that they have completed their family'. The press release thus told a heroic tale about a new technology being tested in the UK that promised to make an important contribution to the emancipation of men and to the reduction of the world population growth – a technology that gave the reader, if he was lucky, the chance to take part in an exciting, important endeavour. To quote the press release once more: 'So the race is on to find suitable couples in the North West.' These attempts to interest the media were very successful. The press release and the press briefing organized by the University of Manchester in July 1993 created hype in the British newspapers. Within two days, more than 40 news articles were published in both the local and national press. Almost all articles opened with the following, almost identical, line: 'Volunteer couples are being sought to take part in the most extensive trial of the "male pill" ever held in Britain.' The press coverage resulted in nearly 350 enquiries, whereas only 30 volunteers were needed for the test. The Manchester clinicians thus demonstrated that they did not need their colleagues in the clinic: alliances with the news media gave them their long-sought access to volunteers for their trials. Despite the reluctance to go public, media contacts have become part of the work of scientists in the field of male contraceptives. Since the late 1980s the enrolment of male volunteers through news media channels has become routine practice in the field of male contraceptives.

Summarising, we can conclude that the scientists and clinicians involved in the trials of contraceptives for men could not easily follow the routine of other clinical testing. The quest for 'healthy patients' could only be solved by approaching institutions outside the medical world, as had happened with the testing of the first hormonal contraceptives for women. There is, however, a difference between the testing of male and female contraceptives. Whereas the major constraint on the testing of hormonal contraceptives for women can be ascribed to political and moral taboos in culture at large, the testing of male contraceptives was constrained by routine practices characteristic of the culture of the medical community itself as well as other cultural norms. Attempts to find male volunteers for clinical trials did not succeed, because male contraceptive research threatened to disrupt the boundaries between medical specialties, as was illustrated by the gynaecologists' refusal to cooperate in the testing. Moreover, no profession was really interested in controlling the fertility of male rather than female subjects. Even family planning clinics, the escape route successfully used by Pincus in the testing of the first hormonal contraceptives for women, could not offer any help, because the family planning clinic's clientele was almost entirely female.[29] In this respect, medical practices reflect and reinforce cultural norms in which the responsibility for contraception is primarily delegated to women. Due to these constraints, the culture of the testing of male contraceptives has developed into a practice in which the medical profession, both in the US and in Europe, closely cooperates with groups outside the clinic, most notably the news media.[30]

## Procedures for getting approval for marketing and testing

Another aspect in which the culture of contraceptive development may differ from the culture of the development of drugs in general is the way in which contraceptives are granted approval for marketing and testing by the drug regulatory authorities. Let us first look at the procedures for obtaining approval for the marketing of the first contraceptive pill for women. The way in which the first oral progestins were approved as contraceptives is an intriguing story. In 1957, the American pharmaceutical firms Syntex and Searle received marketing approval for progestins from the US Food and Drug Administration (FDA), not as oral contraceptives but as drugs for the treatment of menstrual disorders and infertility. The choice to seek approval for the oral progestins as drugs rather than contraceptives can be understood as a political strategy to bypass resistance towards the introduction of the first hormonal contraceptive for women. As Garcia, one of Pincus's colleagues recalled:

> The first application was not as an oral contraceptive but as a gynaecological agent to treat menstrual aberrations, and that was done with political calculation and it wasn't done with any other thing in mind because the contraceptive properties of it were well-known at that point.[31]

However, times were changing. Despite the fact that contraception was technically a forbidden subject in most states of the US, the moral attitudes to contraception and sexuality in general were relaxing in the 1960s.[32] Actually, by late 1959, half a million American women were already using oral progesterone as a contraceptive, although it had been prescribed for them as a drug for menstrual disorders. Both doctors and patients knew the pill's contraceptive power well before it was marketed as such. The FDA, in its first approval of oral progesterone (Enovid) had mandated Searle that the drug should carry a warning to doctors that women would not ovulate while taking the pills, 'a mandate which worked like a "free ad"'.[33] A similar practice existed in European countries. In the Netherlands a combined estrogen-progesterone formulation was first marketed in 1962 for the treatment of menstrual irregularities, carrying a warning that women could not become pregnant while taking this medication. This strategy was chosen to anticipate possible protests from physicians, the media, and the lay public, as well as the mainly Catholic production personnel of Organon, the firm that introduced the pill on to the Dutch market.[34] This practice exemplifies how the activity of a drug may not be dictated by nature, but is the result of a socially-conditioned selection process, in this case religious and moral attitudes towards birth control.[35]

In May 1960, the FDA eventually granted its approval for the marketing of Enovid explicitly for contraceptive purposes.[36] The pharmaceutical firm that put the new contraceptive on the market, G. D. Searle and Company, was very much aware of the novelty of the product and its potential to damage the company's reputation, and remained very cautious. Its executives developed a careful marketing and public relations campaign. Ahead of the launch date for the product, they approached the editors of the *Saturday Evening Post* and *Reader's Digest* and negotiated three major articles, telling the story of 'the new contraceptive that was being tested in Puerto Rico'. Searle soon witnessed the profits from its 'daring decision' to market Enovid as a contraceptive: the company's shares doubled in value in the years following FDA approval.[37] Other American drug companies, such as Syntex and Parke-Davis, did not take this risk. They felt that contraceptives were no suitable business for an ethical firm.[38] Parke-Davis in particular was afraid that the marketing of a contraceptive would ruin their market in Roman Catholic areas.[39] The market, however, was more than ready to accept the new contraceptive.

The procedures for obtaining approval for the marketing of the pill were thus shaped by the political and cultural taboos on contraceptives. To reduce possible resistance towards this novelty in the history of medicines, Pincus, the pharmaceutical firms, and the FDA used a stepping-stone strategy: by approving oral progestins as drugs rather than contraceptives, they facilitated the diffusion of this contraceptive even before the compound was marketed as such. Safety issues did not play a decisive role in the procedures for marketing approval. The first oral contraceptive was introduced before the thalidomide tragedy occurred: pre-marketing regulatory requirements were still very limited, and approval times were very short. Regulatory requirements for contraceptives became more stringent only after the FDA's approval of the marketing of the pill, when the first reports appeared on the increased risks of oral contraceptives for circulatory system diseases and cancer.[40] Both consumer advocates and the women's movement criticized the introduction of the pill and suggested that reproductive science and industry had shown inadequate concern for the health of women.[41] The strong public demand for reduced health risks had two major consequences which eventually led to a decline in industrial activity in contraceptive research and development.

First, the concern about health produced an enormous increase in the number of liability suits, initially against US manufacturers of the Dalkon Shield intrauterine device and later against manufacturers of oral contraceptives. In the 1980s, 'there were more liability suits for oral contraceptives annually than for any other drug category.'[42] In the USA this dramatic increase in lawsuits led to a situation in which liability insurance for manufacturers became temporarily unavailable. Nowadays, the liability costs in the field of contraceptives are higher than for any other drug category.[43] Second, the public demand for reduced health risks led to more stringent rules and procedural regulations for the production and approval of new drugs. This happened generally for all drugs: following the thalidomide tragedy in the early 1960s, drug regulatory requirements became more stringent both in Europe and the United States. Nowadays, there were 'extensive requirements that must be met before a company is permitted to test or market a new drug'.[44] In the US, the role of the FDA shifted from protecting the consumer to guaranteeing the safety of a drug.[45] Consequently, since 1962 the FDA's mandate has not been limited to the approval of new drugs, but has been extended to 'evaluate the efficacy and appropriateness of proposed research designs to investigate new drugs and to monitoring of marketed drugs'.[46]

The regulatory procedures that emerged in the 1960s show a striking difference between contraceptives and other drugs, particularly in the US. For contraceptives, the FDA required much more extensive animal research than for other drugs. Whereas scientists working on curative drugs are free to choose any animal model for research on efficacy and safety, contraceptive researchers had to follow FDA specifications for animal models, type of studies and the length of testing. In response to concerns about the long-term effects of oral contraceptives the FDA has demanded more stringent pre-marketing requirements for long-term animal research, even to the point of specifying animal models. Initially, the FDA requested that contraceptive research should include seven years of testing in beagles and 10 years in monkeys. In reaction to criticism of these guidelines, the FDA simplified the regulatory requirements for contraceptives in 1990 by dropping the requirement for toxicology tests in dogs.[47] Moreover, the FDA introduced requirements for clinical testing for all drugs in which the length of phase I to phase III trials were specified.[48] Owing to severe criticism and pressure from reproductive scientists and pharmaceutical firms, the FDA was forced to make the requirements for testing less stringent. However, procedures for contraceptives have remained much more extensive than for other drugs. These more extensive testing requirements have significantly increased the research and development costs for drugs and contraceptives: within two decades the average research and development cost of developing a new chemical compound has increased from $65 million to $344 million.[49] As a result, most contraceptive research and development has become increasingly dependent on government funding. The more stringent drug regulatory requirements have also led to an increase in the development time for new contraceptives, which eventually shortened the life-time of patents.[50]

The development of new contraceptives for men shows a similar emphasis on safety issues. Because hormonal contraceptives for men are still technology-in-the-making, I can only discuss the procedures for obtaining approval for testing. The way in which scientists involved in male contraceptive research have received FDA approval for clinical trials vividly shows the vulnerable nature of the testing of male contraceptives. The volunteers enrolled in one of the first clinical trials of a hormonal contraceptive compound for men organized by the WHO were a very specific selection of men: hypogonadal men, patients with a deficiency in androgen metabolism.[51] This choice was made not merely to establish the pharmacokinetic profile of the drug in men with low endogenous concentrations of testosterone, but to ensure that the drug would also have an application in clinical medicine, i.e. hormone replacement therapy. The development of a dual drug profile seems to be a normal practice in the testing of male contraceptives. The Population Council and other US agencies have tested male contraceptive agents as drugs for the treatment of prostate cancer. The development of a dual drug profile has been chosen as a strategy to secure FDA approval for testing. Moreover, the strategy to develop a dual drug profile seems to be oriented particularly towards industry. Pharmaceutical companies that do not directly support research on male contraceptives seem much more willing to collaborate in research and development projects aimed at the development of clinical applications such as the treatment of hypogonadism and, even more, the treatment of cancer.[52] Because FDA regulatory requirements for drugs for clinical applications are less stringent than for contraceptives, it is easier to test potential contraceptives for applications other than contraception. Dr Rosemary Thau, the former manager of the Population Council, has vividly described how the choice of trial subjects is a result of negotiations with the FDA:

> We are now testing the LHRH vaccine in men with prostate cancer in our clinic in Texas. The FDA, when we discussed it with them, advised fifty-fifty whether we should start with normal men or in cancer patients. At first they could not make up their mind and then a month later they told us to start with the cancer patients.[53]

As with female contraceptive development, safety is a crucial issue in the development of male contraceptives. The tolerance of risks by regulators and the scientific community seems to be even lower for male contraceptives than for female contraceptives. Or to quote Geoffrey Waites, who was involved in the coordination of the clinical testing of male contraceptives at the WHO:

> I see it very much amongst some of my review groups actually which consist primarily of obstetricians and gynaecologists. I can still remember putting out the table of side effects of the first contraceptive agent we have tested here. There was one case of discontinuation because of liquid changes. This led to an outcry and a lot of comments coming from obstetricians and gynaecologists who were on the case. It did not help me to say that none of the partners of the male trial participants had menstrual disorders, which is the main reason for discontinuation in female trials. More than 30 per cent of women cannot tolerate these side effects. But it did not help me at all to say that.[54]

Moreover, there are important differences between the assessment of adverse effects of contraceptives on women and men. For women, the health risks of contraceptives are calculated against the risks of pregnancy, including maternal mortality and morbidity and psychological problems related to unwanted pregnancies and abortion. For men, the risks of contraceptives are calculated against the condition of healthy men. These differences in assessment of the risks and benefits of contraceptives, and the low tolerance for health risks of contraceptives among the public in general, have led to a situation in which any indication of possible adverse effects has developed into a major disincentive to continuing the development of a specific lead for male contraceptives.

•

## Conclusion

Reflecting on this analysis of the development of contraceptives, we can conclude that contraceptives are a very peculiar type of therapy. The very fact that these pharmaceuticals are used to control fertility rather than for treating acute diseases has created a culture of testing practices that differs from those of other drugs. First, there are major differences in the procedures for enrolling volunteers for clinical trials, at least for the development of new contraceptives for men. The testing of these contraceptives cannot easily follow the routines of other clinical testing. For male contraceptives, the quest for 'healthy patients' requires the creation of networks outside medical institutions. Owing to resistance within the medical community, particularly among gynaecologists, clinicians involved in the testing of new male contraceptives have to rely on cooperation with the media to recruit volunteers. Secondly, there are important differences in the procedures for obtaining approval of testing and marketing by drug regulatory agencies. The ways in which approval was granted for the first oral contraceptive for women, as well as one of the first prototypes for hormonal contraceptives for men, shows the very vulnerable status of these types of pharmaceuticals. In both cases, the actors involved in the testing and marketing procedures adopted very carefully planned 'detour' strategies to bypass possible resistance among audiences and regulatory agencies: the pill was first introduced as a drug for the treatment of menstrual disorders, and the prototype for an hormonal contraceptive for men was approved for testing as a drug for prostate cancer. The culture of contraceptive development can thus be described as a culture of detours that relies heavily on networks with institutions outside the medical world.

## Notes

1. Parts of this paper have been previously published in N. Oudshoorn, *Beyond the Natural Body. An Archeology of Sex Hormones* (London and New York: Routledge, 1994); and N. Oudshoorn, 'Shifting Boundaries Between Industry and Science: The role of the WHO in contraceptive R & D' in J-P. Gaudilliere, I. Löwy (eds), *The Invisible Industrialist. Manufactures and the Production of Scientific Knowledge* (Houndmills, Basingstoke and London: MacMillan Press, 1998), 345–69. I would like to thank T. M. M. Farley, Alvin Paulsen, Rosemary Thau, Geoffrey Waites, Fred Wu for granting me interviews.

2. L. McLauglin, *The Pill, John Rock, and the Church: The Biography of a Revolution* (Boston, MA and Toronto: Little, Brown, 1982), 38; J. S. Segal, 'Contraceptive Research: A Male Chauvinist Plot?', *Family Planning Perspectives*, 4 (1972), 21–5.
3. J. Rock, *The Time has come. A Catholic Doctor's proposals to end the battle over birth control* (New York: Alfred A. Knopf, 1963), 168.
4. A. Q. Maisel, *The Hormone Quest* (New York: Random House, 1965), 114.
5. McLaughlin, *op. cit.* (note 2), 120.
6. P. Vaughan, *The Pill on Trial* (Harmondsworth, Middlesex: Penguin Books Ltd, 1972), 51.
7. Rock, *op. cit.* (note 3).
8. J. Reed, *The Birth Control Movement and American Society: From private vice to public virtue* (Princeton, NJ : Princeton University Press, 1984), 354.
9. Rock, *op. cit.* (note 3), 163.
10. McLaughlin, *op. cit.* (note 2), 41.
11. Rock, *op. cit.* (note 3), 163.
12. McLaughlin, *op. cit.* (note 2), 110.
13. *Ibid.*, 115.
14. *Ibid.*, 121; Vaughan, *op. cit.* (note 6), 36.
15. McLaughlin, *op. cit.* (note 2), 118.
16. A. B. Ramirez de Arellano and C. Seipp, *Colonialism, Catholicism, and Contraception: A history of birth control in Puerto Rico* (Chapel Hill, NC and London: University of North Carolina Press, 1983), 110; McLaughlin, *op. cit.* (note 2), 119.
17. McLaughlin, *op .cit.* (note 2), 119.
18. McLaughlin, *op. cit.* (note 2), 120; Vaughan, *op. cit.* (note 6), 39, 40.
19. Ramirez and Seipp, *op. cit.* (note 16), 107.
20. McLaughlin, *op. cit.* (note 2), 28.
21. *Ibid.*, 127; Vaughan, *op. cit.* (note 6), 55, 56.
22. L. Marks, '"Public Spirited and Enterprising Volunteers": The Council for the Investigation of Fertility Control and the British Clinical Trials of the Oral Contraceptive Pill, 1959–1973', this volume.
23. *Ibid.*
24. Contemporary Medical Archives Centre, Wellcome Library, London, A/FPA/A5/158B. Box 249, as cited in *op. cit.* (note 22).
25. For the report of one of these trials, see World Health Organisation, Task Force on Methods for the Regulation of Male Fertility, 'Contraceptive Efficacy of Testosterone-induced Azoospermia and

Oligospermia in normal men', *Fertility and Sterility*, 65 (1996), 821–9.
26. Interview Alvin Paulsen, Professor in reproductive physiology at the Medical School in Seattle, 18 October 1994.
27. *Op. cit.* (note 26)
28. Interview Fred Wu, Department of Medicine at the University of Manchester, 22 April 1994.
29. For a detailed analysis of how family planning discourse is gradually changing towards including men, see N. Oudshoorn, 'Making Room for Men. Symbolic and material interventions to change family planning towards including men', Paper presented at the Social Studies of Science conference in Tucson, Arizona, October 1997.
30. See G. D. Feldberg, *Disease and Class: Tuberculosis in the Making of North American Society* (New Brunswick, NJ: Rutgers University Press, 1995), who has described a similar situation for vaccines where testing also took place largely outside the medical institutions.
31. Garcia, as cited in Anonymous, 'Historical perspectives on the scientific study of fertility', transcript from the Conference on Historical Perspectives of the Scientific Study of Arts and Sciences (Boston, MA , 5 May 1978), 60.
32. Vaughan, *op. cit.* (note 6), 52, 53; McLaughlin, *op. cit.* (note 2), 137, 138.
33. I. C. Winter, Searle's executive, as cited in McLaughlin, *op. cit.* (note 2), 139.
34. A. A. Haspels, 'Hormonen en de Pil', *Cahiers Biowetenschappen en Maatschappij*, 10 (1985), 19–27.
35. H. J. H. W. Bodewitz, H. Buurma, G. H. de Vries, 'Regulatory Science and the Social Management of Trust in Medicine', in W. E. Bijker, T. P. Hughes, T. J. Pinch (eds), *The Social Construction of Technological Systems. New directions in the sociology and history of technology* (Cambridge, MA: MIT Press, 1987), 19.
36. Maisel, *op. cit.* (note 4), 142.
37. B. Seaman, *The Doctor's Case against the Pill* (New York: Peter H. Wyden, 1969), 179.
38. McLaughlin, *op. cit.* (note 2), 137.
39. Anonymous, *op. cit.* (note 31), 36, 37.
40. A. Gelijns and C. Pannenborg, 'The Development of Contraceptive Technology. Case studies of incentives and disincentives to innovation', *International Journal of Technology Assessment in Health Care*, 9 (1993), 210–32, especially 227; B. Seaman and G. Seaman, *Women and the Crisis in Sex Hormones. An investigation of the dangerous uses of hormone, From birth control to menopause and the*

*safe alternatives* (Brighton, Sussex: Harvester Press, 1978).
41. Gelijns and Pannenborg, *op. cit.* (note 40), 227; Seaman and Seaman, *op. cit.* (note 40).
42. Gelijns and Pannenborg, op. cit. (note 40), 227; C. Djerassi, 'The Bitter Pill', *Science*, 245 (1989), 356–61.
43. Djerassi, *op. cit.* (note 42), 357.
44. R. O. Greep, 'Some Reflections on Male Reproductive Biology and Contraception', in C. H. Spilman, T. J. Lobl and K. T. Kirton (eds), *Regulatory Mechanisms of Male Reproductive Physiology. Sixth Brook Lodge Workshop on problems of reproductive biology* (Oxford and Amsterdam: Excerpta Medica. New York: American Elsevier Publishing Co., 1976), 352.
45. L. Diller and W. Hembree, 'Male Contraception and Family Planning: A social and historical review'. *Fertility and Sterility*, 28 (1977), 1271–9, especially 1275.
46. Greep, *op. cit.* (note 44), 352.
47. Djerassi, *op. cit.* (note 42), 357.
48. C. Djerassi, 'Birth Control after 1984', *Science*, 169 (1970), 941–51.
49. Estimates, Mercke & Sharpe in World Health Organisation, Special Programme of Research, Development and Research Training in Human Reproduction, *Inter-Agency Consultation on Meeting the Challenges of the 1990s in Human Reproduction Research* (Geneva, 1990), 14.
50. Gelijns and Pannenborg, *op. cit.* (note 40), 227.
51. World Health Organization, Special Programme of Research, Development and Research Training in Human Reproduction, *Annual Technical Report 1992* (Geneva, 1993), 10.
52. Interview Dr Rosemary Thau, then Director of Contraceptive Development at the Population Council in New York, 16 April 1993.
53. *Ibid.*
54. Interview, Geoffrey Waites, manager of the WHO's Task Force on Methods for the Regulation of Male Fertility, 14 February 1994.

# 7

## Contrasting cultures of contraception: Birth control clinics and the working-classes in Britain between the wars

### *Kate Fisher*

In October 1929 Mrs Jenkins was given a contraceptive sponge at Dr Marie Stopes's caravan clinic when it visited Cymmer in the Rhondda in South Wales. Five months later she was visited by Nurse Fowles. Apparently a successful customer, Mrs Jenkins reported that she and her husband 'find it a great benefit in every way'. However, she also enthusiastically added that 'many around here who did not come to the caravan got their own sponges or crocheted nets and are being helped'.[1] Such instances of 'make your own birth control' and of neighbourly innovation and self-help were exactly what Marie Stopes was trying to counter by setting up clinics. Indeed, she warned her nurses of the dangers of giving contraceptive devices to uneducated women who do not

> understand the responsibility of not handing on the method to ignorant women who may be unsuitable for it. ... [The] poor class women... are certain to hand on to their neighbours the advice you give, and it is not safe for them to use the cap without proper examination.[2]

In this chapter I compare working-class people's use of birth control with the expectations and beliefs of those who set up and ran birth control clinics. Using evidence gathered in oral history interviews I argue that clinics frequently failed to appreciate the complex attitudes towards contraception held by those they hoped to advise. They struggled to convince many potential patients to accept their particular principles but did not attempt to tailor their clinics to make them more attractive to the working-class communities they targeted.

I have studied the impact of birth control clinics as part of a wider oral history of contraceptive use, using a sample of men and women married during the inter-war years from South Wales and Oxford. I have interviewed a total of 107 people, 59 from South Wales (41 women and 18 men) and 48 (31 women and 17 men) from Oxford. Three of these also took part in a group interview, which included 12 other women. Most were widows or widowers, but there were 13 interviews with couples.[3] Interviews lasted up to four hours and covered various questions about marriage, family, courtship, and sexual attitudes, and concentrated in particular on birth control practices. Dates of birth ranged from 1899 to 1925.[4]

Two people were interviewed as the result of a newspaper appeal for information on birth control clinics. However, the response to this appeal was disappointing, moreover I was interested in interviewing a more random sample in order to investigate a wide range of contraceptive practices. All but these two interviewees were obtained through visits to old people's homes, day centres and social clubs. All interviewees were guaranteed anonymity, and interviews took place in private, generally in a respondent's own home. Very few of those I met declined to be interviewed.

The majority of interviewees were unaware of birth control clinics, even when one existed in their own small town, even though they went regularly to the premises for other sorts of welfare services – ante-natal clinics, dentists and so on. Only 14 of the total sample had attended a birth control clinic (six from South Wales and eight from Oxford) at one time or another during their married lives. The bulk of this chapter will examine the limited appeal birth control clinics had for the few respondents who knew about clinics or attended them.

### 'It was too much of a palaver'

Clinics demanded regular attendance, and the contraceptive methods provided were novel and tricky to learn how to use. Stanley neatly summarised the feelings of many when explaining why his wife rejected the cap: 'a doctor or somebody skilled had to fit it, and they could be very painful. And they didn't work very well.'[5]

Clinics provided medical methods, which patients had to be taught how to use. Many women found cervical caps and sponges rather difficult to insert, and teaching patients to use them correctly proved a major difficulty.[6] Marie Stopes uncharitably noted that 'there is always a percentage of extremely stupid and unreliable women whom it is difficult to instruct.'[7] In fact, her preferred method of birth control was the most complex available, required an elaborate fitting procedure, and was, moreover, by the clinics' own reckoning, unsuitable for many. Sylvia Dawkins, a family planning doctor interviewed by Television History Workshop explained the complex procedures of examination and the difficulties experienced in determining which method was suitable and finding the right size:

> If you gave a barrier method you had to instruct the people how to use it. You fitted them with, say a diaphragm, instructed them, asked them to go home and practice putting it in and out, come with it in, so that we could sure they got it right, you see, and knew what they were doing. Then we gave them the cap, and we didn't on the first occasion because you couldn't fit them properly the first occasion, they were tense. When they'd come back with the cap in they were relaxed and you found the size wasn't anywhere near right.[8]

Those who had been physically affected by frequent pregnancy and/or poor gynaecological care found the cap difficult to use. Nurse Williams wrote to Marie Stopes after the caravan stopped in Swansea in May 1929 that 'the uterine conditions of the mothers on the whole is not good. The sponge and the sheath being practically the only suitable methods'. Many others were nevertheless given caps. Gertrude, for example, who attended a birth control clinic in Aberdare, was tried first with a cervical cap, which appears to have been entirely unsuitable, despite the clinic's apparent determination to try to fit one:

> ...couldn't wear what the woman did, I couldn't hold it. I went, I don't know how many times they tried to fit me, and you had to go on the table and be examined and all that, see, before they would er. But I couldn't, I wasn't, I should have been stitched and I wasn't, so I couldn't hold it.[9]

Clinic records are dotted with similar examples. Mrs Jones, for example, 'is very stout and found it awkward to place and remove sponge' and Mrs Davies 'was too tender to use a sponge' as she had been 'badly lacerated after severe labour and delivery'.[10] Sometimes those who had problems inserting caps and sponges were given other methods, such as the sheath.

However, patients were expected to keep trying. Many were sent away, sometimes with written instructions, and were told to practice and come back for further instruction. It is hardly surprising that some lost patience.

> *When your doctor told you not to have any more children, he gave you a cap, and you said you didn't get on with that.*
> Couldn't be bothered.

> *Tell me more about that. Why didn't you like that?*
> Well, I found it awkward to fix. And I go back to the clinic, and I got fed up with trying to fix it properly.[11]

Similarly, Enid Charles' survey of contraceptive practice among primarily middle-class women found that the 'most frequent source of dissatisfaction' with the cap 'is fitting and adjusting'.[12] Norman and Vera Himes found, in a follow up survey of 58 patients, only 55 per cent were using the appliance and of these only 18 people (31 per cent) were found to be using the device satisfactorily.[13] Similarly, Lella Secor Florence found that only 50 per cent of the women who attended her clinic in Cambridge successfully used the method provided.[14]

Patients were also required to return for regular checks. It proved difficult to persuade many women that they needed continued medical supervision of their contraceptive practices.[15] In north Kensington it was found that 'hundreds of them were never heard from after their first or second visits'.[16] While many may have continued using the methods provided others, such as Margaret, found the requirement to keep attending the clinic a disincentive to continued use.

> Oh yes, when I went I went, she was a private one, and er he said, you know, I'd got to be fitted with, and I was fitted with a cap. [*Mm*] So,
> *And what was that like?*
> Well, it was a bit uncomfortable, you know, I'd to keep going back and having it checked, and er....[17]

Even conscientious and content users found it difficult to keep attending. At first, Eva who started going to Marie Stopes' clinic in Cardiff soon after it opened in 1937, would re-visit regularly: 'Every now and again – I would say, "Well I've had this x amount of time, do you think it's time I had a new one?"' However, she did not maintain this level of devotion to the regimen and eventually stopped using the method in favour of another: 'After a while we stopped going [to the clinic] so often. I stopped using it after the war.'[18]

Another hurdle, as one clinic reported, was that 'the working woman has a deep-rooted resistance against seeing the doctor on any account, and she is dismayed at the prospect of an examination.'[19] Many clinics were aware that the 'medical aura' of birth control clinics was off-putting and did what they could to change the ambience in birth control clinics.[20] Marie Stopes instructed her nurses to 'rub in the homely atmosphere' when informing others of the clinics[21] and in Leicester the medical staff 'didn't wear a uniform' in order to create a 'friendly non-medical approach to the whole thing'.[22] However, the medical associations of birth control clinics were unavoidable. Indeed, for many women, it was medical need that prompted attendance. Local authority run clinics were in fact only supposed to provide birth control advice for those who had medical reasons for avoiding pregnancy. For all but three of the respondents who attended birth control clinics there was a specific and urgent medical need to avoid pregnancy. Many were sent to the clinic by a doctor or other medical authority. Gwen, for example, was told by the nurses at her maternity hospital not to have any more children. She then received a referral from her doctor, which she took to a local birth control clinic.

> *And did you only have one child?*
> Only the one child. Well, he told me that it wasn't...I shouldn't have any more actually. He give me something, you know, to prevent it and I thought, well, I mean, my mother died when I was 9 months old. She never got out of bed after I was born, and, er, I thought I'd rather look after my one child instead of having two, and somebody else looking after him perhaps.
> *So what did they give you to prevent you having more children?*
> Well, of course this is years ago, and they gave me a cap (*Whispers*)
> *And tell me exactly what they said. And who was it? Was it the nurses at the hospital? Or did you have to go to a clinic, or?*
> Well, it was funny really. I went down to Lizzie Bain...'cos they thought the strain would be too much. And then I had a letter from a doctor in Abersychan, and I went up there and they said, it would be advisable that I didn't have any children for at least say, about 5 or 6 years, and then I could go back but I didn't want to risk it. So they told me to use this particular thing.[23]

Others, such as Eva, were motivated to seek out clinics themselves after strict admonitions from a doctor to avoid pregnancy.

> Well, I'd been quite ill before he was born and after and then when he was about eight months old all I had a very bad bout of tonsillitis and the doctor came up and he said, 'You are absolutely at rock bottom and whatever happens you mustn't have any more family.' Well when I went down the surgery I saw another young doctor and I said to him, 'Well that's all very well doctor, but what am I supposed to do?'....

Yet, clinics were so clearly associated with the medical establishment that when Eva's husband found out about the existence of a Marie Stopes clinic she worried that she might need a doctor's referral to go there, despite her pressing medical need:

> And, he came home one day, full of excitement, he said, 'Well I understand that there's a family planning clinic out in Splott and you can just go there - you don't have to be sent by the doctor or anything - you just go there.' So we had a little talk about it, and I said, 'Well I'll go out on the bike and scoot around,' because it wasn't advertised in any way. And I went into Railway Street and went up and down and I did spot it.[24]

Fundamentally, clinics remained unashamedly and unequivocally medical in their approach to birth control. Clinics primarily sought to ally themselves with a modern medical approach and with healthcare services and to distance themselves from other outlets of birth control information, which they saw as disreputable, quack or commercial. Clinics promoted new 'scientific' approaches to contraception, provided advanced appliances, and rejected all traditional forms of birth control, especially withdrawal and abortion. Marie Stopes was particularly sensitive to the possibility that her 'constructive birth control' might be confused with lay practices. She warned her nurses that 'birth control work must be so carefully distinguished from abortion... our enemies are always on the look-out to associate the control of conception with the destruction of the embryo'.[25] The central aim to appear clinical, safe, and clean was clearly at odds with the desire to seem motherly. This tension was played out in clinic spaces in which rooms, decorated in a style aping a contemporary domestic sitting room (with flowery or pastel wall paper) were filled with tables full of gleaming medical equipment. Photographs of babies (reminiscent of family portraits?) hung next to framed copies of the medical qualifications of the staff.

Perhaps the biggest challenge faced by birth control campaigners was convincing women that the strange new methods they promoted were safe and reliable. Evelyn Fisher, who worked at Marie Stopes' clinic in London, failed to get a clinic in South Wales set up in the late-1920s because she found 'the women were afraid to use' caps because the 'idea was totally new'.[26] Reports from clinics are full of similar cases, such as Mrs Heard who 'couldn't fancy the idea,'[27] Mrs Williams who was 'too frightened to try' and Mrs Thomas who was 'too nervous to use sponge'.[28] Patients had two main worries: first that caps and sponges would not prevent pregnancy and secondly that caps and sponges were harmful.

Elizabeth and her husband were clearly concerned that the cap might not be safe. Her husband was unwilling to abandon withdrawal and she recalled telling him:

> 'Oh you can leave it there now because I got a cap or something', you know, and then, 'You sure it's safe?' 'Well, they said in the clinic it's safe.'[29]

Lella Secor Florence found that 'sometimes, even after instruction at the Clinic, a patient will write in great anxiety to know whether it is possible for the pessary to get lost inside, or whether this or that story she has been told about the ill-effect of contraceptives is true'.[30] Clinic records also provide similar cases such as Mrs Watkins who 'only used the method once or twice, as she feared she could not remove it' and Mrs Jug who did not use the cap 'for fear of causing cancer'.[31] Similarly, Leslie gave the following explanation why his wife did not attend the clinic in Pontypridd that his sisters went to:

> Ooh, my wife never went any like that. Oh no, no, no. But she didn't believe in anything like that.
> 
> Why was that?
> 
> Oh well, she don't know, she didn't believe in it. Perhaps, I was so much of a dead nut against it, causing cancer, things like that.[32]

### 'Just used our own methods'

It is crucial to recognise that birth control clinics were competing with an existing and extensive culture of contraception. It was particularly because clinic culture came into conflict with existing beliefs, expectations and preferences about contraceptive behaviour that women were often unconvinced of the benefits of birth control clinics. Clinics were not simply rather demanding in terms of time and effort but also required a significant shift, on the part of the woman patient, away from familiar methods of birth control, generally accepted and/or trusted, in favour of a novel appliance method. This was not an easy transition for many women. Traditional methods of birth control, especially withdrawal, remained important in working-class lives, even to those who attended birth control clinics. Clinic workers found a lot of people, like Mrs Jones, who 'did not bother to use' the method she had been given, as she 'felt quite safe with coitus interruptus'.[33] Even those happy with the method provided often used it sporadically, 'only when they went all the way'.[34] Lella Secor Florence also found husbands 'do not seem to mind withdrawal – they prefer this method, with its freedom from preparation.'[35]

For many withdrawal worked according to a simple principle and seemed more reliable than an internal, unseen, and unfelt barrier method. Elizabeth is a good example:

> *Which do you prefer of those? [methods tried]*
> Withdraw, oh yes, you knew you were safe then, you know.[36]
> 'Cos it was a worrying time though they got protection.
> *So would you trust withdrawal more than caps?*
> Definitely, oh yes. Yeah.
> *Why was that?*
> I don't know, you felt safer, you know, not so messy, no.[37]

She also hints at the common finding that withdrawal was for many the preferred method of contraception - it was 'natural', interfered least with the spontaneity of sex, required the least preparation and was seen as the least messy. Enid Charles also found distaste for contraceptive devices among her respondents and a preference for coitus interruptus because it involved no trouble, preparation or expense.[38]

None of the people I interviewed preferred the methods that were provided by clinics and almost all stopped using such methods in favour of tried and trusted ones at some time during their contraceptive careers. Only three people used caps for a significant period. Over half rejected caps immediately or after only a few years. Thus the increasing availability of 'medical' methods of birth control did not necessarily lead to more satisfactory use of birth control, nor were traditional methods merely retained reluctantly in 'ignorance' of more advanced methods favoured by the clinics.[39] Most of those I interviewed were perfectly satisfied with traditional methods, and did not see the need to attend birth control clinics. Those who knew about birth control clinics but did not attend were largely satisfied with their existing contraceptive practices. Annie, for example, was encouraged to attend the Oxford clinic, but she was happy with the method she had and had no interest in going.

> *Had you heard of any other methods than condoms?*
> Well, I did hear something once. They wanted me to go to some clinic, but I wouldn't go. Why bother!
> *What clinic was this?*
> I dunno. It's something. Shouldn't tell you.[40]
> *And who wanted you to go?*

> Well, somebody, something said to me one day, but I can't remember now. But I didn't go. I thought, no, I'm all right.
>
> *And why didn't you want to go?*
>
> Because I was all right as I was.[41]

Many women did not distinguish between clinics and other sources of birth control information despite the attempts made by clinics to distinguish themselves from all lay and traditional approaches to family limitation. Rather, some women tried to adapt clinic teaching to fit in with existing cultures of contraception. Many expected to be able to receive abortions at birth control clinics. Horrified nurses lectured patients on the immorality of the practice: 'We have had two requests for abortion this week and both seemed to think that the clinic existed for the purpose. The unlawful side of it had not struck them at all. The other said, "Surely you are going to do something for me." I had to explain to her very plainly that we did not teach how to destroy life'. One of the women I interviewed was similarly convinced that Marie Stopes used knitting needles to bring her friend on when she attended the clinic in Splott, Cardiff.

> *Had you heard of a woman called Marie Stopes?*
>
> Marie Stopes. She was in London, I think, yeah, a lot of people used to write to her and she used to send them pills and things like that, Marie Stopes.
>
> *And what were the pills for?*
>
> To try and bring your periods back on, you know. I'm sure there was a Marie Stopes in Splott somewhere.
>
> *There was?*
>
> There was! I thought, too, yeah. There was a Marie Stopes in Splott, she had an old shop made into a clinic, aye, aye, yeah...
>
> *And did you know anyone who went there?*
>
> Yeah, friend of mine went there, I don't know, she never had any children, so she must have come on...
>
> I know she used to give tablets to the people, like. I think she used a knitting needle and all, yeah, I'm sure my friend had a knitting needle, come to think of it.[42]

The importance of traditional approaches can similarly be seen in the tendency of many to misinterpret the advice provided in clinics and in Marie Stopes' books in an attempt to accommodate such advice with existing beliefs about contraception. Joe and Delia, for example, claimed to have used withdrawal as a result of reading the advice given in a Marie Stopes book, despite the fact that Marie Stopes felt that 'in any normal marriage its use is to be condemned' as 'this method has without doubt done an incredible amount of harm' to the 'nervous systems of both man and woman'.[43]

> But I did buy this book, a lady doctor who wrote it. It was well known then and we read it, and it gave a good advice in it.
> *So what sort of advice does it give?*
> I can't remember now. I think it was mostly talking about using condoms, such as there was then, and the man wasn't allowed to let his sperm go into the woman. That was the main thing.[44]

A clear distinction between types of birth control information was impossible to maintain. As shown in Willem de Blécourt's discussion of the elaborate and contradictory meanings the term 'hygienic' acquired, all providers of birth control advice attempted to give legitimacy to their own endeavours with reference to each other, and in particular, through the borrowing of particular vocabulary. For example, when Marie Stopes's clinic was stationed in Bolton she complained to the police that a leaflet for aphrodisiacs and 'corrective medicines pour les dames' had printed her name on the top left hand corner of the letter heading. 'This kind of thing has happened before when we sent our free clinic,' she wrote. 'These traders follow us with their objectionable literature.' She added that her project was to do 'all she can to get rid of this type of trader'.[45] Inevitably, various forms of birth-control information were forced to co-exist uneasily. Apparently contradictory messages were blurred, conflated and open to multiple interpretations. Clinic campaigners could not distance themselves from traditional approaches, but had to compete with various contemporary cultures of contraception.

### 'I prefer the man to help'

There was one intrinsic belief central to birth control clinics that ran counter to existing working-class traditions of fertility control and that I shall argue lay behind many women's dissatisfaction. The emphasis in all clinics was to give women the responsibility and power to control contraceptive use. Clinics were for mothers only and the methods provided were for female use (except in unusual circumstances). Clinics presented themselves as battling against men and their propaganda portrayed them almost as refuges where women who had been mistreated by either male doctors or husbands could go. Such stories of suffering were prominent in clinic literature as were arguments in favour of female methods, such as cervical caps: vaunted because they could be used without the knowledge of the husband (although in practice in cramped working-class homes this must have been nearly impossible). Although many women benefited from this approach, such as Mrs James, who said on leaving the Splott clinic, 'Thank God, I can keep myself safe now and not have to trust to him,'[46] there is reason to believe that this anti-male stance may have alienated a number of other women from attending, and done little to encourage husbands to send their wives. Oral testimony suggests that husbands played a very significant role in all aspects of contraceptive use: in initiating discussions about birth control, in determining which methods to use, in making sexual advances and in deciding how frequently contraception would be used, in finding out about methods, and in obtaining any appliances used. The vast majority of those I have interviewed, both women and men, have asserted that men were expected to take 'responsibility' for birth control.[47] Ernest, for example, was adamant that it was 'the man's duty':

> Oh well, we used, we used to use the err French letters we used to call em, I don't know, what's the official thing called? What was the expression? Sheaths. The sheath, that's right. It was the man's option... It was the man, it was the man's job.[48]

There was a clear 'male culture' of contraception. Men were the accepted actors in birth control; they were expected to obtain what was needed and to use them. Women were not eager to challenge this role.

> But all we knew about was the French letter, up to the fella, you never heard much about what you could do with yourself, no pills then. And I wouldn't, I don't think I'd've taken them then. I prefer the man to help. I think they should do. The men are free today, aren't they? They rely on the girl having the pill, they don't do anything.[49]

Clinics demanded action on the part of women that ran counter to their expected marital and sexual roles. Many women preferred male methods of contraception and rejected female ones, precisely because they did not want to take responsibility for contraception. Doris, for example, presented her husband's role thus:

> *So what did you use, in order not to get pregnant, during those 12 years?*
> Oh, he used something. Not me.
> *What did he use?*

> Well, the usual, whatever you call 'em, French letters we used to call them.
> *And where did you first find out about those?*
> Oh, that was up to him... oh, men knew all about those things long before they got married, don't worry.

She later revealed that she had, in fact, used a female method, but she preferred leaving it to her husband.

> Yeah, I did use some sort of pessary in the beginning. I forget what they were, so long ago. Gosh. But um, he started using something then, see, didn't bother.
> *So which did you prefer, you preferred French letters to pessaries?*
> Oh, yeah.And why was that?I thought it was safer. He had all the stuff then, I didn't. (laughs)[50]

The practicalities of using a female method of birth control meant that women had to anticipate or prepare for sex. Lella Secor Florence, for example, found in her clinic that many women were resistant to using caps because they were 'an unwomanly invitation to pleasures which are supposed to have been designed for her husband alone'.[51] Such an open embracing of sexual activity was clearly behind a number of respondents' dislike of birth control clinics and the methods they provided. Gwen was clearly very unhappy with the cap because she had to play a proactive role in sex and much preferred withdrawal because it meant she simply 'trusted him'.

> What was it like to use? Well, it wasn't very, you know (pause) I don't like talking about it really, but you had to put it in so long, you know, you didn't have intercourse until you put it in - so long - and then take it out and all that business. It was horrible, really.
> *So what didn't you like about it? Was it,*
> I didn't like it at all. I don't (pause) I mean, we had been married two and a half years and didn't have any children, so, er, I thought it was quite safe anyway. Fortunately we never had any more anyway.
> *So what had you done during those two and a half years to try and not get pregnant?*
> No, I didn't try. I trusted him really. (laughs)
> *And what did you trust him to do? What did he do that?*
> Oh! (faintly, as if sharp intake of breath)
> *You see I don't really know.*
> Withdrawal they call it, don't they? (pause)[52]

Working-class culture saw women as responsive to male initiative and defined sex as 'for men'. Such a culture fostered male responsibility for obtaining and using contraception and strong preferences for 'male' methods as opposed to female ones.

## Conclusion

There is a general tendency in historical studies of contraception to assume that attitudes towards methods remain constant or are self-evident. Frequently it is assumed to be obvious that 'traditional' methods, such as withdrawal, abortion and also abstinence, must have been unpalatable, or at least chosen only because they were the only methods available. It is assumed that the increasing availability of 'modern', 'better' and 'more reliable' methods of birth control during the course of the twentieth century can only have led to more satisfactory and probably more frequent use of birth control. My research suggests that for some, tried and trusted traditional methods of birth control were preferred over 'new', supposedly 'safer' 'appliance' ones. Hetty, who tried a number of different methods, illustrates the main points raised here. Hetty did not like the cap she was given, nor did she trust it. She preferred a method which left all responsibility in the hands of her husband.

> *Three methods you used – French letters, caps, and Rendells pessaries – perhaps you could compare the methods.*
>
> Well I should say the French letters, or condoms as they call them now are from my point of view, because the cap wasn't very successful where I didn't seem to be able to cope with that and with that you've got to be so sure that you've got it in correctly which I, I don't know, it's a hit and miss method isn't it really, when it comes to it. And the pessaries were messy, it was sort of gelatine stuff, or something, I don't know quite what was in them, but they were horrible, at least I thought they were. And um 'cos if you use anything like that you needed to um have a douche thing afterwards, it was too much of a palaver wasn't it really, come to think of it, absolutely. It made a, it made a thing of it didn't it really, instead of just being pleasurable.[53]

Predominately, the women I have interviewed were largely uninterested in birth control clinics. Those that did attend generally did so only after specific referral from a doctor or after insistence from a health official that severe steps be taken to avoid pregnancy. Those that did attend were frequently put off by clinic rigmarole and unhappy with the method provided. Most preferred alternative methods, such as withdrawal or condoms. Also, they did not necessarily perceive 'scientific' methods of birth control provided at birth control clinics as safer or more reliable than traditional methods. A considerable amount of distrust of 'modern' methods remained, as did faith in the efficacy of withdrawal and condoms. Above all those I have interviewed preferred methods which left the main responsibility for birth control with the husband. The sexual connotations of birth control meant that women were reluctant to be seen as too actively or conspicuously involved, while men were more prepared to take on the responsibility for birth control because they were the main instigators of sex. Men were expected to take the active role in all elements of sexual behaviour, including contraception. Many women were not keen to challenge these roles or this male culture of contraception. Thus, they were frequently largely unhappy with 'female' methods of birth control, and largely indifferent to birth control clinics. They were put off, not by the principle of family limitation, but by the social and moral beliefs that underpinned the delivery of birth control advice in birth control clinics.

## Notes

1. Fowles to Stopes, 22 March 1930 in Marie C. Stopes papers in the Department of Manuscripts at the British Library (hereafter BL), Add Mss. 58622.
2. Stopes to Williams, 1 May 1929, BL Add Mss. 58621.
3. All had been married.
4. The research was funded with the assistance of a Wellcome Trust Studentship.
5. Stanley, bc3ox#38. (private collection – those respondents who have given consent will have their tapes deposited in a suitable archive in the near future using these codes. 'sw' indicates the respondent was from South Wales and 'ox' that they were from Oxford. Any respondent without an 'sw' or an 'ox' in the code was interviewed in South Wales).
6. Deborah Cohen, 'Private Lives in Public Spaces: Marie Stopes, the Mothers' Clinics and the Practice of Contraception,' *History Workshop Journal*, 35 (1993), 105.
7. Marie Stopes to Victor Roberts, 12 December 1924, Marie Stopes papers in the Contemporary Medical Archives Centre at the Wellcome Library, (hereafter CMAC): PP/MCS/C.15.
8. Derek Jones and Sharon Goulds (eds), *In the Club? Birth Control This Century* (Television History Workshop in Association with Channel Four, 1988).

9. Gertrude, bc3sw#27.
10. British Library, Add Mss. 58622.
11. Dorothy, bc3ox#30.
12. Enid Charles, *The Practice of Birth Control. An Analysis of the Birth-Control Experiences of Nine Hundred Women* (London: Williams & Norgate, 1932), 53.
13. Norman E. and Vera C. Himes, 'Birth Control for the British Working Classes. A Study of the First Thousand Cases to Visit an English Birth Control Clinic', *Hospital Social Service*, 19 (1929), 578–??, 612.
14. See Lella Secor Florence, *Birth Control on Trial* (London: George Allen & Unwin, 1930), 97, 143, 157.
15. Some women had to travel considerable distances to get their nearest clinic. Oxford had two clinics (opened in 1926 and 1935), and although south Wales was especially targeted by the National Birth Control Association and had succeeded in getting 17 clinics established by 1939 difficulties were still posed by the inaccessible landscape of small isolated villages situated along steep valleys. On birth control clinics in south Wales see Kate Fisher, '"Clearing Up Misconceptions": The Campaign to Set Up Birth Control Clinics in South Wales Between the Wars', *Welsh History Review*, 18 (1998), 103–29.
16. Himes, *op. cit.* (note 13), 610.
17. Margaret, bc3ox#18.
18. Eva, bc1#1.
19. Florence, *op. cit.* (note 14), 26.
20. Angus McLaren also argues that the 'few clinics that were established had difficulty in attracting working-class women who were intimidated if not repelled by their male, middle-class, medical aura'. While I am less convinced that clinics were perceived as 'male', his identification of the rift between middle class birth controllers insistence on 'scientific' birth control and the examination of all women and the views and approaches to contraception and abortion of the working-class people they targeted is pertinent. See Angus McLaren, *A History of Contraception from Antiquity to the Present Day* (Oxford: Blackwell, 1990), 227.
21. Cohen, *op. cit.* (note 6), 113 n.8.
22. Shirley Arcott, *Mothercraft and Maternity. Leicester's Maternity and Infant Welfare Services 1900–1948* (Leicester: Leicestershire Museums, Arts and Records Service, 1997), 63.
23. Gwen, bc3sw#18.
24. Eva, bc1#1.

25. Marie Stopes to Jean Peterson, 5 July, n.d. ?1937?, CMAC/PP/MCS/C.24
26. Alan S. Parkes and Dee King, 'The Mothers' Clinic', *Journal of Biosocial Science*, 6 (1974), 168.
27. British Library, Add Mss. 58622.
28. British Library, Add Mss. 58622.
29. Elizabeth, bc3sw#12.
30. Florence, *op. cit.* (note 14), 144.
31. BL Add Mss. 58622.
32. Leslie, bc3sw1. Marie Stopes also declared that caps caused cancer, excepting her own 'pro-race' version. See Ruth Hall, *Marie Stopes. A Biography* (London: André Deutsch, 1977), 260.
33. BL Add Mss. 58622.
34. Fowles to Stopes, 10 January 1930, BL Add Mss 58622.
35. Florence, *op. cit.* (note 14), 102.
36. Gigi Santow has also argued that the safety of withdrawal is generally underestimated. Gigi Santow, 'Coitus interruptus in the Twentieth Century', *Population and Development Review*, 19 (1993), 770–2.
37. Elizabeth, bc3sw#12.
38. Charles, *op. cit.* (note 12), 52.
39. Some studies in developing countries similarly find that 'the social, economic and cultural context in which fertility regulation decisions are made …technology is often less important than reproductive preferences and the complex interplay of characteristics of families, communities and social and cultural factors.' Axel I. Mundigo, James F. Phillips and Aphichat Chamratrithirong, 'Determinants of Contraceptive Use Dynamics: Research News on Decision and Choice', *Journal of Biosocial Science*, 11, supplement, (1989), 15.
40. It is difficult to know how to interpret this statement. Perhaps it reveals an opposition to 'birth control' or maybe, like others, she suspected illegal abortions were available in birth control clinics.
41. Annie, bc3ox#27.
42. Elizabeth, bc3sw#12.
43. Marie Stopes, *Contraception. Birth Control Its Theory, History and Practice* (London: G.P. Putnam's Sons, first published 1923, third edition, reprinted 1932), 69.
44. Joe and Delia, bc3ox#29.
45. Marie Stopes & Co. to Bolton Police, 5 July, 1932, CMAC/PP/MCS/C.20
46. Gordon to Stopes, 29 April 1938. BL Add Mss 58625.
47. See Kate Fisher, '"She was quite satisfied with the arrangements I made": Gender and Birth Control in Britain 1920–1950', *Past and*

*Present*, in press.
48. Ernest, bc3sw#2.
49. Louisa, bc3ox#14.
50. Doris, bc3sw#6.
51. Florence, *op. cit.* (note 14), 68.
52. Gwen, bc3sw#18.
53. Hetty, bc3ox#12.

# 8

### 'Public spirited and enterprising volunteers': The Council for the Investigation of Fertility Control and the British clinical trials of the contraceptive pill, 1959–1973

## Lara Marks

On the eve of the launch of the first large clinical trial of the oral contraceptive pill in Britain in 1960, one concern uppermost in many of the organisers' minds was how British women would compare with those who had taken part in earlier trials in Puerto Rico, Haiti and the United States since 1956. Initial trials in these three countries had proven that the effectiveness of the pill depended not only on each woman's physical tolerance of the drug, but also on their ability to remember to take it every day. Women in Puerto Rico, for instance, were found to be more persistent in taking the medication than those in Los Angeles.[1] As one organiser of the British trials asked, to what extent would British women, even those who were 'the most public spirited and enterprising volunteers... stand up to the necessity of remembering to take a pill every time they clean their teeth in the morning'?[2] One of the purposes of the British trials was to find an easier regimen for taking the pill. Investigations elsewhere had shown the difficulties women faced in remembering when to take and stop the pill.[3]

The central question for those running the British trials was whether the high dose of the hormones in the original formulation of the pill could be reduced so that it would continue to be an effective contraceptive, while having fewer unpleasant adverse effects. The search for lower dose pills also stemmed from a recognition that the variety of women's physiques required different formulations. Preliminary tests in Britain, for instance, had shown that the average housewife in Devon tolerated the pill in larger doses than women in London, because they were at least 'a stone if not two stones heavier'. Similarly, smaller doses of the pill were more effective in Japanese women than others, because they were so much lighter in weight.[4] In reducing the dose of the pill the British trials also aimed to reduce the cost of oral contraceptives.[5]

The most intriguing feature of the British clinical trials was the degree to which they were more centrally organised than in the USA. This is particularly striking, given that before 1964 Britain overall had a much weaker system for regulating and monitoring pharmaceutical drugs than the USA. While the American government had established a Food and Drugs Administration (FDA) to regulate the safety of drugs as early as 1906, the equivalent in Britain, the Committee on Safety of Drugs (CSD), was instituted only in 1964, after the thalidomide disaster of 1959 to 1962. Similarly, the social and political taboos surrounding contraception in those years meant that the British government wanted nothing to do with the oral contraceptive and its clinical testing. Had pharmaceutical companies desired it, therefore, they could have released the pill on to the British market without any prior clinical testing or government approval.[6]

Yet the pill was subject to much more rigorous and coordinated testing than many other British pharmaceutical products during those years. Part of this stemmed from the special role played by a voluntary agency, the Council for the Investigation of Fertility Control (CIFC). From its establishment in 1957 until 1974, when its private funding diminished, the CIFC undertook trials on 63 different types of oral contraceptives.[7] These trials helped lower the dose of the pill. While the CSD took over some of the responsibility for testing the toxicity of the pill after 1964, the CIFC continued to play a significant role in monitoring oral contraceptives throughout the late 1960s and early 1970s, their major contribution being to assess the overall effectiveness and tolerance of new low-dose pills. In later years, the CIFC also became instrumental in long-term follow-up studies of the pill.[8] This paper explores the complex dynamics that allowed the CIFC, a voluntary body, to become the main tester and self-appointed approver of the earliest oral contraceptives in Britain.

**The Council for the Investigation of Fertility Control**

Founded in 1957, the CIFC was established as a result of a donation to the Family Planning Association (FPA) by Captain Oliver Bird. Originally a businessman in the food industry and a conservative MP, Bird had a strong interest in family planning and was keen to fund research that would help develop a simple and effective contraceptive to help curb population growth.[9] The aim of the CIFC was to organise and run clinical trials of new contraceptives.

Although under the auspices of the FPA, the CIFC was treated as autonomous from the parent organisation. Organisational distance from the FPA was seen as important in terms of obtaining further research funds. It was also seen as a safeguard against patients in FPA clinics being used as easy targets for the CIFC's trials.[10] Those sitting on the CIFC's committee nevertheless included leading campaigners in the family planning movement, such as Mrs Margaret Pyke, as well as experts in the reproductive field, such as the biologist Dr Alan Parkes, the endocrinologist Dr Gerald Swyer, and the medical practitioner Dr Margaret Jackson.[11] From May 1960, CIFC also had a special Medical Advisory Council. This consisted of leading medical practitioners concerned about the long-term effects of steroid contraception on health, including Sir Russell Brain[12], Sir Charles Dodds, and a number of experts in endocrinology and gynaecology, such as Professor Sir Dugald Baird. From the start all oral contraceptives tested by the Council in large scale trials had first to pass the scrutiny of this Medical Advisory Council.[13]

## Preliminary trials

The CIFC was not the only one to launch trials of oral contraceptives in Britain. For instance, G. D. Searle, the pharmaceutical company that had sponsored and tested the first pill in the Caribbean and the USA, launched its own small study in Britain in 1958. Conducted among upper and middle-class patients visiting the well-known private birth-control clinic run by Helena Wright[14] in London, this investigation contrasted later trials set up by the CIFC, in that it was initiated and run by Searle and focused on one particular compound. One of the reasons Searle had initiated the trial with patients from Helena Wright's clinic was the frustration its officials had perceived as a bureaucratic delay on the part of the CIFC.[15] While the day-to-day business of the trial was carried out by the doctors at Wright's clinic, Searle masterminded the organisation of the trial and the information supplied to the patients.[16]

The CIFC's officials were wary of launching a trial of the pill without their own prior screening of the product. Many of the procedures the CIFC adopted for testing oral contraceptives were rooted in the long tradition of monitoring new contraceptives within the FPA as a whole. From the 1930s the FPA had been at the forefront of instituting stringent scientific testing of all contraceptives and had established its own list of approved products.[17] The CIFC thus had its own standards and criteria for the safety and efficacy of contraceptives. Not reliant on the finance of any particular company, the Council also had the freedom to identify and test new contraceptive compounds at its discretion.[18]

Anxious about the harmful effects of the pill, the Council explicitly decided to delay launching large-scale trials in Britain until enough evidence had been collected in the USA. In 1957 the CIFC began to test all potential pills from a number of pharmaceutical companies in rats and mice.[19] The pills were tried for their toxicity as well as their hormonal and teratogenic effects and impact on fertility.[20] Once passed in animals, these substances were then screened in women. Started in 1958, this work was conducted by Dr Gerald Swyer from University College Hospital in London, and by Dr Margaret Jackson in Exeter.

Not specifically aimed at evaluating the drugs for their oral contraceptive value, the preliminary tests were designed to evaluate each new substance in terms of human tolerance, the degree to which it inhibited ovulation, and its impact on the secretory function of the endometrium. The purpose of these tests was also to find the optimum dose that would postpone menstruation and prevent breakthrough bleeding. As had been the case in trials elsewhere, before treatment and for six months thereafter, each woman had to undergo various cancer tests, vaginal smears, endometrial biopsies, gonadotrophin assays, chromosome counts and liver function tests. Initially the substances were tested in five to ten women. Most of these women were attending a hospital for some medical reason. Only once the substances were proven safe in these women were they put forward for a contraceptive trial. Then the substances were further tested in 25 women for an indefinite period.[21]

The preliminary trials conducted by Searle at Wright's clinic indicated that the CIFC would have difficulty in controlling the organisation of the pill trials in Britain. Most importantly, Searle's trial showed that pharmaceutical companies did not have to rely on the Council for conducting trials. The CIFC was therefore in a tenuous position. The one advantage that the CIFC had was the fact that it was under the auspices of the FPA, and therefore had access to a major supply of potential contraceptive users. This gave it a strong bargaining position with the pharmaceutical industry. During the Council's early years the majority of women who wanted contraceptive advice and devices were visiting family planning clinics, because few general practitioners, gynaecologists or obstetricians wanted anything to do with contraception. One British doctor, Dr A. Hill, summed up the attitude of many of his colleagues when he argued in 1962 that, 'medicine's calling is to guard against illness... and to treat established diseases through appropriate remedies.' He regarded the prescription of oral contraceptives as a 'debasement' of the medical vocation, and 'a misapplication' of medical 'knowledge and totally unworthy of a great profession'.[22]

## Organising large trials

Having conducted preliminary tests, by 1959 the CIFC was ready to launch trials on a much wider basis. However, one of the problems confronting the Council was that it did not have the machinery to conduct large scale trials outside central London.[23] It was reluctant to rely on FPA clinics, for fear of being accused of using family planning patients as 'involuntary guinea-pigs'.[24] Still operating in a climate in which contraception was seen as socially and morally unacceptable, the CIFC's organisers realised that they had to be careful about the way they enlisted volunteers and publicised the trials.[25]

Before launching large trials with the pill, the CIFC's officials tested public opinion by setting up pilot spermicide trials in 1958. Advertised in newspapers, these trials were designed to gauge the degree to which volunteers would come forward to take part in contraceptive investigations. The Council's leaders were stunned by the response – over 900 letters from people willing to participate in the trial. The reaction seemed to confirm the fact that the trials could 'be freely discussed without offence or unpleasant repercussions'. Moreover, it appeared that there were a large number of couples who were 'genuinely anxious to assist' in the trial. The replies also indicated a more general desire by many for 'a simpler contraceptive' and a general distaste for the methods then currently available.[26]

On the basis of the response the Council set up a postal trial with spermicides. Volunteers were divided into groups so that different spermicidal products could be tested and compared. A similar spermicide trial was also launched with volunteers from the Birmingham FPA clinic.[27] The spermicidal trials also established guidelines for the recruitment of volunteers and how to run a randomised controlled trial.[28] Those running the spermicide investigations saw the trials as helping to find people who were 'trial minded' who would be good subjects for later oral contraceptive trials.[29]

Despite the success of the spermicide trials, the CIFC ran into difficulties in mounting pill trials. The Council's workers had originally intended to rely on appeals for volunteers through different clinics and newspaper advertisements rather than to set up any specific trial in any individual family planning clinic. However, these plans were immediately thwarted, when organisers of a Birmingham family planning clinic allowed Searle to use their clinic for a large-scale trial without first gaining approval from the Council's headquarters. The incident not only challenged the Council's central authority, but raised ethical and financial questions about whether the CIFC and its FPA associates should be involved in a trial that was financially assisted by a manufacturer.[30] After much negotiation and compromise matters were resolved; the Birmingham FPA was allowed to run the trial, but all planning and organisation were subject to the scrutiny of the CIFC.

The Birmingham affair set a precedent for future trials. The CIFC made it clear that no individual clinic could undertake a clinical trial for any pharmaceutical company or any other organisations and individuals without first gaining approval from the Council's headquarters. Part of this stemmed from the strong desire of the CIFC's leaders to keep central control of the trials. Their reasoning was that their medical experts had more knowledge about the pill and its effects than most medical practitioners in Britain at that time. The CIFC's officials saw the strict regulations and safeguards in the trials as necessary not only for the safety of volunteers, but also in limiting any accidents in the running of the trials, which might reinforce the social and political taboos already surrounding contraception.[31] The need for caution was strengthened by the scandal just beginning to emerge over thalidomide in 1960. The Council's workers were also wary that any publicity concerning the trials might unrealistically raise public expectations.[32]

The episode with the Birmingham clinic showed the fine balancing act the CIFC's organisers had to perform. They not only had to win officials in family planning clinics to their side, but could not force their rules on the pharmaceutical industry. This had been illustrated in the case of the trial set up at Wright's clinic as well as in Birmingham. Soon after Birmingham, Searle had also approached a Slough family planning clinic to undertake a trial for them.[33] These incidents showed the weakness of the Council's negotiating position.

Despite these incidents, the CIFC had a strong bargaining tool, in that it was the body responsible for deciding whether the pill could be added to the FPA approved list of contraceptives. Without the CIFC's approval, pharmaceutical companies could not have their oral contraceptives officially used in family planning clinics, which initially constituted a major share of the consumer market. The CIFC's approval was also seen as important for oral contraceptives to be marketable abroad.[34]

One way the CIFC won family planning doctors to their cause was to allow individual medical practitioners to use family planning clinic facilities to carry out clinical trials. In this way no individual clinic could be seen to be running a trial and doctors within a clinic would gain access to potential volunteers for trials. Those running the trials were expected to work with patients who had specifically volunteered for the trial and to inform each patient of the unknown effect of the product being tried.[35] By 1963, ten of the 240 FPA clinics were holding special sessions for new oral contraceptives being tried by the CIFC, the results being coordinated by the Council's headquarters in London. Within two years trials were being held in Slough, London, Brighton, Exeter, Liverpool, Leicester, Leeds, Manchester and Sheffield. That year 2600 women were participating in the trials, and the number of women testing each product varied between 300 and 600.[36] The CIFC's sources do not reveal the total number of women on which they based their approval of each product, but the numbers of women involved with these trials compared favourably with other pharmaceutical drugs being tested at this time.[37]

## Recruiting women volunteers

The spermicide trials had shown the enormous potential for recruiting volunteers for contraceptive trials. As soon as the newspapers had announced the Birmingham trial they had received over 500 requests from women, many of whom initially had to be turned away.[38] Women continued flocking to join the trials. In 1961 the CIFC launched a television campaign, which led to an avalanche of volunteers, many of whom had to be rejected.[39]

Many of the women coming forward as volunteers were keen for any form of contraception. The anxiety that women faced during these years of another pregnancy, and their willingness to take a gamble in taking a product that was still so new and unproven is illustrated by a letter that was received by the CIFC in 1962 from a woman living in Chelmsford, Essex:

> A friend has just passed on to me your letter in the *Pictorial*. It seems to be an answer to my prayer, and I do hope I am not too late in writing.
>
> I have 5 children – age 13 and a half, 10, nearly 6, nearly 3 and a half, and 11 and a half. We did not 'plan' no. 4 and definitely did not want any more after he was born, for financial reasons. So I went with my doctor's letter to my local women's clinic. However, in spite of all their recommended precautions no. 5 arrived.
>
> My midwife suggested oral contraceptives so I went to the

Family Planning Clinic in Chelmsford. The doctor accepted me as a suitable patient – but I could not possibly afford the cost. She got in touch with my own doctor and asked him to let me have the 'PILL' on H.H [NHS]. He refused. I have his letter, after a most unfortunate visit. He disagrees entirely with the whole idea. So I was at a dead end and just hoped I would not become pregnant for the sixth time, before I received help.

Is there any more you need to know? I'm crossing my fingers you'll need me as a volunteer, please.[40]

Initially, the Council's trials represented the only chance for women to get the pill. Few general practitioners, for example, were willing to prescribe the pill when it first came on to the market. Family planning clinics also offered the pill only on an extremely limited basis. The high response of women volunteering posed an ethical dilemma for the CIFC's workers, for they did not know where else to refer them.[41] In many cases the pill trial brought women into contact with family planning services for the first time, having previously been shy of seeking help.[42] Before the pill the only method available had been the cap, which not only demanded an intimate familiarity with one's own body, but entailed an extensive vaginal examination. By contrast the pill necessitated less medical scrutiny and was taken by mouth.

As had been the case in previous trials carried out in other countries, all women accepted for the CIFC's trials had to be married, and healthy and to have proven their fertility before the trial. A more detailed list of all the criteria British women were expected to satisfy is given in Figure 8.1.[43] These women were expected to commit themselves to staying in the trial for at least six months. Each woman was also required to sign a consent form along with her husband. The Council's officials undertook this procedure to ensure that a woman's decision to be in a trial was a joint decision, for they saw family planning as a collective decision between a husband and wife.[44] The form, approved by the Medical Protection Society, indicated that the drug was experimental and could not be guaranteed to prevent pregnancy. All women were carefully informed that the pill could have adverse effects. Figure 8.2 shows the information the women were given on starting in a trial. Each woman was expected to take pills on a set number of days after their periods, marking carefully on a chart when they took the tablet, had intercourse, and had a period.[45]

*Figure 8.1:*
*Criteria for volunteers participating*
*in the CIFC's trials, 1960*

1) Residence within easy access to the clinic.
2) Age under 35 years.
3) At least one living child of present marriage and not more abortions than children.
4) Average frequency of coitus not less than once weekly.
5) No other form of contraception to be used.
6) Menstrual cycle limit 23 to 32 days in year prior to starting the trial.
7) Expressed intention of volunteer to continue the trial for a minimum of 6 months.
8) No history of illness of husband or wife likely to have altered fertility since first child.
9) Satisfactory general health of volunteer, determined by history.
10) Satisfactory findings on examination of breasts, abdomen and pelvic organs.
11) Maximum weight of volunteer (partly clothed) 11 stone.
12) Consent form to be signed by wife and husband.

Source: 'Proposed trial of Searle Contraceptive Tablet',
2 May 1960, CMAC SA/FPA/A5/157/1, Box 249;
and 'Proposed Trial of Searle Contraceptive Pill', 23 March 1960,
in CIFC Minutes, SA/FPA/A5/154.

## Aims of large trials

From the start the CIFC did not intend to run a 'straight forward repeat' of trials run elsewhere.[46] The main objective of the trials was to adjust the dose of the original pill so that its adverse effects could be limited while continuing to provide contraceptive effectiveness. Initially all tablet doses were decided by the manufacturers and not the CIFC.[47] Some work had already been carried out in Puerto Rico and Japan in lowering the dose of the pill, for it had been found that the intensity of adverse effects experienced depended on the dose of the drugs. In these trials the dose of progestogen (semi-synthetic progesterone) had been reduced by a quarter. While this had diminished the amount of nausea women suffered, it had resulted in more break-through bleeding. Investigators had found that some of the break-through bleeding could be controlled by increasing the

*Figure 8.2:*
*Information for volunteers*

> Once each month a healthy, fertile woman produces an ovum, or egg, from the ovary (usually called ovulation). If this ovum is fertilised by a spermatozoon from the seminal fluid, pregnancy results. Further egg production does not, however, occur during pregnancy. This is prevented by certain chemical substances, known as sex hormones, which are produced in large amounts by a healthy woman during normal pregnancy. It is now possible to prevent ovulation in this way by taking tablets by mouth. If ovulation is prevented in this way month after month, pregnancy cannot occur, even though sexual intercourse takes place normally and no other form of contraception is used. Extensive tests have shown that it is safe to take the tablets for 2 years at least. Approximately one thousand women have used the tablets and when the tablets are known to have been taken as described no cases of pregnancy have been reported. Many women have decided to have children after using the tablets for periods of up to 2 years. Pregnancy occurred within a short time and the children born have all been quite normal. Amongst the women who have taken the tablets but have failed to take them regularly, some have become pregnant and the children born have also been normal.
>
> The best method and dosage to ensure regularity of the monthly periods while taking the tablets is now being studied. The effectiveness of the tablets in preventing pregnancy is already known.
>
> Most women find that their periods are normal and regular provided that the tablets are taken regularly as instructed. Women whose periods have previously been irregular tend to develop a regular 28 day rhythm when taking the tablets. Women accustomed to heavy losses can expect the flow to be less troublesome while taking the tablets. Some women, however, find their normal rhythm may be altered on first using the tablets. Bleeding may occur earlier than expected but this is not harmful. We believe that this type of irregularity may settle down during the first few months. We do not expect any other difficulties. It is possible, however, that a few women will experience reactions. We already know that such reactions usually decrease and disappear on continuing the tablets. Women who have used the tablets for any length of time have found this method to be highly satisfactory and usually prefer it to other methods of contraception.

*Source: CMAC file: FPA/A5/157/1, Box 249; also CIFC notes, 80, file: A5/154*

dose of oestrogen while decreasing the progestogen. Much depended of the weight of the women as to the effects they experienced while taking the pill. What was clear from these studies was that more research was needed to perfect the pill.[48]

The first pill trial, started in Birmingham in June 1960, tested the same compound that Searle had provided for the Puerto Rican trials. A key goal of the trial was to find a means of lowering the doses of oestrogen with progesterone in the pill.[49] Soon after the Birmingham trial started, investigators discovered that many of the volunteers experienced unusual menstrual cycles, and, worse still, that some of them were falling pregnant even when taking the pill as directed. This resulted partly from the fact that the manufacturer had unintentionally mislabelled the pills, with the result that the first batch of pills distributed contained only one-third of the originally intended oestrogen. The accident revealed the importance of the dose of oestrogen on inhibition of ovulation.[50] Pregnancy had partly occurred because the lower dose of oestrogen had merely delayed and not suppressed ovulation. While this was traumatic for the women who became pregnant, the error of the trial nevertheless provided valuable information for the investigators, because it showed the lowest dose to which oestrogen could be reduced before its preventive effect was diminished. In September the remaining women on the trial were switched to pills containing higher doses of progestogen and oestrogen.[51]

Testing the effectiveness of various doses of hormones in pills continued to be important in the trials that followed the Birmingham trial. One of the earliest considerations for the CIFC's trials was whether the dose and hormonal components of the pill could be altered to prevent the problem of break-through bleeding. Early trials in Puerto Rico had shown that oestrogen was an important factor in controlling break-through bleeding. Break-through bleeding had proven most problematic when the pill had consisted solely of progestogen. Early investigators had decided to add 1.5 per cent of oestrogen to the pill precisely to stop the bleeding.[52] However, the problem, had not been totally resolved.

Break-through bleeding proved to be one of the most difficult problems the British investigators faced in reducing the dose of the pill. In 1961, for instance, 20 per cent of volunteers participating in the CIFC's trials experienced break-through bleeding.[53] While such bleeding was not seen as dangerous or a cause of ill-health it 'upset' the patient. As Dr Jackson explained,

> They do not like having odd spots of bleeding perhaps on four or five successive days and then a gap of two days and then two days bleeding, and so on. This upsets them, they do not like it, and they say, 'Please, we would rather not take your tablets', so it is important if you are going to find a method which is effective that you have one which is not going to upset the patient for any reason of that sort.[54]

As had been tried elsewhere,[55] the CIFC's investigators attempted to solve the problem by doubling the dose of the pill on the days women experienced the spotting. Another was to ignore the spotting but to stop taking the drug when bleeding occurred and treat it like a normal menstrual period, resuming the pill on the fifth day as usual.[56] Some formulations caused more break-through bleeding than others.[57] By 1964 various trials had shown that the type of oestrogen component used in the pill affected break-through bleeding.[58]

From 1963 the Council began to test a new dosage system for oral contraceptives, known as the sequential pill. Previous pills had consisted of tablets with the same balance of oestrogen and progesterone throughout the month. In the sequential regimen women took tablets containing only oestrogen for the first couple of weeks of the cycle, followed by pills containing both oestrogen and progestogen for the remainder of the cycle.[59] Part of the reasoning behind this regimen was that it would be cheaper to manufacture and was physiologically closer to women's hormonal cycle. Soon into the trials, however, the sequential method was found to have a higher pregnancy failure rate than the original combined pill. On account of this, in 1964 the CIFC decided not to pursue large-scale trials with the sequential pills.[60] Further trials with higher doses of oestrogen had better success rates.[61] Later trials also investigated progestogen-only pills, as these were thought to cause fewer thrombotic complications, already thought to be associated with oestrogen.[62]

In testing for different formulations and doses of the pill the CIFC and other UK investigators had an advantage over researchers working in other countries, for British rules governing the setting of the dosage of drugs were fairly relaxed. This allowed the CIFC more freedom to do preliminary trials with different doses of the pill than was the case elsewhere. In the USA, for instance, where the initial development of the pill had occurred, experimental trials with the dose took longer to pursue, because the FDA insisted on setting the dose of the pill at a very early stage. The flexibility of British regulations was also particularly good for investigating sequential pills, which required studying not only different doses but also patterns of therapy, such as whether the method worked best with 15 or 11 days of oestrogen followed by 11 or 10 days of combined oestrogen and progestogen.[63]

In addition to trying out new chemical substances, the CIFC's investigators also tried various methods for administering the pill. Initially they pursued the same routine as had been tried in Puerto Rico and elsewhere. The regimen expected women to take the pill for 20 days from the fifth day of the start of their menstrual period.[64] Like other researchers, those at the CIFC were keen to find a different regimen for dispensing the pill, because many women were confused by this routine.[65] The Council's trials therefore explored different regimens for taking the pill. The CIFC helped to establish the routine of taking the pill for 21 days, with a seven day break. This schedule was easier for women to follow, because it involved stopping and starting the pill on the same day of the week, and did not necessitate calculations in relation to their menstrual cycles.[66] Another regimen that was tried was to put seven dummy tablets in the packaging of the pill so that women could continue to take the pill for the whole month without a break.[67]

The overall strength of the CIFC was that it could coordinate a number of trials with different pills and did not depend on any one pharmaceutical company for funding. What the CIFC offered were trials conducted on a uniform basis with several pills which could then be compared with each other on a more rational and scientific basis.[68] The CIFC's trials were used for surveying a range of products in terms of effectiveness as well as negative reactions.[69] These trials made it clear that the type of hormone and dose used in different pills affected adverse effects, such as breast discomfort, nausea, headaches, and weight gain.[70] They also showed that certain pills suited some women and not others. Much depended on the metabolism of the women and their medical and menstrual history.[71]

The CIFC was also in a good position to follow its patients over a long period of time because they had access to a highly selected group of women who had participated in trials from early on. Such women could provide information on the biochemical and physiological characteristics of those who took the pill for long periods of time.[72] Overall, however, the CIFC was unable to gather any significant data from the long-term studies. Part of this stemmed from the fact that the percentage of women remaining in each trial varied between products.[73] This rendered the numbers statistically insignificant for understanding the association of the pill with rare events, such as blood clots. Such investigations also provided only minimal information on the impact of the pill on more common adverse effects, such as nausea.[74] While this research never provided fruitful results, the population base built up by the CIFC's trials later provided fundamental research data for the first British epidemiological studies of the pill.

### The CIFC's relationship with the pharmaceutical industry

Despite its success, the CIFC was continually struggling financially. One of the ways its staff tried to survive was to gain sponsorship from pharmaceutical companies. This, however, did not come without conflict. In 1963, for instance, Searle representatives registered a complaint when a CIFC's publication indicated that women experienced more nausea on one of its pills than those of other manufacturers. Searle not only argued that the evidence had been distorted, but also queried the methods used by the CIFC for determining the comparisons between the products.[75] On another occasion, Searle refused to fund the full costs of a trial that entailed regular cervical smears every six months. For the Council's workers these smears were useful in understanding the rate of pre-cancer cells and not cancer deaths. However, Searle representatives did not see this research as important to their own interests. They also saw the high costs of the smears as unjustified, because it would only pick up a minimal number of problematic cases, and because these cases were unlikely to be missed in the process of routine clinical examination.[76]

Other tensions emerged in 1964, when Searle officials asked the CIFC to release data prematurely from a double-blind study that they had helped to sponsor. From the perspective of the Council's staff this contravened the agreement made between them and the pharmaceutical companies which had made it clear that no analysis would be made until well after the close of the trial, which was to last two years.[77] In later years comparative double-blind studies continued to be a source of contention between pharmaceutical companies and the CIFC.[78]

Friction also surfaced over the funding of long-term trials. From the perspective of pharmaceutical companies such research cost too much and yielded little information that was of direct relevance.[79] By 1966 pharmaceutical companies were refusing to continue to pay for such work. Cynically, one official from Ortho Pharmaceuticals wrote to the CIFC,

> Having presented a bill for £1,750 to our Board of Directors, for clinical trial of our oral contraceptive, I find the only really valid

reason for this claim is to maintain the product on your approved list. The cost of the clinical evaluation can be no greater than one-third of this amount, and when presenting the matter in this light, it certainly gives a most undesirable picture of the FPA – and one which is completely undeserved.[80]

Such incidents underlined the major difficulty the CIFC's investigators faced in retaining their own organisational and administrative independence while accepting financial support from pharmaceutical companies. While the CIFC carried the administrative and organisational burden of the clinical trials, pharmaceutical companies were expected to contribute towards the cost of the clinical trials of their own products. This was not an insubstantial sum. In 1963 manufacturers granted £19,001 for clinical trials, 85 per cent of the CIFC's total income (£22,419).[81] Grants from pharmaceutical companies continued to be a significant part of the CIFC's budget until the late 1960s. In 1968, for instance, manufacturers' grants came to a total of £18,227, 99 per cent of the Council's income.[82] With this amount of investment pharmaceutical companies were adamant that they should have a voice in the research planning and organisation of the trials. They also saw themselves as having the appropriate methodological expertise for the trials.[83]

While in the early 1960s the CIFC had been in a strong bargaining position to demand such money from pharmaceutical companies, by the late 1960s circumstances had altered. One of the major changes had come with the establishment in 1964 of the CSD, which took over responsibility for screening pharmacological and toxicological data provided by manufacturers on all drugs, including the pill. This radically weakened the position of the CIFC. While the Council remained responsible for testing the efficacy of oral contraceptives, it was no longer the main agency responsible for testing for the safety of new pills before their use in clinical trials.[84]

In December 1969 the Council's authority was challenged more directly by the government, when it decided to phase out the high oestrogen pills the CSD had identified with thrombotic complications. Before this episode all oral contraceptives provided in family planning clinics had had to pass the CIFC's investigations before they could be included in the FPA 'Approved List' and distributed. In 1969, however, with a large number of the high oestrogen oral contraceptives excluded from prescription by the government, the FPA was forced to include three oral contraceptive pills on the list that had not been previously tested by the CIFC. As a result of this, the CIFC was no longer the sole agency responsible for deciding which pills could be distributed in family planning clinics.[85] From this moment on all pills that were accepted for the FPA's Approved List had to be proven effective contraceptives with no serious or unacceptable adverse effects. Trials other than those conducted by the CIFC were sufficient for establishing this issue.[86]

In addition to having their power undermined by government decisions, the Council's position was further weakened by the shift in the distribution of oral contraceptives. By 1970 over 80 per cent of oral contraceptives were being prescribed by general practitioners. This contrasted with the situation in the early 1960s, when family planning clinics had been the main providers of the pill. Manufacturers therefore no longer relied on the CIFC and its connections with family planning clinics to find volunteers for their trials. In some instances pharmaceutical companies preferred to approach general practitioners to secure results from quick trials.[87] The CIFC had thus lost its strong bargaining position in terms of providing patients as well as determining the types of trials pursued. On the whole manufacturers were now less likely to cooperate with the CIFC and were more concerned with using the FPA as 'a source of patients for trials in which' they could 'brief the doctors, collect and process the data and decide which preparations be tested.'[88]

## Conclusion

In the end the CIFC was forced to bring its work to an end owing to lack of financial support. By 1968 the original capital of £11,000 that had been used to establish the CIFC had fallen to £3,540 and was only expected to last another year.[89] In 1970 the Council had a deficit of over £8,000. Aided with some money from the FPA, it managed to struggle on for a couple more years.[90] Finally, however, in 1973 the Council was forced to disband. Although the Council became obsolete, it had been crucial in the initial testing of the pill in Britain. With minimal government regulation for testing the efficacy and safety of drugs in Britain during the 1950s the CIFC filled a vital vacuum in terms of monitoring and testing the pill. Although pharmaceutical companies were testing of their own accord in this period, the CIFC was crucial, in that it was independent from the pharmaceutical industry. This allowed the CIFC's investigators the freedom to test each product without bias. The Council also played a key role in helping to adjust the dose of the pill as well as the regimen of taking the drug. In later years the trial population built up by the CIFC laid the foundations for the British epidemiological work, which established the links between high oestrogen pills and thrombotic disease.

Starting at a time when contraception was highly taboo both socially and politically, the CIFC had also been important in supplying the pill. As the woman writing from Chelmsford in 1962 demonstrates, the CIFC trials were the one means by which women could initially obtain the pill free. However, once contraception became easily available the CIFC was no longer so significant. By the time the CIFC folded, contraception had become such an accepted part of life that the National Health Service began to take over its provision. By 1974 not only had the FPA come under the auspices of the NHS, but all women were now entitled to free contraceptives, including oral contraceptives. The pill contrasted with other medications at this time, which were increasingly being subjected to a small prescription charge. In many ways such acceptance of the pill can be attributed to the work of the CIFC.

## Acknowledgements

This paper could not have been written without the archival support of Lesley Hall and other staff from the Contemporary Medical Archives Centre, Wellcome Library. I would also like to thank Jean Infield, Joan Nabarro, Denise Pullen, Geoffrey Venning and Aviva Wiseman for recalling their work in testing the pill, and the women who were willing to share their experiences while participating in the trial. I am also indebted to Wendy Neil, Rosalind O'Brien, Helen Wickham and Maridowa Williams for their research help and to Suzanne White Junod for her comments on an earlier version of this paper. Research for the article was assisted by a Wellcome Award from the Wellcome Trust.

## Notes

1. Notes from Mrs Clifford Smith to Dr Pyke, 4 March 1960, SA/FPA/A/161/1, Box 251. All files with reference to SA/FPA can be found in the Contemporary Medical Archives Centre, Wellcome Library, London. For more information on these earlier trials see L. Marks, '"A Cage of Ovulating Females": The Early Clinical Trials of the Oral Contraceptive Pill', in S. de Chadarevian and H. Kamminga (eds), *Molecularizing Biology: New practices and alliances, 1910s–1970s* (Amsterdam: Harwood Academic, 1998); P. Vaughan, *The Pill on Trial* (London: Weidenfeld & Nicolson, 1972); J. Reed, *The Birth Control Movement and American Society* (Princeton, NJ:

Princeton University Press, 1978); N. Oudshoorn, *Beyond the Natural Body: An Archaeology of Sex Hormones* (London: Routledge, 1994).

2. 'The Pill', *Eugenics Review*, May 1960, SA/FPA/A5/161/1, Box 251; E. Mears, 'The Clinical Application of Oral Contraceptives', paper read to 'Symposium on Agents Affecting Fertility', held at Middlesex Hospital Medical School, 24 March 1964, SA/FPA/A5/158B, Box 249; 'Trials of Oral Contraceptives', c.1960, SA/FPA/A5/161/1, Box 251; IPPF Press Conference, 30 March 1960, SA/FPA/161/4, Box 251, 7.

3. Dr M. Jackson at IPPF Press Conference, 30 March 1960, SA/FPA/A5/161/4; 'Report of a Medical Conference of FPA Medical Officers and Nurses', 19 November 1960, SA/FPA/A(/167, Box 253.

4. A. Maisel, 'At last a pill for birth control', *Reader's Digest* (March 1961), 37–41.

5. H. Hill, 'Report from the Clinical Trials Committee Concerning Proposals for the Future Medical Policy of Trials of Hormonal Contraceptives', 20 September 1968, SA/FPA/A5/160/2, Box 250; Interview with G. Venning by L. Marks, 16 October 1996, tape and notes. Telephone conversation with Dr Parkes, 28 December 1956, SA/FPA/127, Box 245; letter from O. Bird to M. Pyke, 15 March 1957, SA/FPA/A5/126, Box 245.

6. CIFC Fact Sheet, November 1970, SA/FPA/A5/160/3, Box 250. In 1955 the Ministry of Health had specified that it did not want any involvement with contraception, and preferred contraceptive services to be kept in the hands of a voluntary body such as the FPA. See 'Family Planning in Practice', *The Times*, 17 July 1959.

7. Memo: 'Future of CIFC Trials', 23 April 1969, SA/FPA/A5/160/2; CIFC Fact Sheet, November 1970, SA/FPA/A5/160/3. Both in Box 250.

8. Meeting between representatives from CIFC and Manufacturers of Pharmaceutical Products, 12 November 1970, SA/FPA/A5/160/3, Box 250.

9. Between 1900 and 1946 Oliver Bird had been director of his family's company, the food firm, Alfred Bird and Sons, Ltd. He had also been a Conservative MP for Wolverhampton West. Bird was able to finance the project by selling his oil shares in Trinidad. See obituaries in *Birmingham Post*, 19 April 1963; *Manchester Guardian*, 12 June 1963; *Solihull, Warwick News*, n.d; M. Pyke to O. Bird, 9 July 1956; all in SA/FPA/A5/130, Box 246; and Notes for Dr Parkes' visit to Captain Bird, 13 February 1957, SA/FPA/127, Box 245; Deed of declaration of trust between Margaret Amy Pyke and Judith Anne

Burrell and Dr Alan Stirling Parkes,' 1957, SA/FPA/A5/126, Box 245.
10. OBT meeting, 5 April 1957, SA/FPA/A5/128, Box 245; CIFC Minutes, 15 January 1960, 75, SA/FPA/A5/154, Box 248; CIFC Minutes, 29 June 1966, 51, SA/FPA/A5/129, Box 245; E. Mears to D. D. Reid, 28 September 1960, SA/FPA/A5/162.3, Box 252.
11. Deed of declaration of trust between Margaret Amy Pyke and Judith Anne Burrell and Dr Alan Stirling Parkes', 1957, SA/FPA/A5/126, Box 245.
12. Sir Russell Brain had formerly been president of the Royal Society of Medicine. He had left this position in order to head the Family Planning Association 'because he felt birth control to be the most important immediate world problem.' McCormick's Notes on Conversation with Dr Pincus, April 16 1958, Margaret Sanger's Papers, Sophia Smith Library, Northampton, Massachusetts, USA.
13. Press Cutting, n.d, in FPA/A5/161/4, Box 251; General Secretary to Mrs A.K. Court, 23 April 1960, SA/FPA/A7/110.3, Box 288; E. Mears to M. Davies-Westerman, 2 June 1964, SA/FPA/A5/161/3, Box 251.
14. Helena Wright had become a key family planning doctor during the interwar years. Right to the end of her career she preferred barrier methods, and in the 1970s officially stated her distrust of the pill. See B. Evans, *The Freedom to Choose: The Life and Work of Dr Helena Wright* (London: Bodley Head, 1983), 231–3.
15. Interview with G. Venning. The cautious attitude of British doctors also infuriated the early American developers of the pill. See K. McCormick to G. Pincus, 27 July 1964, and G. Pincus to K. McCormick, 4 August 1964, Pincus Papers, Library of Congress (henceforth GP-LC).
16. Interview with J. Nabarro by L. Marks, 9 December 1996, notes, 2, 3 and interview with Venning, notes, 2.
17. 'The FPA Approved List', n.d., SA/FPA/A5/167, Box 253; E. Mears to A. Parkes, 30 October 1959, SA/FPA/127, Box 245.
18. *Ibid.*
19. This included Schering and the British drugs houses as well as Searle. CIFC Minutes, 16 October 1958, 35, SA/FPA/A5/154, Box 248.
20. 'Screening test for oral contraceptives', 3 August 1960, SA/FPA/A5/162.3, Box 252. After 1964 the Committee on Safety of Drugs took over the responsibility for scrutinising the data on harmlessness supplied by manufacturers on oral contraceptives, but the CIFC continued to scrutinise the pill for efficacy. E. Mears,

'Future of the CIFC', 6 May 1964, SA/FPA/A5/158B, Box 249.
21. E. Mears to Sir R. Brain, 12 September 1961, SA/FPA/A5/158B, Box 249; 'Report presented to Medical Advisory Council', 25 July 1962, SA/FPA/A5/161/4, Box 251; 'Report of Work of the CIFC for OBT', in CIFC Minutes, 18 July 1963, 122A and Doctors' Meeting, 16 October 1962, 3 in SA/FPA/A5/155, Box 248. See also L. Marks, *op. cit.* (note 1).
22. *British Medical Journal*, ii (1962), 52. For more information of the medical profession's response to the pill see L. Marks, *Sexual Chemistry: A History of the Contraceptive Pill* (Newhaven and London: Yale University Press, 2001), chapter 5.
23. Draft letter from Mr Stallabrass to Mr G. G. Robertson, n.d., SA/FPA/A5/161/1, Box 251.
24 CIFC meeting, April 5 1957, SA/FPA/A5/128, Box 245.
25. Unsigned letter to A. Parkes, 19 June 1958, SA/FPA/127, Box 245; Secretary's Report, 1958 in CIFC Minutes, 16 October 1958, 35, SA/FPA/A5/154, Box 248.
26. Secretary's Report, 1958, in CIFC Minutes, 16 October 1958, 35, and CIFC Minutes, 16 April 1959, 43, SA/FPA/A5/154, Box 248.
27. CIFC Minutes, 16 April 1959, 43, SA/FPA/A5/154, Box 248. The products used included Delfen, Bymeston Foaming tablets, Eli Lilly Lubricating jelly, GP solubles and Volpar Foaming tablets.
28. CIFC Minutes, 16 April 1959, 43; 16 October 1958, 35, SA/FPA/A5/154, Box 248.
29. M. Pyke to O. Bird, 25 June 1958, SA/FPA/A5/130, Box 246.
30. Memo from Mrs Clifford Smith, 15 January 1960, CIFC Minutes, SA/FPA/A5/154, Box 248.
31. Questions were already surfacing in parliament about whether adequate precautions were being taken to guarantee the safety of women taking part in clinical trials with the pill. See CIFC Minutes, 10 March 1960, 96, SA/FPA/A5/154, Box 248.
32. Unsigned letter to O. Bird, 7 August 1958, SA/FPA/A5/130, Box 246; Letter from A.J. Clifford Smith to FPA branch and clinic secretaries, 11 March 1960, SA/FPA/A5/161/4, Box 251. For more information on thalidomide see Henning Sjöström and Nilsson, *Thalidomide and the power of the drug companies* (Harmondsworth, Middx.: Penguin, 1972) Similar fears about raising unrealistic expectations were also present in the campaigns with cortisone. See D. Cantor, 'Cortisone and the Politics of Empire: Imperialism and British Medicine, 1918–1955', *Bulletin of the History of Medicine*, 67/3 (1993), 463–93.
33. Interview with Venning, notes, 3. Some of the tensions between the

CIFC and pharmaceutical companies can be seen in a memo from CIFC Minutes, 15 January 1959, 74–5, SA/FPA/A5/154, Box 248.
34. CIFC Meeting, 14 January 1964, SA/FPA/A5/158B, Box 249; CIFC Minutes, 29 June 1966, 51, SA/FPA/A5/129, Box 245.
35. CIFC Minutes, 15 January 1959, appendix, SA/FPA/A5/154, Box 248.
36. 'The FPA Approved List', n.d., SA/FPA/A5/167, Box 253; E. Mears to A. Parkes, 30 October 1959, SA/FPA/127, Box 245.
37. For comparisons between the testing of the pill and other drugs see L. Marks, S. W. Junod, 'Women on Trial: Approval of the First Oral Contraceptive Pill in the United States and Great Britain', *Social History of Medicine* (unpublished paper).
38. *Birmingham Mail*, 28 June 1960, SA/FPA/161/4, Box 251.
39. E. Mears to S. J. Hadfield, British Medical Association, 16 April 1962, SA/FPA/A5/161/2, Box 251.
40. Letter from a woman from Chelmsford, Essex, to Dr Mears, 22 November 1962, SA/FPA/A5/158a, Box 249.
41. E. Mears to S. J. Hadfield, British Medical Association, 16 April 1962, SA/FPA/A5/161/2, Box 251. In 1961 the pill was available in family planning clinics only for the purposes of clinical trials and training doctors. E. Mears to M. C. R. Sinclair-Loutit, 10 November 1961, SA/FPA/A5/161/2, Box 251.
42. Interview with D. Pullen, 16 December 1996 by L. Marks, transcript.
43. For the criteria used in earlier trials see Marks, *op. cit.* (note 1).
44. Interviews with J. Infield by L. Marks 29 January 1996, transcript, and interview with Pullen.
45. CIFC Minutes, 10 March 1960, SA/FPA/A5/154.
46. CIFC Minutes, 1 October 1958, SA/FPA/A5/154, Box 248.
47. E. Mears letter to *British Medical Journal*, n.d, *c.*1963, in SA/FPA/A5/159, Box 249.
48. G. Pincus to E. Rice-Wray, 6 April 1956, GP-LC, Box 22; *Proceedings of a Symposium on 19-Nor Progestational Steroids* (Chicago, IL: Searle, 23 January 1957), John Rock's Papers, Countway Library. 'The Pill', *Eugenics Review*, May 1960, SA/FPA/A5/161/1, Box 251; 'Oral Contraceptives', *c.*1960, SA/FPA/A5/167, Box 254.
49. Report of a discussion with Dr Parkes, Dr Venning, Mrs Clifford Smith, Dr Mears and Mrs Pyke, 10 March 1960, SA/FPA/A5/161/1, Box 251; 'Oral Contraceptives', *c.*1960, SA/FPA/A5/169, Box 254.
50. Some oestrogens are more potent than others. No trials, however,

were ever conducted to see which type of oestrogen was most effective. Interview with Venning, notes.
51. CIFC Clinical Trial Committee, Minutes, 13 October 1960, SA/FPA/A5/160, Box 250; E. Mears to editor of the *Guardian*, 6 November 1961, SA/FPA/A5/161/2, Box 251.
52. *Proceedings of a Symposium on 19-Nor Progestational Steroids*, (note 48); 'Oral Contraceptives', c.1960, SA/FPA/A5/167, Box 254.
53. E. Mears at Second Medical Advisory Council, 4 October 1961, SA/FPA/A5/161/4, Box 251.
54. M. Jackson at IPPF Press Conference, 30 March 1960, SA/FPA/A5/161/4, Box 251.
55. Study of long-term administration of 17 ethinyl-19 nortesterone in fertility control (preliminary report)' n.d, GP-LC, Box 45.
56. Statement of the use of oral contraceptives', prepared for publication in *Lancet*, July 1960, SA/FPA/A5/161, Box 251; E. Mears, 'Clinical Application of Oral Contraceptives', 1964, SA/FPA/A5/158B, Box 249.
57. Untitled information leaflet, 5 November 1963, SA/FPA/A5/159, Box 249.
58. 'Memo to all Members of the CIFC', 11 January 1963, SA/FPA/A5/157/1, Box 249; E. Mears, 'Clinical Application of Oral Contraceptives', 1964, SA/FPA/A5/158B, Box 249.
59. CIFC Minutes, 20 June 1963, 99, SA/FPA/A5/155, Box 248.
60. G. I. M. Swyer, 'Fertility Control: Achievements and Prospects', 2 February 1967, OBT lecture, SA/FPA/A5/135, Box 246; CIFC Minutes, vol. 2, 10 August 1964, SA/FPA/A5/155, Box 248; Fourth Meeting of Doctors Conducting CIFC Oral Contraceptive Trials, 30 June 1964 and Meeting of CIFC Clinical Trials Subcommittee, 10 August 1964, and CIFC Minutes, 19 May 1964 and Mears, 'Clinical Application of Oral Contraceptives', 11, all in SA/FPA/A5/158B, Box 249.
61. CIFC Minutes, 19 September 1967, 147; and 5 May 1965, 60, SA/FPA/A5/156, Box 249.
62. 'CIFC Progestogen only trials', April 1972, SA/FPA/A5/160/4, Box 250.
63. E.Mears, 'Future of the CIFC', 6 May 1964, SA/FPA/A5/158B, Box 249.
64. Memo from N. G. Newsbury to Mrs Clifford Smith, n.d, SA/FPA/A5/161/1, Box 251; Memo from N. G. Newsbury, CIFC Minutes, March 1960, 79, SA/FPA/A5/154, Box 248; 'Proposed trial of Searle Contraceptive Tablet', 2 May 1960, SA/FPA/A5/157/1, Box 249.

65. 'The Pill', *Eugenics Review*, May 1960, SA/FPA/A5/161/1, Box 251.
66. E. Mears to D. C. Macdonald, 18 June 1962, SA/FPA/A5/161/2, Box 251.
67. E. Mears, 'Clinical Application of the Oral Contraceptives', 4, an unpublished paper read to a Symposium on 'Agents affecting Fertility' held at Middlesex Hospital Medical School, 24 March 1965.
68. 'Clinical trials of oral contraceptives: Review of arrangements between manufacturers of oral contraceptives and CIFC', 17 December 1971, 2, SA/A5/160/3, Box 250.
69. E. Mears, *op. cit.* (note 67).
70. Unlabelled document, 5 November 1963, SA/FPA/A5/159, Box 249.
71. E. Mears, *op. cit.* (note 67).
72. 'Memo re long-term trials', SA/FPA/A5/157/1, Box 249; CIFC Minutes, 24 January 1967, 136, SA/FPA/A5/156, Box 249; CIFC Minutes, 19 September 1967, 147, SA/FPA/A5/156, Box 249; Memo to Clinical Trials Committee from the Medical Officer, Christine Butler, 9 March 1972, SA/FPA/A5/160/4, Box 250.
73. Between 1962 and 1967, for instance, the number of women who remained on the Anovlar trial from the time it had been set up had fallen to 27 per cent. By contrast 58 per cent of women had remained on the Lyndiol trial in the same time span. Similarly, of the women who had started Conovid in 1960 65 per cent remained on trial in 1967. 'Long-term Trial of Approved Products', in CIFC Minutes, 12 January 1967, SA/FPA/A5/156, Box 249.
74. 'Memo re long-term trials', SA/FPA/A5/157/1, Box 249.
75. CIFC Meeting, 21 October 1963, 21 November 1963, SA/FPA/A5/158B, Box 249; Minutes of the First Meeting of the Complaints Subcommittee of the CIFC, 21 November 1963, SA/FPA/159, Box 249; E. Mears, 'Memo regarding Searle's complaints', SA/FPA/A5/159, Box 249; CIFC meeting, 14 January 1964, SA/FPA/A5/158B, Box 249. The standard used was trying the pill on 100 women for a period of six months.
76. Letter from G. Venning to CIFC, 30 April 1964, and CIFC Meeting, 19 May 1964, SA/FPA/A5/158B, Box 249.
77. CIFC Meeting, 14 January 1964, SA/FPA/A5/158B, Box 249.
78. Extraordinary General Meeting of the CIFC, 28 September 1972, SA/FPA/A5/157/3, Box 249.
79. Sir T. Fox, notes re meeting with Searle, 8 June 1965, SA/FPA/A5/162.2, Box 252; CIFC Minutes, 19 April 1966, SA/FPA/A5/156, Box 249.

80. 'Memo re long-term trials', 2, SA/FPA/A5/157/1, Box 249.
81. E. Mears, 'Report on the work of clinical trials committee of CIFC', 18 July 1963, SA/FPA/129, Box 249.
82. C. Brook to N. Raphael, 1 May 1969, SA/FPA/A5/129, Box 245.
83. Meeting of Members of CIFC Clinical Trials Sub-Committee with G. Venning, 29 October 1959, SA/FPA/A5/160, Box 250; CIFC Minutes, 13 December 1962, 46, SA/FPA/A5/155, Box 248; H. Nelson Barrett, 'Brief Resume of the Work and Objects of the OBT', 6 May 1969a SA/FPA/A5/129, Box 245. Interview with Venning, notes.
84. H. Hill, 'Report from the Clinical Trials Committee Concerning Proposals for the Future Medical Policy of Trials of Hormonal Contraceptives', 20 September 1968, SA/FPA/A5/160/2, Box 250; 'Clinical Trials of Oral Contraceptives: Review of Arrangements between Manufacturers of Oral Contraceptives and CIFC, 17 December 1971, SA/FPA/A5/160/3, Box 250; CIFC Fact Sheet, November 1970, SA/FPA/A5/160/3, Box 250.
85. CIFC Fact Sheet, November 1970, SA/FPA/A5/160/3, Box 250.
86. *Ibid.*
87. G. Venning at meeting between the CIFC and Pharmaceutical Representatives, 12 November 1970, SA/FPA/A5/160/3, Box 250.
88. Clinical Trials Committee, 29 June 1972, SA/FPA/A5/160/4, Box 250. 89. Mrs H. Nelson-Barrett, 'Brief Resume of the Work and Objects of the OBT', 6 May 1969, SA/FPA/A5/129, Box 245 and in SA/FPA/A5/152, Box 247.
90. Information for CIFC from Secretary, Caspar Brook, 13 June 1972, SA/FPA/A5/160/4, Box 250; Extraordinary General Meeting of CIFC, Minutes, 28 September 1972, SA/FPA/A5/157/3, Box 249.

# 9

## 'Hygienic articles, patent medicines and rubber goods': Markets and meanings in early-twentieth century Netherlands.

### Willem de Blécourt

Remedies are not just pharmaceutical substances. They have form, colour, wrappings and labels, which contribute as much to their meaning, and to the ways they are perceived and used, as do the physiological effects that are ascribed to them. When the category 'remedy' is approached culturally, it does not have to be medically defined, or to be confined to particular substances. Operations, rituals, or indeed any sort of health-enhancing practice can be considered remedial, too. On a non-medical level, boundaries between remedies and cures are often blurred. Nor can curative and preventive measures always easily be discerned from each other. The question of whether contraceptives fall into the category of 'remedy' is linked to all these considerations. Should they be considered as an extraordinary remedy, because in preventing a pregnancy, 'a normal condition is being impeded'?[1] Or do we have to take the point of view of the user for whom a pregnancy is undesired and therefore abnormal? In this article I shall illustrate and elaborate these remarks by focussing on a very peculiar group of remedies, the so-called 'hygienic articles'.

The transmission of remedies took place in the context of particular medical markets. A medical market, however, is not just an economic category, it is also a heuristic device that facilitates the conceptualisation of health care. At least, the concept of a medical market is used in this way among Dutch social and cultural historians of medicine.[2] Although the historians highlight different aspects, they agree that the medical market should encompass the field of health and illness in its totality in any historical period and area. From the patient's point of view the medical market comprises all the available possibilities of finding a cure. This implies that the patient's definition of illness is decisive and that questions involving selection and choice of treatment are of particular relevance. Issues facing the healer include personal popularity, specialisation of treatment, and competition among healers. Looking at medical markets also involves analysing processes, ranging from the first discussions about illness to the final reactions to cures. Here healers and patients constitute the focal points, not the remedies, drugs or instruments they apply.

The study of remedies thus provides a different approach to the medical market, and thereby a new dimension to the discussion about it. But remedies do not create their own demand, or their own meaning; there are still human agents involved. Besides healers and patients, a new group consisting of the producers and suppliers of remedies enters the stage. As a result, the interaction models have to be extended from two to three actors. Or, when the services from doctor and druggist overlap, it has to be determined what sort of authority was ascribed to the different kinds of specialist. Looking at 'hygienic articles' brings this abstract discussion about the medical market down to earth. Furthermore, 'hygienic articles' draw attention to the opposites of illness and health, or misfortune and well-being, which have not always been noticed by medical historians. What are they?

### Advertisements

For the reader of early-twentieth century Dutch newspapers 'hygienic articles' would have been a familiar term. The oldest advertisement for 'hygienic articles' I have come across dates from 1907. Although at the time the name 'Hygëia' was used by an Amsterdam depot, the designation 'hygienic articles' only appeared a little later.[3] From then onwards advertisements proliferated. In the early years of the century a Maison Adler from Amsterdam advertised 'hygienic articles',[4] as did many other firms in the capital. Newspapers such as the *Nieuws van den Dag* carried advertisements for 'hygienic articles' from the firm Boersma of the Heerenmarkt ('near the Central Station'), the firm Cramer of the Sarphatistraat ('next to the Weesperpoort station'), the firm Lafrene ('near the Central Station'), and many others.[5] In Amsterdam cards were distributed, too:

> Dear Madam, I kindly take the liberty of drawing your attention to my institution. I am always available to give all desired information about the articles I have available. I also gladly inform you about the hygiene of married life. Yours sincerely, Miss W. DEKKER. registered midwife, Leidscheplein 2, corner of Leidschestraat, Amsterdam.[6]

Another 'maison' with the name of Jasinski, even boasted of a chemical laboratory 'Hygiëa'.[7] In 1919 in The Hague a company with the name of 'de Noorderpost' offered 'hygienic articles, patent medicines and rubber goods'.[8] Also the hygienic articles of Dr Stakman and Dr Stopes were brought to public attention.[9]

> The Blue Cross is and will ever be the eldest and most trusted address in this town for hygienic articles, patent medicines and rubber goods,

ran an advertisement in the *Rotterdamsch Nieuwsblad* at the end of the 1920s. 'Hygienic articles, patent medicines, syringes, rubber goods', advertised a certain Maison Santé in the same paper.[10]

This array of announcements can easily be supplemented, based as it is on a selection of a random sample from Dutch newspapers. If the right newspaper is consulted, it can safely be assumed that there was at least one advertisement for hygienic articles in every issue between about 1910 and 1940.[11] Already by 1906 it was remarked about one of the Sanitas company advertisements that hardly a day passed without it appearing in several newspapers.[12]

The main question addressed in this paper is, what exactly was advertised? What kind of wares did the firms, houses and companies supply? What kind of afflictions were they meant to remedy? What did the term 'hygiene' mean in this context? In looking for answers I will analyse a historical phenomenon, in this case hygienic shops and their inventory, by way of the publicity they generated. Textual traces are among the few remnants left for the historian to build this story on.

The process, however, is not as straightforward as it may seem. By the early-twentieth century the term 'hygiene' had restricted and elaborate meanings. The public had been confronted with news about international 'hygienic' exhibitions in Paris (in 1900), Berlin (1908) and Dresden (1911). Amsterdam was only to follow in 1921. There were also discussions about racial hygiene. Less newsworthy but probably more effective in influencing changes in public practice were sanitary programmes of clean drinking water, sewers, refuse collection and many other preventive health measures. Women were especially targeted by an army of (semi-) official health visitors, inspectors and district nurses promoting household hygiene. In the Netherlands, as elsewhere in western Europe, most of those officials were connected to local clinics or to one of the 'societies of the cross'. The White Cross, for instance, provided help in case of epidemics. The aim of the Green Cross was to improve home nursing and to popularise hygiene.[13] Women were also inundated with 'hygienic pamphlets', dealing with all kinds of preventive health-measures they could adopt at home and apply to their children.[14]

Undoubtedly, hygienic shops were linked to these general developments in preventive health care. But they also differed from them, in the sense that they gave their own interpretation to the concept of 'hygiene'. Notwithstanding their visibility in daily life, hygienic shops have curiously not been at the forefront of historical research. Social historians of medicine have devoted more attention to public than to publicised hygiene.[15] Few studies on abortion and contraception mention the shops or the hygienic articles.[16] 'Hygienic articles', it is noticed, were often an euphemism for contraceptives.[17] That, however, is only a part of the story. The study of 'hygienic articles' not only leads us to contraceptives, but also to the whole shadowy realm of abortion, contraception and sexually transmitted diseases. In short, to aspects of sexuality. As such, the story presented here should be taken as only a first cultural probe into these topics.

### Sources

An important source on hygienic products and shops stems from their critics. Most important are judicial files and reports by opponents of 'quackery'; hygienic shops left very few substantial texts of their own. Most of the relevant reports of court proceedings and verdicts were drawn up in the course of prosecutions based on sections 251bis and 451ter of the Dutch penal code, which were in operation since 1912. Section 251bis concerned abortion and section 451ter the open display and distribution of articles to prevent pregnancy. A third series of legal documents pertaining to hygienic products resulted from prosecutions based on the Medical Act of 1865. Sections 30 and 31 declared it illegal for unqualified persons to sell remedies weighing less than 50 grams. Professional qualifications were dealt with in section 436 of the penal code. Conclusions about the range and distribution of 'hygienic articles' remain tentative if only based on the available judicial sources. Since the violation of articles 451ter and 436 concerned misdemeanours rather than crimes, they were in the first instance dealt with by the Dutch lower courts, the condition of whose archives prevents any systematic research. Moreover, information from the prosecution cases is naturally biased towards their original purpose, the crime of abortion, or the illegality of advertising contraceptives or remedies, rather than the people who provided them and the businesses they ran, or those who actually bought the products. The prosecution cases nevertheless provide a cross-section of 'hygienic articles' and of the shops where they were sold.

## 'Hygienic articles, patent medicines and rubber goods'

In their turn the editors of the *Monthly journal of the Dutch Society for the Repression of Quackery* (the *Monthly against Quackery*) made yet another selection of the available information. This Society, founded in 1880 and unrelated to the Dutch professional medical societies, acted as a consumer organisation combating health fraud. Its aim was to inform the general public about the intentions of unscrupulous healers (including licensed physicians) and about unsubstantiated claims of cure. Because of its public function, the *Monthly against Quackery* was extremely reluctant to discuss abortion, contraception and sexual diseases. 'Our paper is no medical paper and it comes to the attention of all kinds of male and female readers,' stated the editors in defence of the decision to use euphemisms such as 'secret disease' (Dutch: *geheime ziekte*) without explaining them. The journal portrayed itself as 'too decent' to quote from a Sanitas pamphlet, since its aim was to be available for 'everyone, young and old'.[18] Thus, combating quackery boiled down to showing the divergence between promise and fulfilment in the case of morally less thorny remedies. An analysis of Sanitas pills proclaiming to ease difficulty in urinating concluded:

> Urotropine is indeed prescribed by doctors in case of disease of the urinary passages ...but it is only without danger when under medical supervision.[19]

In other cases remedies were revealed as ineffective or simply too expensive.

Hygienic shops also produced their own, albeit textually meagre sources. Advertisements are one example. Some of these also point to books. One 'expert' directed her public to 'Our illustrated book, in which all hygienic remedies are discussed, also the newest ones'.[20] Sanitas advertised with: 'Secret D.... The book for "MEN" with all information and description of the diseases[,] and the book for "WOMEN".[21] The Noorderpost offered '"For women", the corrected and extended Book with all Information and Advice'.[22] 'WOMEN', announced Miss Edeling in Rotterdam, 'my booklet (36 pages) provides you with advice and [information on] all hygienic products'.[23] This probably looked momentous, although it only concerned thin brochures or pamphlets.[24]

The three different sources all have their specific limitations and grant only partial views of a market whose outlines remain nebulous. However, the picture can be made a little sharper when we look at what the sources tell us about the most prominent chain of hygienic shops.

## Sanitas

The Sanitas chain was the oldest of the specialist hygienic shops, notwithstanding other claims. As early as 1902 there was a Sanitas store in Amsterdam, selling 'pills for women'.[25] From 1905 at least the main depot was located in The Hague. The formula proved successful, for in 1916 there were branches in Amsterdam, Haarlem, Leiden, The Hague, Rotterdam, Dordrecht, Utrecht, Arnhem, Nijmegen and Groningen.[26] The chain was set up by a certain Van Dijk ('a man of ill-fame'), who, according to an article in the *Telegraaf*, had died by 1922, when the business went bankrupt. As the newspaper article explains, the policy was to found as many branches as possible (by 1920 there were probably as many as 30). Branch managers had to put in fl.2000 as guarantee and they were paid a set weekly salary of fl.35. They also received 5 per cent commission on all goods sold. This scheme failed when turnover dropped below costs. For a while the deficit was obscured by finding new managers who paid the guarantee and by selling existing shops to old branch managers; but these were merely makeshift measures that only resulted in a (temporarily) higher density of sales outlets and consequently even lower turnover.[27] Nevertheless, parts of the organisation survived. While some of the shops changed hands (for instance, two Sanitas shops in The Hague were taken over by the firm Schneider & Kolsteeg), others, like those in Amsterdam and Amersfoort, kept the name.[28] In 1927 the 'pharmaceutical wholesale business' Sanitas Novum operated from Heerlen in the province of Limburg, with branches in Roermond and Utrecht.[29] Sanitas also distributed its wares among druggists.

As a merchandising strategy, all Sanitas shops had a similar design. A visitor in 1915 noticed 'much similarity between kinds of products, wrapping, etc.'.[30] This was copied by other companies. The director of the Noorderpost, Jakob Brommet, had started his career as a branch manager of Sanitas in Groningen. In around 1914 he opened his own shop there and branched out to Amsterdam, Rotterdam and The Hague.[31] He took the Sanitas concept with him, 'using everything he had seen and learned when he had worked for Sanitas as a branch manager'.[32] By the end of the 1920s he had added shops in Utrecht and Leeuwarden to his chain.

Other hygienic shops seem to have been merely local. Apart from the Noorderpost the town of Groningen had a shop by the name of the 'Seinpost' (literally: 'signpost'). Both names referred to mail order businesses. Others stayed within the domain of health and echoed

Sanitas by labelling themselves with Latin-sounding names starting with an S: 'Sanitum', 'Salutair', 'Securitas'.[33] It shows the appeal of Sanitas, as well as the medical respectability attached to the Latin language. Again others tried to enhance their status by adding the word 'Maison' to their own name; whereas the Rotterdam 'Maison Santé' played safe by connecting to both traditions.

### Contraceptives

One of the meanings of 'hygienic articles' alluded to contraceptives. As it was illegal to display them, subterfuges were needed, especially in labelling. The regulation in section 451ter concentrated on the nature of the display. Contraceptives as such were not offensive, it was only their public exhibition that was considered to cause moral offence among adults and to be highly morally corruptive of adolescents.[34] The problem was how to define public display. Did wooden boxes with the word 'never-rip' printed upon them in a shop window present a case for prosecution? Several times shopkeepers were acquitted because the contents of the box had stayed hidden from the public gaze.[35] This argument centred on the formal question, which of course did not diminish its impact. In contrast, other judges and lawyers took a moralistic stance. They stressed that the wrapping was insubstantial and based their decision on the presumed awareness of the purpose of the objects.[36] Others disagreed. According to one Attorney General even those without any command of English knew what the word 'never-rip' hinted at.[37] These debates reveal a certain disdain for discussing contraceptives openly. Lawyers stuck to the designation 'preservatifs', a French rather than a Dutch word. 'Gummiwaren' (rubber goods), which had more of a Dutch ring to it, or more specifically 'sanitaire gummiwaren' was initially ranked as an innocent collective noun.[38] By the end of the 1920s, however, the moralistic approach had gained the upper hand. Judges now accepted a direct and meaningful link between labelled box and contraceptives. English was no longer an obstacle, the brand name 'never-rip' ('silk finish, guaranteed for one year') had become generally known.[39]

A broader assortment of contraceptives was displayed in the *Books for Women*. So far, my research has only unearthed one copy, namely a brochure from the hygienic shop, The Salamander, in Groningen.[40] Other 'books' will have been similar. The brochure was written by an 'expert' (Dutch: *deskundige*, see below) purporting to deal with 'hygienic remedies for women'. On the inner title page the brochure advertised 'hygienic articles and rubber goods for men and women'.

It opened with a plea for Neo-Malthusianism. While the 'book' was careful not to associate directly with the Neo-Malthusian League, its case was supported by referring to the work of Johannes Rutgers, its founder and long-term driving force, among others. The unknown author juxtaposed the helplessness of the professionals (doctors, judges, priests and philanthropists) to prevent large families and the population increase, with the dire necessity of solving these problems, which all professionals accepted. It was furthermore suggested that publications of a more scientific nature were always available and that they proclaimed contraceptives as totally harmless. Any notion that they were unsafe and detrimental to one's health was described as a prejudice of the lower classes. Next the female reproductive organs were discussed. From this the most effective way of contraception was to prevent the sperm from reaching the womb. Thus introduced, the contraceptives were presented: the irrigator that every woman should possess, the sperm-killing paste, the diaphragm, the pessary, the douche and the syringe. The male contribution was distilled in a brief remark about the dangers of withdrawal before ejaculation because it caused headache, dizziness and insomnia. A whole page was dedicated to the theme of condoms, of which six different brands were on offer.[41] Although the published judicial texts on contraceptives (concerning 451ter) seem to show a virtual monopoly of one brand, promotional material demonstrates otherwise.[42] Apparently 'never-rip' functioned as a front for other condoms precisely because it was English.

The brochure *For Women* was composed of different texts for each product, with slight variations of style and presentation. Descriptions of uses of the wares were as plain and detached as possible with occasional references to the medical doctors who had invented them, such as the German gynaecologist 'Mensinga' and 'Dr. Mary [sic] Stopes'. While the text mentions the continuous presence of competent 'deskundigen' in the shop, abortion is not mentioned anywhere. The hygiene discussed in the brochure is the hygiene of sexuality. 'Hygienic articles' stands exclusively for 'contraceptives'. The wares protect women from pregnancy and diseases, they are clean, antiseptic and, by implication, rational and modern. The brochure also issued a warning against 'so-called addresses, which, by their cheap prices, try to draw the public.' The title of 'deskundige' was not protected and everyone could pose as one. Prospective clients should always be careful. In this way, the brochure followed the lead of the Neo-Malthusian League, drawing a sharp distinction between contraception, which was favoured, and abortion, which was publicly decried. Yet the very same terms used for contraceptives were also applied in offers of abortion services.

**Abortion**

In the early-twentieth century the expanding Dutch abortion market was primarily operating underground. It was forbidden to advertise abortion services openly. Women who had undergone an abortion were not prosecuted, since they were needed as prime witnesses for the prosecution, but they ran the risk of becoming socially stigmatised. Abortionists on the other hand were liable to be prosecuted, the more so after the implementation of the Morality Acts of 1911. One of the unforeseen effects was a manipulation of daily speech. Certain terms acquired, for the initiated, specific connotations referring to abortion, whilst officially retaining their more innocent meanings. The language of abortion was even more concealed than that of contraception. For instance, the expression 'the restoration of menstrual regularity' depended for its meaning on context, speaker and addressee, and could refer directly, or not, to abortion. This way of speaking was widespread throughout Europe. The substitution of 'seamstress' for abortionist seems to have been more specifically Dutch. Most of the time, however, speech was extremely indirect and only made sense if one already knew what it was about.[43] One of the more direct ways of mentioning abortion was to refer to 'hygiene'. When, for instance, several women in The Hague were asked by the police (and later in court) how they had found their abortionists, they said they had been directed by advertisements about 'hygienic articles'.[44] 'It is curious, how the interest in hygiene has risen lately,' a reader wrote to the main Dutch judicial weekly. 'Especially the sale of hygienic articles has soared.' This reader's astonishment was a pretence, however, because he had noticed that many of the people advertising hygienic wares had called themselves 'deskundigen' before.[45] He thus replaced one oblique reference with another. The title of 'deskundige' had been introduced by the Neo-Malthusian League for their consultants, but had then been adopted by commercial abortionists. Since the two groups overlapped, this was quite logical.[46] Thus the reader actually emphasised that abortionists were hiding behind the label of hygienic articles. Indeed, many of the proprietors of the Amsterdam firms were prosecuted for having procured abortions.

The 'deskundigen', especially those who were trained by the Neo-Malthusian League, were supposed to give advice on birth control and to provide contraceptives. Notwithstanding the permeable boundaries between abortion and contraception, the latter is hardly mentioned in court reports based on section 251bis of the Dutch Penal Code. The dissemination of information on methods of birth control and family limitation was in itself not punishable, and the Supreme Court interpreted the title of 'deskundige' in its broad, innocent, sense.[47] This fact was immediately used by the abortionists. 'In case the police interrogate you,' a 'deskundige' advised one of her clients, 'just tell them that I placed a cap'.[48] In the context of the prosecution of abortionists, contraception figured merely as an excuse used by the prospective suspect.

The Amsterdam 'deskundigen' may have been instrumental in substituting 'hygienic articles' for 'abortion services', but they did not have a monopoly on the term. According to an 1918 editorial of the *Monthly against Quackery*, shops and so-called 'laboratories', which were mainly occupied with the distribution of 'deplorable and dangerous quackeries', had mushroomed recently.[49] The first shops that came to the editor's mind were Sanitas and the Noorderpost, the two most high profile chains of 'hygienic' shops in the Netherlands. But in this case 'quackery' did not refer to abortion indirectly. The names of these two companies turn up only occasionally in the abortion files. Some Sanitas chain branch managers were convicted for having promoted abortion: in Groningen by selling a syringe and liquid, in Amsterdam by referring a client to an abortionist, and in Delft by performing an abortion.[50] On the whole, the keepers of the hygienic shops have to be distinguished from the 'deskundigen'. The former were foremost salesmen and only abortionists in the sense that they were sometimes convicted because they had sold abortifacients to women seeking an abortion. In most areas the Sanitas shops merely figured as the places that provided abortion instruments to 'deskundigen' and other abortionists. Selling douches or catheters was only illegal when the customer wanted them to use for an abortion, otherwise there were no prohibitions as the instruments could be used for other purposes as well. The articles could also be obtained from special druggists, such as the 'people's apothecary', Spetter, in Rotterdam.[51]

If the content and meaning of 'hygienic articles' is only to be derived from judicial documents on abortion, then it is narrowed down to 'abortion'. In that context 'hygienic articles' did not even denote specific abortifacients or abortion techniques. The article for sale was abortion and the 'deskundigen' and their 'firms' thus had consulting, rather than just opening, hours.

## Medicines

A third area in which 'hygiene' could provide a linguistic cover for practices that the moral majority deemed unspeakable consisted of sexually transmitted diseases. Of the several measures that could impede the operation of hygienic shops, policing the sale of medicines seems to have had the lowest priority. This was probably due to the fact that each product had to be analysed chemically to establish whether it contained ingredients from list C, which could only be legally sold by pharmacists if the product contained less than 50 grams. Samariter Crême, for example, was sold by Sanitas and among others advised to counter a drain of 'life force'. This medicine contained calomel (mercurous chloride), which figured on list C.[52] The 'zekerheids pastilles' from the same company contained boric acid.[53] A second reason for the low level of this particular kind of prosecution will have been the high number of offenders. According to a report from pharmacists, the Netherlands counted over 3000 chemists who were selling some kind of patent medicine with illegal ingredients. In contrast the number of unqualified salesmen was relatively small, estimated 'far below a hundred'.[54] The fact that druggists and branch managers of Sanitas in small towns, such as Steenwijk and Arnhem, were reported to sell medicines illegally, does however indicate the geographical extent of this phenomenon.[55]

The *Book for Men* dealt with venereal diseases, but the *Monthly against Quackery* concealed this (so far, the *Monthly against Quackery* is the only source to reveal anything at all about this particular pamphlet).

> In agreeable language... the different so-called secret diseases are described in a quasi-scientific way; it really looks like a booklet that could be given to youngsters.

But it was all pretence. 'The effects of the diseases are extremely exaggerated,' warned the *Monthly against Quackery*. It only served to make the remedies on offer extra appealing. According to the *Monthly against Quackery*, the pamphlet aimed at making sufferers buy the remedies without consulting a licensed doctor. It promoted self-help and thus invited danger. This is about as far as the anti-quacks' textual analysis went, they had more expertise in chemical analysis. As they had to keep silent about the ('secret') purpose of the remedies, all they could reveal was that one remedy was meant to help in case of 'lack of power, dreams, and loss of life-force'.[56] This can be interpreted as impotence and premature ejaculation. Male sexuality, it can be concluded, was threatened by venereal disease and unproductive loss of semen.

The total stock of hygienic shops went beyond contraceptives. In their public presentation the shops may have stressed (non-) procreative issues, among others, by displaying Neo-Malthusianism in their windows,[57] but they had much more for sale. Even in the brochure *For Women* a few pages are filled with the pictures of bandages, trusses, elastic stockings and all kinds of nursing articles (without explanatory texts). Still other wares can be perceived from advertisements. Because the Sanitas company offered a blueprint for the later shops, I have used their advertisements for an overall view. Of course texts like 'All articles for Women and Men. Largest assortment, reasonable prices. Illustrated Books and price list' mainly conveyed the name of Sanitas to those who already knew what kind of articles were being offered.[58] Other texts are more precise.

One of the regular schemes was to offer a reward of 1000 guilders to every sufferer who was not healed totally 'after having followed the treatment correctly'. This was offered in the case of Kawasan 25350, a remedy meant to ease painful urination, and also in the case of 'Dr Roland's Drink', a Belgian concoction supposed to cure epilepsy.[59] The authority of mainly foreign physicians was also evoked in the case of the American 'enforcement pills' of Professor Janson (against wet dreams) and those of his colleague Professor Dr Spencer.[60] Dr Pieter's name was attached to trusses.

As was the case with the brochures, most of the remedies Sanitas offered were meant for men or for women. 'All rubber goods for gentlemen, brand Venus' was obviously aimed at men,[61] although the incorporation of condoms in the *Book for Women* leads to the suspicion that women were supposed to buy them (and to fit them?). Presumably women would have washed them out when re-use was in order. As far as can be seen mainly men were supposed to suffer from venereal disease and (sexual) enfeeblement. Women, on the other hand, were addressed in texts offering douches and syringes and even more in advertisements showing bust developers (with illustration) and 'Pasta de Beauté' for erasing skin irregularities such as freckles, pimples, black heads and 'red spots'. 'Oriental power powder' was proclaimed against leanness and contributed 'to obtain full and pretty bodily forms'. 'Bust shapers' (also with illustration) not only gave women an elegant figure but were also pleasant to wear.[62] A similar obsession with appearances is shown by a hair-dye advertisement ('absolutely harmless'). And when obesity struck, then defattening pills would surely help.[63] Women's 'hygiene' was individually oriented and for important parts directed at her appearance, her sexuality and her procreative functions. Men's interest in 'hygiene' was only evoked in case of trouble.

**Distribution**

The complaints of the Society for the Repression of Quackery about the proliferation of hygienic shops at the end of 1910 not only points to a heightened awareness of the trade, but also to a real increase.[64] This occurred on two levels: within the big cities in the West and in provincial towns all over the Netherlands. 'Until very recently only a few of these shops existed, operated by the Sanitas company,' lamented the Health Committee of The Hague in 1922. 'Now one can see these shops in every part of the town'.[65] The nationwide spread of Sanitas and the Noorderpost has already been mentioned above. However, the final picture of the distribution of hygienic shops and sales outlets on the Dutch medical markets will remain vague, as it is not always clear from the sources whether it concerned specialist hygienic shops, druggists who sold hygienic products on the side, or 'deskundigen' and others who sold merchandise from private addresses.

There was also a marked difference in the localities in which specific 'hygienic' products could be obtained. Women from the Dutch countryside, for instance, who sought abortion from other women had to travel to the bigger market towns. The published judicial texts on contraceptives indicate the availability of condoms in the big cities of Amsterdam, Rotterdam and The Hague. But if reports seem to show a wider distribution of patent medicines than of contraceptives, it does not follow that the countryside was totally deprived of the latter. It was always possible to obtain the merchandise by travelling to market places, by mail order, or from travelling salesmen. To what extent people did so is uncertain, but the information was certainly disseminated to even widely remote places. Thus, the Noorderpost distributed cards advertising 'hygienic articles, patent medicines and rubber goods' in Rinsumageest, a small village in the province of Friesland.[66] A commercial male abortionist from the town of Utrecht had his address cards distributed in Baarn.[67]

Only a thorough and time consuming analysis of newspaper advertisements covering the different regions in the Netherlands could establish how exactly the business in hygienic products fluctuated over the years. So far, only disparate evidence is available, such as the statement by an abortionist from The Hague in 1929, who declared to a policeman that 'the trade in hygienic articles didn't prosper, as he didn't know how he would make a living in the long run'.[68] On the basis of current material, no conclusions can be drawn about a possible increase or decrease in the popularity of contraceptives, abortion or venereal disease remedies. There are also no contemporary Dutch surveys available.[69] However, the evidence of the availability of the various 'hygienic' products offers a contradiction to the dearth of sexual education material that can be found in contemporary textbooks.[70] Dutch morality prospered on a foundation of its antithesis. At the same time, hygienic shops fitted neatly into the general Dutch culture. Their spirit of enterprise and salesmanship was recognised and validated (if not secretly admired) and the gender norms as portrayed by 'hygienic' advertisements were totally in line with dominant opinion.

## Meanings

The term 'hygiene' in the early-twentieth century did not solely refer to cleanliness or to other preventive health measures as they appeared in the official medical propaganda. 'Hygiene' not only covered public works and household matters, but also the individual body. Female bodies were affected rather differently than male bodies. As it turned out, 'hygiene' incorporated a range of activities within the sexual sphere that were otherwise unspeakable. These different meanings of 'hygiene' were clearly interrelated. When people used 'hygiene' in its restricted, sexual meaning, they toyed with its elaborated, public meaning. This is particularly evident in Amsterdam where one of the authors of social hygienic pamphlets was the physician H. Pinkhof. He was also a declared opponent of Neo-Malthusianism in general and abortion in particular.[71] By adopting the term 'hygiene', the 'deskundigen' thus played a mean trick on their main enemies, also because the *Nieuws van den Dag*, where many of their advertisements appeared, featured many an article on the then fashionable orthodox medical hygienic measures. Other examples of adaptation occurred when the so-called 'societies of the cross', known for their repositories of nursing articles, were imitated in different colours, such as the Blue Cross, quoted earlier in this paper. The Sanitas company had a white cross within a black circle printed with its advertisements. Following the official hygiene offensive at the turn of the century, pharmaceutical manufacturers, distributors and retailers were quick to appropriate the general acceptance of the positive image of hygiene. Public hygiene was connected to modernity and rationality and in these they strove to implicate their version of sexual hygiene.

Apart from adaptation, plain copying took place. 'Deskundigen' raided the repertoire of the Neo-Malthusian League, enterprising merchants imitated the Sanitas formula, and druggists tried to get a share of the pie too. It showed the strength and appeal of the initiatives and probably the real underlying need for remedies to regulate sexuality and procreation.

Specific settings will have determined when particular meanings of 'hygiene' were thought of and which kinds of categorisation were applied. Those who advertised contraceptives, abortion or remedies for venereal disease were certainly aware of the subtle distinctions between one kind of 'hygiene' and another. Most of the clients probably also knew this, as did the people opposing them. After all, only some of the salesmen of 'hygienic articles' were abortionists and not every abortionist sold contraceptives or beautifiers. But the exact composition of the different groups in terms of social, economic and religious characteristics remains largely unknown. While it is possible to obtain some data on the supply side of the market for hygienic products, questions about demand for the respective wares and its possible fluctuations are largely unanswerable. Judicial sources may have captured some of the abortionists' clients, but the buyers and users of the other 'hygienic' products remain unknown.

It is, however, possible to reach some tentative conclusions about whether the distinction between the different meanings of 'hygiene' was situated between medical and lay use of the term. Presumably medical personnel mainly used the public meaning of 'hygiene' and refrained from evoking its sexual connotations, except when they fought advertisers. Dutch doctors, after all, were on the whole dismissive about abortion, although during the interbellum there was a very modest move towards the acceptability of abortion not just on medical but also on social grounds.[72] Opinions about contraceptives and venereal diseases were hardly less moralistic and puritanical. Precisely because sexual issues could not easily be discussed openly (and if people did try to do so they were immediately contradicted), the distinction between 'hygiene's' open public meaning and its hidden sexual counterpart arose. Yet in practice things were not as clear-cut as this. As I have not fully researched the medical literature on the use of the word 'hygiene', the final remarks of this article are restricted to a single example, the Dutch book, *Hygiene for Women*.

Its author was a gynaecologist, who, according to the blurb, had lectured on the topic to thousands of women within 'het Gooi', a region south-east of Amsterdam. Although not mentioning his disdain of abortion or contraception explicitly, he did fulminate against such practices as irrigation of the vagina, a widespread method of birth control, which in his opinion would endanger a woman's life. He called women who wanted to avoid pregnancy 'mentally deranged'. A woman's life, he wrote, revolved around procreation and the education of her offspring. A woman was defined by her bodily functions.

> She is almost constantly involved in reproduction, whether she wants it or not, or whether she knows it or not. It is her 'natural duty'.[73]

Nevertheless, even though the author's use of the term 'hygiene' differed from that of unmentionable establishments, it was still sexual. This gynaecologist was probably considered as liberal by his contemporaries, since he dared to discuss parts of the female body that most members of his public found it necessary to hide even during the sexual act.[74] The gender division underlying the different meanings of 'hygiene' ran straight through the boundary between doctors and those without an official medical education.

## Notes

1. Margaret Stacey, *The Sociology of Health and Healing. A Textbook* (London and New York: Routledge, 1991), 216.
2. Willem de Blécourt, Gerrit van Vegchel (eds), *De medische markt*, special issue, *Focaal*, 21 (1993); Willem de Blécourt, Frank Huisman, Henk van der Velden (eds), De medische markt, special issue, *Tijdschrift voor sociale geschiedenis*, 25(4) (1999).
3. See *Maandblad tegen de kwakzalverij*, 27(9) (1907). There are no examples of 'hygienic articles' among the advertisements presented as evidence by the Amsterdam Society for the repression of Neo-Malthusianism to the municipal counsel, see: *Adressen van de afdeeling Amsterdam der vereeniging tot bestrijding van het Nieuw-Malthusianisme* (Amsterdam: June 1907).
4. *Het Leven*, 7 (1912), 36, 72.
5. *Nieuws van den Dag*, (2 January 1915, 3 and 10 March 1917).
6. *Tijdschrift voor Praktische Verloskunde*, 20 (1916), 184.
7. *Maandblad tegen de kwakzalverij*, 34(12) (1914).
8. *Haagsche Courant*, (8 July 1919).
9. *Haagsche Courant*, (4 July, 8 August 1925).
10. *Rotterdamsch Nieuwsblad*, (1 July 1929).
11. I have not consulted newspapers later than 1939, but the hygienic shops seem to have survived into the early-1960s.
12. *Maandblad tegen de kwakzalverij*, 26(2) (1906).
13. Myriam Daru, 'Hygiënisering en moralisering van de

*'Hygienic articles, patent medicines and rubber goods'*

gezondheidszorg', in: Rineke van Daalen, Marijke Gijswijt-Hofstra (eds), *Gezond en wel. Vrouwen en de zorg voor gezondheid in de twintigste eeuw* (Amsterdam: Amsterdam University Press ,1998), 31–51. Compare with Perry Williams, 'The laws of health: Women, medicine and sanitary reform, 1850–1890', in Marina Benjamin (ed), *Science and Sensibility. Gender and scientific enquiry, 1780–1945* (Oxford: Blackwell, 1991), 60–88.

14. Godelieve van Heteren, 'De troost voorbij: medische instructies voor het kinderlijk leven in de negentiende eeuw', in Willem de Blécourt, Willem Frijhoff, Marijke Gijswijt-Hofstra (eds), *Grenzen van genezing. Gezondheid, ziekte en genezen in Nederland, zestiende tot begin twintigste eeuw* (Hilversum: Verloren, 1993), 203–52, especially 230–1.
15. Compare with Dorothy Porter (ed.), *The history of public health and the modern state* (Amsterdam and Atlanta: Rodopi, 1994).
16. See, for instance, Cornelie Usborne, *The politics of the body in Weimar Germany. Women's reproductive rights and duties* (London: MacMillan, 1992), 80. Compare with the overview of the American literature in which 'hygienic articles' should have figured, but hardly do: Susan E. Cayleff, 'Self-help and the patent medicine business', in Rima D. Apple (ed.), *Women, health, and medicine in America. A historical handbook* (New Brunswick: Rutgers University Press, 1992), 303–28, especially 314.
17. Angus McLaren, *A history of contraception. From antiquity to the present day* (Oxford: Blackwell, 1990), 185; James Woycke, *Birth Control in Germany* (London and New York: Routledge, 1988), 50.
18. *Maandblad tegen de kwakzalverij*, 23(5) (1903); 25(11) (1905); 51(8) (1931).
19. *Maandblad tegen de Kwakzalverij*, 38(2) (1918).
20. *Maandblad tegen de Kwakzalverij*, 27(9) (1907).
21. *Nieuws van den Dag*, (1 May 1915).
22. *Ibid.*
23. *Rotterdamsch Nieuwsblad*, (11 May 1925).
24. Compare the leaflets distributed by the Neo-Malthusian League. See: Gé Nabrink, *Seksuele hervorming in Nederland* (Nijmegen: SUN, 1978), 106–7.
25. *Maandblad tegen de kwakzalverij*, 22(12) (1902).
26. Advertisement in *Nieuwe Rotterdamsche Courant*, (19 May 1916), reprinted in *Maandblad tegen de kwakzalverij*, 37(2) (1917). See Nabrink, *op. cit.* (note 24), 112.
27. *Maandblad tegen de kwakzalverij*, 42(4) (1922), from the *Telegraaf*. Compare *Maandblad tegen de kwakzalverij*, 37(3) (1917), in which a

Frans van Dijk, director of the 'NV Binnen- en Buitenhandelsmij', is mentioned. A statement of a branch manager can be found in RAGr, arr. Groningen, inv.nr. 332, nr. 391.
28. RANH, arr. Amsterdam, inv.nr. 95, nr. 970 (1920); RAU, arr. Utrecht, inv.nr. 297, nr. 11 (1926).
29. *Weekblad van het Recht*, (11621) (1927); (12067) (1930); Nederlandsche jurisprudentie (1927) 1456–8; (1930) 145–6. Compare RAL, arr. Maastricht inv.nr. 20, nr. 337 (1928); inv.nr. 23, nr. 344 (1929).
30. *Maandblad tegen de kwakzalverij*, 35(11) (1915).
31. In Groningen, Brommet's older sister was branch manager, RAGr. arr. Groningen, inv.nr. 317, nr. 239 (1914); inv.nr. 335, nr. 148 (1918).
32. RANH, arr. Amsterdam, inv.nr. 744, nr. 821 (1916).
33. Het Leven, 14 (1919), 894; *Haagsche Courant*, (5 July 1922; 5 August 1925).
34. *Nederlandsche jurisprudentie*, (1913), 1056.
35. *Weekblad van het recht*, 11184 (1924).
36. *Weekblad van het recht*, 10930 (1922).
37. *Nederlandsche jurisprudentie*, (1927) 48.
38. *Nederlandsche jurisprudentie*, (1925) 1231; see also *Weekblad van het recht*, 11621 (1927).
39. *Weekblad van het recht*, 11737 (1927).
40. *Ons inlichtingenboek voor de vrouw* (Groningen: De Salamander). The pamphlet is not dated but was probably issued in the 1930s. The company had a shop in Rotterdam as early as 1925, *Rotterdamsch Nieuwsblad*, (7 May 1925).
41. To name: Venus, Never-rip, Tip Top, Amulette, Transparent, and Salamander.
42. On the basis of my material, no conclusions can be drawn about a possible increase in the popularity of contraceptives. There are no contemporary Dutch surveys available either. For details about the USA, see Andrea Tone, 'Contraceptive consumers: Gender and the political economy of birth control in the 1930s', *Journal of Social History*, 29 (1996), 485–506.
43. See Willem de Blécourt, 'Cultures of abortion; daily practice in The Hague, early twentieth century' in Franz Eder, Lesley Hall, Gert Hekma (eds), *Sexual cultures in Europe* (Manchester: Manchester University Press, 1999), 195–212.
44. RAZH, arr. Den Haag, inv.nr. 458, nr. 222 (1912); inv.nr 460, nr. 412 (1912).
45. *Weekblad van het recht*, 9810 (1915).

46. Nabrink, *Seksuele hervorming*, (note 24) 125; H. Q. Röling, 'De tragedie van het geslachtsleven'. *Johannes Rutgers (1850–1924) en de Nieuw-Malthusiaanse Bond* (Amsterdam, Van Gennep, 1987), 202–3.
47. *Weekblad van het recht*, 9348 (1912).
48. RAZH, arr. Den Haag, inv.nr. 466, nr. 1136 (1912).
49. *Maandblad tegen de kwakzalverij*, 38(1) (1918).
50. RAGr, arr. Groningen, inv.nr. 332, nr. 391 (1918); RANH, arr. Amsterdam, inv.nr. 95, nr. 970 (1927); RAZH, arr. Den Haag, inv.nr. 597, nr. 668 (1925).
51. RANB, arr. Breda, inv.nr. 511, nr. 6715 (1916); inv.nr. 692, nr. 1122 (1925).
52. *Maandblad tegen de kwakzalverij*, 35(11) (1915). Calomel was used as a prophylactic against syphilis, compare Annet Mooij, *Geslachtsziekten en besmettingsangst. Een historisch-sociologische studie* (Amsterdam: Boom, 1993), 108.
53. RANH, *kantongerecht* Haarlem, inv.nr. 115, nr. 1009 (1916). 'Zekerheid' can be translated as 'safety' and as 'certainty' and 'confidence'.
54. *Maandblad tegen de kwakzalverij*, 36(4) (1916), from *Pharmaceutisch Weekblad*, (1) (April 1916). Obviously complaints of apothecaries about patent-medicines were part of the repertoire used in their struggle with druggists. This does not imply that the number of 3000 is exaggerated; it rather obscures that apothecaries also sold patent-medicines.
55. *Maandblad tegen de kwakzalverij*, 33(12) (1913); 35(1) (1915).
56. *Maandblad tegen de kwakzalverij*, 35(11) (1915).
57. *Maandblad tegen de kwakzalverij*, 22(12) (1902).
58. *Het Leven*, 9 (1914), 2, 36, 72, 100, 133, etc.
59. *Haagsche Courant*, (8 April 1915); *Maandblad tegen de kwakzalverij*, 26 (1906), 2. The 'san' in Kawasan was derived from 'santal', as is shown by an earlier advertisement, *Het Leven*, 9 (1914), 5, 134. The remedy was thus epistemologically linked to the 'Santal pearls of Dr. Dumon', also advertised in case of problems in the urinary passages and venereal disease, *Maandblad tegen de kwakzalverij*, 23(5) (1903); 25(10) (1915). These 'pearls' were also for sale at druggists known for their dabbling in 'quackeries', compare with the advertisements in the *Telegraaf*, (8 May 1916).
60. *Nieuws van den Dag*, (1 April 1915); Het Leven, 9 (1914), 3, 66.
61. *Nieuws van den Dag*, (13 June 1915).
62. *Haagsche Courant*, (7 April 1915), 2, 3.
63. *Het Leven*, 9 (1914), 1, 34.

64. The Netherlands remained neutral during World War One and the Dutch armed forces were only mobilised. An increase in military demand of hygienic articles will only have had an indirect effect on the Dutch market.
65. *Tijdschrift voor sociale hygiene*, 24 (1922), 329–34, quotation on page 332.
66. RAF, arr. Leeuwarden, inv.nr. 378, nr. 83 (1929). At the time Rinsumageest was well known for its (irregular) healer Jan Monsma, see: Willem de Blécourt, 'Duivelbanners in de noordelijke Friese Wouden, 1860-1930', *Volkskundig bulletin*, 14 (1988), 159–87, especially 174–6. Brommet's cards, however, were distributed among the inhabitants of the hamlet. Whether they were also handed out to Monsma's foreign patients is not indicated.
67. *Nederlandsche jurisprudentie*, (1926), 1392.
68. G. A. Den Haag, gemeentepolitie, inv.nr. 2558, nr. 78. The abortionist could have lied, of course.
69. Compare Andrea Tone, *op. cit.* (note 42).
70. Compare with H. Q. Röling, *Gevreesde vragen. Geschiedenis van de sexuele opvoeding in Nederland* (Amsterdam: Amsterdam University Press, 1994).
71. Jan de Bruijn, *Geschiedenis van de abortus in Nederland* (Amsterdam: Van Gennep, 1979), 71–7.
72. *Ibid.*, 109–12.
73. W. F. Bijvoet, *Hygiëne voor vrouwen* (Amsterdam: Kosmos, 1937). Quotes on pages 10, 17, 31, 32, 70, 71, 82, 89.
74. The publisher, Kosmos, also issued books written by medical consultants of the Aletta Jacobs clinic in Amsterdam, as well as books about how to deal with venereal diseases and about naturopathy.

# 10

## Streptomycin in postwar Britain: A cultural history of a miracle drug

*Alan Yoshioka*

'Miracle drugs'. We have all heard of them, and many of us recognise names such as insulin, penicillin, streptomycin, or cortisone. A search on the Web for the phrases 'miracle drug' or 'wonder drug' turns up several thousand matches each.[1] But what is a miracle drug? All too often the label is prosaically taken for granted as a cliché expressing the power of scientific medicine. I suggest in this paper that the term 'miracle drug' needs to be considered in a broader context. I propose that the cultural phenomenon of the miracle drug is symptomatic of the persistence of magical thinking during an era in which rationality is highly regarded. That the meanings of the substances are, as it were, caught in a tension between 'evidence-based medicine' and something much more primal.

At a recent historical conference on alternative healing, the question was asked whether we might find a continuous though changing current of 'therapeutic pluralism'; according to this view, 'magical and medical-scientific thinking and acting' by both patients and healers developed in interaction with each other.[2] Consider the analogy historian Barry Smith has drawn: 'Quacks offered salvation through a new set of private rituals.... Thus the justice of providence was restored in a world otherwise devoid of miracles and the intercession of therapeutic saints.'[3] It may be worth looking for further connections between cultural phenomena in the fields of spirituality and science: is it not curious that a long-running and heated religious dispute over the nature of miracles lost its steam between the 1930s and the 1960s, coinciding with arguably the all-time zenith of public trust in doctors and modern medicine?[4] The forms of faith that were practised during a period of relatively quiescent religious belief deserve examination, even if this requires us to assume that such impulses were sublimated.

But the core of this paper is a less ethereal matter: a narrative of the manipulation of the lay public's images of one miracle drug, streptomycin, in the immediate aftermath of the Second World War. A postgraduate student named Albert Schatz first isolated streptomycin in 1943, under a screening program directed by his supervisor, Selman Waksman, at Rutgers University in New Jersey.[5] This substance became the second clinically significant antibiotic (after penicillin), and was the first effective chemotherapeutic treatment for tuberculosis. As we shall see, the British government deliberately created a toxicity scare in order to limit demand for the drug, which was very expensive and at the time had to be imported from the United States. Waksman remarked in his book-length history of tuberculosis that in Britain 'possible reactions from the use of this drug were kept in mind and even overemphasised',[6] and social historian Linda Bryder repeated this same point without substantive elaboration,[7] but otherwise this episode is absent from the literature on streptomycin.

Although we have a shortage neither of books with 'miracle' in the title,[8] nor of historical literature on certain individual exemplars of the category of the 'miracle drug',[9] there has been relatively little historical examination of what these drugs might have in common. And almost all that we know about the history of the antibiotic drugs, which are a potent symbol of modern medicine, comes from the example of penicillin.[10] There has also been a focus on discovery and early research, to the exclusion of study of the diffusion and use of these products.[11] The first half of the paper, the story of lay images of streptomycin, illustrates a conflict between bureaucratic-scientific rationalities and subjective considerations of the value of the drug. In the second half of this paper, again using examples mostly from postwar Britain, I attempt to draw out some other aspects of the cultural significance of the concept of 'miracle drugs'.

Much further comparative work is desirable to assess the applicability of this admittedly speculative analysis to other drugs, countries and periods. (See the papers in this volume on oral contraceptives, interferon and taxol.) As well, further research is required to bring out the sociological specificity of the assertions made here in general terms. What roles did doctors play in mediating the interaction between scientific and magical understandings of the power of such substances? Might gender differences in the reception of miracle drugs echo the preponderance of women among users of alternative therapies such as homoeopathy?[12] To what extent can we differentiate between 'miracle' and 'wonder' drugs – terms used interchangeably in this paper – and to what extent might these terms be linked to Catholic and Protestant sensibilities respectively?[13]

David Masters' *Miracle Drug: The Inner Story of Penicillin*, published in 1946, breathlessly declared:

> [T]hat the main secret was eventually wrested from this humble mould by this team of Oxford scientists of whom Sir Howard Florey was the inspiration and leader was something in the nature of a miracle. But it was not wrought by pressing a button or waving a magic wand. It was achieved by the application of scientific knowledge and the unremitting toil of many brilliant scientists and above all by their refusal to be beaten by difficulties which seemed to be insuperable.[14]

In that era, not only contemporary popularisers but, it seems, lay members of the public were more than ready to ascribe miraculous properties to drugs such as streptomycin.

## Lay images of streptomycin

> The news of the finding by Feldman, Hinshaw and others, in America, that streptomycin was active against the tubercle bacillus not only in the test-tube but also in the living body naturally caused great excitement throughout the world – an excitement which was intensified when it was shown by these workers that the drug could at least prolong life in certain acute forms of human tuberculosis, such as tuberculous meningitis and acute miliary tuberculosis, which hitherto had proved almost invariably fatal within a short period. The story rapidly found its way into the newspapers on both sides of the Atlantic, and streptomycin was hailed as a 'miracle drug', in terms of hyperbole which too often omitted reference to its limitations and possible ill-effects.[15]

Early in 1946, Sir Edward Mellanby was asked, as the Secretary of the Medical Research Council (MRC), to nominate a speaker for the annual Harben Lectures at the Royal Institute of Public Health and Hygiene.[16] He chose William Feldman, a leading researcher from the Mayo Clinic in Minnesota, on the recommendation of Ernst Chain, a Nobel laureate the previous year for his contribution to the discovery of penicillin. Mellanby described streptomycin as an 'exciting' development, one in which 'scientific and medical men would take a great interest', and he even urged the Institute to move their date ahead several months so that Feldman could visit in June.[17] But his enthusiasm toward the visit soon cooled to the point that he was 'not sure that this was really wise', and privately he blamed Chain.[18] This came after the Chief Medical Officer of the Ministry of

Health remonstrated with him, most likely saying that to stir up public interest in streptomycin would be politically dangerous on the grounds that demand for the drug would be impossible to satisfy.[19] A particular focus was the treatment of tuberculous meningitis: a Mayo Clinic paediatrician concluded from a literature search (performed just before the development of streptomycin) that worldwide, only 62 patients with confirmed cases of this condition had ever recovered.[20] To put this figure into context, in 1945 alone, over 500 patients died of tuberculous meningitis in the UK, and most of these were infants or young children; in total, the various forms of tuberculous disease were blamed for some 25 000 deaths annually in Great Britain.[21]

On Saturday, 21 September 1946, *The Times* and the *British Medical Journal* (*BMJ*) both carried a press release from the Ministry of Supply; it appeared a week later in the *Lancet*.[22] It announced that pilot-scale streptomycin production was underway in Britain, under the auspices of the Ministry and in collaboration with the MRC among others, and that it was hoped that preliminary clinical trials would begin before the end of the year. The Ministry's Chief Information Officer firmly believed that frank and authoritative statements would clear up speculation and misinformation, so it is quite likely that the press release in September on streptomycin was his personal initiative.[23] Mellanby wrote to a friend who had remarked on the *British Medical Journal* statement, 'I had no previous knowledge of the statement appearing in the medical press about streptomycin, nor should I have approved of it if I had known it was going to be inserted.'[24] His apprehension was well-founded. The first request for streptomycin had come to the MRC in September 1945, from a surgical member of the Council's penicillin clinical trials committee. During the first half of 1946, enquiries trickled in at a rate of less than one a month. Eight written requests arrived in the last week of September following the Ministry's announcement, and twenty during October, and the pace continued to accelerate thereafter, due also to a series of radio broadcasts beginning in November, described below.[25]

Miracle drugs excite economic demand that often strains the capacity of the ordinary channels of distribution, whether that be through direct or insured purchase or a national health service, such as the UK was about to implement at the time of our story. Until 1949 the USA was the only nation producing substantial quantities of streptomycin, and therefore the drug was in extremely short supply in Britain. Since the vast majority of ordinary citizens were unable to obtain streptomycin through official channels, and the demand was great, it is not surprising that some of them found alternative means of procuring the substance. Shipments of streptomycin from the USA to Britain ranged from smuggling rackets, at one end of the spectrum, to donations to hospitals and gifts to family members, at the other end; because many were clandestine, there is no way to determine the scale of such activities.[26] The American media had been explicit about the threat.[27] Of course, black-market drugs were extremely expensive and might well be adulterated, since the ordinary person had no reliable way of recognising this unfamiliar new article. Fake penicillin in Berlin, made from dextrose or yellow face powder, was reportedly selling for $375 an ampoule in 1946.[28] Graham Greene's novella and film *The Third Man*, written in 1948 using reports from *The Times*'s correspondent in Vienna, eloquently illustrates this issue.[29] In the story, children with meningitis (of an unspecified type) were treated with black-market penicillin, heavily diluted with filler. The children ended up 'off their heads' and could not even benefit from full-strength penicillin because the infections had become drug-resistant. In the famous Ferris wheel scene of the movie, the villain Harry Lime told his school friend Martins that for the life of each of the human 'dots' moving far below them, he could earn £20,000 – 'free of income tax, old man'.[30]

The cultural clash between those who would see wondrous properties inherent in some substance and those who would insist on evidence, is clear around the issue of the range of ailments to be treated. Bureaucratic rationality generally favours release of the drug only under careful control; it abhors the waste that, it is feared, would result if the drug were to come into general use before sound knowledge were obtained of its properties. Attempts by authorities to persuade the public that streptomycin was 'not a cure-all' were not successful, and administrative controls were used in order to enforce what they considered rational distribution. Early in 1946, the committee responsible for distribution of the drug in the USA effectively barred its use in treatment of ulcerative colitis, lupus erythematosus, leukaemia, cancer, fever of unknown cause, rheumatic fever, and rheumatoid arthritis.[31] Otosclerosis, a condition involving growth of bone in the inner ear, was among the diverse ailments presented in the British files of enquiries, which are a rich source of information on the perceptions of streptomycin by the members of the general public.[32]

*Alan Yoshioka*

The Medical Research Council's efforts focused on procuring – and on keeping unfragmented – a sufficient supply of streptomycin to run clinical trials that would establish conclusively the relative usefulness of the drug in conditions such as pulmonary tuberculosis. At least there was solid laboratory evidence of its effectiveness in tuberculous animals.[33] Animal modelling, according to the understanding that prevailed in elite scientific circles, gave reasonable grounds for hope that streptomycin would be useful in human tuberculosis. In other conditions, such as various cancers, there was also uncertainty about the value of streptomycin, but it was of a different order in the eyes of scientific officials. No one had bothered to *prove* that the drug was useless in these latter conditions, but for the administrators, the onus lay on applicants to show that their request to try the drug was based on more than blind hope. Especially while the drug remained in very short supply, officials would attempt to ensure that it was allocated with as little waste as possible, according to what they considered the best scientific evidence. This policy of course came into direct conflict with the views of some members of the public. For them the main issue was to obtain some treatment that might possibly help them or their loved ones. If the scientists weren't able to say that streptomycin would definitely help, at least they couldn't say for sure that it wouldn't. And what some patients knew undeniably was that nothing else had worked for them. If a slim hope was more comfort than no hope at all, the value of streptomycin might be incalculably great. Those members of the public who had great resources at their disposal could go to correspondingly great lengths in an attempt to procure the drug.

The status of streptomycin is well illustrated by the enquiry from Sir Charles Hambro, a powerful industrialist, banker, and wartime senior civil servant. On the morning of Saturday, 12 October 1946, he telephoned MRC headquarters, anxious to obtain a small supply of streptomycin for the treatment of his young grandson, who was suffering from acute leukaemia. Hambro had consulted two specialists, who, according to the telegraphed summary of their letter to the British Ambassador in Washington, 'confirm that only cure worthy of trial is streptomycin otherwise chance recovery hopeless'.[34] The Ambassador was reminded, 'You will appreciate also that time factor is of maximum importance.'[35] Hambro's claim that streptomycin in leukaemia would be of 'great interest to the profession as a whole'[36] cannot have been taken very seriously by the MRC. While he surely had faith in the expert status of these medical men, the MRC administrators would have had cause to doubt whether an eminent paediatrician and a radiologist had any more claim to special knowledge about streptomycin than did the medical superintendents of provincial sanatoria. A bibliography of more than 5000 publications on streptomycin, later compiled by Waksman's department, indexed none of Hambro's experts and only a single paper on leukaemia, which did not appear until 1951.[37] The MRC headquarters received word a few days after Hambro's call that he had personally obtained 10 grams of streptomycin from the USA. Ten grams of streptomycin at that time would have cost anywhere up to $150 on the legal market, although one cannot imagine this being a barrier to a man of his means, even allowing for an exorbitant mark-up on the black market.

So how might a patient in need bypass the system of controls and designated hospitals, and locate a supply of genuine streptomycin that had been imported privately? The solution, which emerged rather anarchically, was a series of emergency broadcast appeals, and it was the BBC News Service that was thrust into the coordinating role. The BBC evening news on Friday, 1 November 1946, carried a broadcast appeal for streptomycin for what it called an urgent case: a young boy was critically ill with tuberculous meningitis in the Royal Surrey Hospital in Guildford. Landsborough [later Sir Landsborough] Thomson, the MRC's second-ranked administrator, later received a report that a firm in Tottenham had supplied the hospital with a small quantity of the drug within a couple of hours. Further information, he wrote, was that the child had died immediately after receiving an injection – although, Thomson noted, not necessarily as a result of it.[38] The next day Philip Hart, a physician who was soon to become Director of the MRC's new Tuberculosis Research Unit, told Thomson that the material had been a single bottle containing one half gram of streptomycin, which the firm's parent company in Philadelphia had sent as a standard in case it were to start manufacture in Britain.[39]

Many individuals close to the MRC and Ministry of Health reacted indignantly to such radio broadcasts, of which there were many more over the following months. A letter from the microbiologist C. H. Andrewes strikingly illustrates the tone of such correspondence:

> One expects ill-informed and sensational items from the less responsible elements of the Press, but something rather better from the BBC. They go to a lot of trouble to get scientific advice for some

of their feature programmes... but are apparently [sic] quite lacking in guidance where news bulletins are concerned.... I do not venture to suggest the best remedy but feel that the mystery disease affecting the B.B.C. news department cannot be incurable.[40]

Sir Weldon Dalrymple-Champneys of the Ministry of Health agreed that it was 'improper of the BBC to broadcast appeals for a substance which was not available'.[41] But if in fact the substance had genuinely been completely unavailable, then the radio appeal would of course have failed. As one of the Ministry of Health officials explained to the news editor of the BBC, 'The broadcast "S.O.S." may, however, have the unfortunate effect of giving the impression that supplies are already available over here and can be obtained for treating specific diseases. This is far from being the case.'[42] One Member of Parliament remarked, during a debate in April 1947, 'It seems fantastic that a person's life should depend on whether or not a particular hospital has a radio set.' Aneurin Bevan, the Minister of Health, replied,

> I have already said that the advice I have received does not go to show that patients' lives are necessarily dependent on the supplies of this drug. I very much deprecate false hopes being raised among poor people and sick people by appeals of this sort.[43]

The officials' predictions that the radio appeals would stir up demand turned out to be well-founded. The incident was widely reported, for example in the *Daily Express* story 'Car races rare drug to boy', and even in a Belgian journal.[44] Four days after the first broadcast, a Ministry of Health official said they were 'daily being pestered with requests',[45] and suggested that a joint statement from the MRC and the Ministry be published in the *Lancet* and *British Medical Journal*.[46] A statement was indeed produced, but before they were able to take action, a new piece of American research added fuel to the fire.

An authoritative report from the Mayo Clinic in the *Journal of the American Medical Association* (*JAMA*) on 30 November 1946 declared that four of their nine patients with tuberculous meningitis had survived for several months.[47] Among the patients whose tuberculous meningitis was arrested, blindness of one patient was attributed to the disease itself, while in the case of a deaf patient, they wrote, 'there is a question whether the deafness is due to the streptomycin'; a third patient was reported to have 'profound disturbances of cerebellar function', but the fourth was described as 'clinically well, ambulatory and free of all symptoms', five months after having been admitted with 'severe symptoms of early tuberculous meningitis'.[48] This new paper, cautious as it was, stood in stark contrast to a highly unfavourable report that a group from the Radcliffe Infirmary in Oxford had rushed into print about four months earlier, on the use of streptomycin in several types of meningitis.[49] As both sides agreed, there was little point in instituting treatment of tuberculous meningitis unless it was begun promptly, since bacteriological confirmation of a presumptive diagnosis of the condition would take weeks, by which time it would be too late. Whenever a child was suspected of having tuberculous meningitis, the incentives to get treatment quickly were high; the public's search for emergency supplies became more frantic.

The radio appeals increased the public's perceptions that there were stocks of the drug to be had in Britain, and provided a method by which cooperating institutions, reacting to explicitly humanitarian entreaties, could voluntarily exercise control over distribution, thus interfering with central administrative attempts to maintain a rule-bound system of distribution. The government's fulfilment of its scientific and industrial objectives – to say nothing of those in public health – depended on its maintaining control over its own supplies, which in turn required the capacity to resist the demands of petitioners. It was relatively easier to turn people away if the government could plausibly maintain the impression that no other member of the public was able to get the drug either, on the grounds that it was all allocated to scientifically necessary clinical trials. But if appealing to rationalist principles of distribution could not dampen the demand for the drug as much as the MRC and Ministry of Health wished, there was a more plainly intelligible argument at their disposal: that the drug was dangerous. The government thus deliberately created a toxicity scare in order to stem a tide of public requests that it could not meet. Against the backdrop of a major public health problem, these centrally directed cultural images of streptomycin reflected the constraints of economic crisis and a rapidly accumulating body of American research on the new drug.

Back in May 1946, Landsborough Thomson first applied an argument that would eventually become a key element of the Medical Research Council's letters of refusal of appeals for streptomycin. He placated one supplicant, the Medical Officer of Health for Cardiff, with the statement, 'It is perhaps poor consolation, but I may mention that the first reports of the value of streptomycin in tuberculosis seem to have been rather too optimistic, and the indications are that its chief uses may be in other conditions.'[50] Thomson wrote similarly to a doctor in Guildford in July, 'I may add that in spite of some rather optimistic reports, present indications are that streptomycin is *not dramatically successful* in the treatment of tuberculosis.'[51] From the summer onwards it became increasingly common for official replies to frame the success of the drug in terms that ensured that the criteria remained unfulfilled. That is, the MRC consistently used negative-sounding phrases that were intended to discourage demands for the drug. For example, it seems likely that Thomson inserted the word 'dramatically' because by July 1946 he could no longer truthfully have written a bare, 'present indications are that streptomycin is not successful in the treatment of tuberculosis'. A stencilled statement that the MRC began sending to enquirers in October 1946 illustrates particularly well the Council's pessimistic framing of American research findings. This standard statement concluded,

> The evidence from such trials as have already been made in America leaves it at present quite uncertain whether streptomycin is likely to *prove* of *great* value in tuberculosis, and it may eventually prove that its chief uses lie in the treatment of certain other conditions.[52]

Around the end of October, again through framing that was pessimistic to the point of being deliberately misleading, the MRC began to say about streptomycin, 'it certainly "works ill" in some clinical forms of the disease'.[53] Of course, the warning a few months before from the American authorities, on which the MRC apparently based its claim, probably had also been tailored to discourage requests for the drug.[54] Then for the issue of the *British Medical Journal* dated 14 December, the MRC at last provided the previously suggested leading article on tuberculous meningitis treated with streptomycin (but took pains to conceal its authorship). It declared, 'there seems to be a very real risk that, even if the infection is controlled (as has only very rarely happened), the patient will usually be left mentally deficient, deaf, blind or otherwise a hopeless invalid.'[55] The *Lancet*, on the other hand, did not publish any statement of this kind. Instead, within a few weeks, it published a report from the Kent County Council's Tuberculosis Chemotherapy Unit, which declared,

> Our experiences were free from the hazards and perils which have characterised previously reported trials [such as that from the

Radcliffe Infirmary group], and have convinced us that streptomycin, of the purity which we used, can be administered in safety at the dose levels which we adopted.[56]

But the allegation of danger from the use of streptomycin in tuberculous meningitis would often be repeated to the public in the coming months. A statement made in Bevan's name, appearing in *The Times* on 23 January 1947, warned, 'in the very small number of patients with tubercular meningitis whose life has been prolonged by the treatment there has nearly always been permanent serious mental derangement, blindness or deafness.'[57] This provoked a much sharper response than the similar statement in the *British Medical Journal* had done in mid-December. Waksman cabled Sir Jack Drummond, Director of Research at the manufacturer Boots, to get an explanation. Although American officials advised Waksman to ignore the matter,[58] he also contacted the British Commonwealth Scientific Office in Washington, whose chief cabled London that the American authorities were 'seriously concerned' about the statement on toxicity.[59] A testy response was cabled back to Washington:

> In view of scarcity of streptomycin in this country great embarrassment has been caused by exaggerated press claims for its value which go beyond evidence as yet available especially for tuberculosis. It has accordingly been necessary to inform British public that treatment is still in experimental stage and not free from danger. Facts regarding the latter are drawn from American medical reports.[60]

A senior MRC official explained to the British Foreign Office that the statement by the Ministry of Health 'was intended to discourage broadcast appeals for the drug'.[61] Thomson, under pressure from the Ministry of Health, blamed the Americans for having first played up the publicity about streptomycin.[62] Drummond took the position that the Minister's statement was fair even if it erred on the side of being over-cautious.[63] Hinshaw, when asked by the British United Press for the American reaction, said he could add nothing to the Mayo Clinic's *JAMA* paper from late November 1946.[64] Meanwhile, continuing to take an independent line after *The Times*'s warning appeared, at the end of January 1947 the *Lancet* published a leading article that summarised the positive Mayo findings in tuberculous meningitis. Though it denied that chemotherapy was a 'shortcut to cure'[65] – an illustration of the delicate balancing act that was required – the journal asserted, 'In spite of transient and permanent toxic effects, uncertainty regarding the development of drug-resistance by tubercle bacilli, and difficulty of purification and production of streptomycin, these early reports give great hope for the future.'[66]

The Ministry's continued interventions failed to prevent a succession of similar radio broadcasts for many more months.[67] The British Medication Association's Charles Hill, acting as a mediator between the Ministry of Health and the BBC, chaired a conference – which the MRC boycotted.[68] The toxicity scare of the winter of 1946/7 appears to have reduced the use of streptomycin during the following few years. In 1950, once British manufacturers were producing ample supplies, the Ministry of Health published a report that noted, with some concern,

> There appears to be a belief prevalent amongst many medical practitioners that streptomycin treatment does no more than prolong life or produce 'recovery' as a physical and mental wreck. This is not true.[69]

Of patients treated early in the disease, some 40 per cent 'made a complete recovery except in some instance for minor disabilities which at the time of assessment did not interfere with their leading a normal life'.[70] Responsibility for such confusion on the part of practitioners can be laid squarely back at the door of the Ministry of Health itself. The Ministry biased the presentation of reports on the outcome of streptomycin treatment of cases of tuberculous meningitis. With the full cooperation of the MRC, it deliberately insinuated that unfavourable clinical outcomes were a side effect of the drug, rather than the results of the disease. It is possible that the deception resulted in higher mortality from certain forms of tuberculosis during the late 1940s than would have occurred in Britain if the American research findings had been relayed without distortion. On the other hand, the private justification for this strategy was that streptomycin could not have been made available in sufficient quantity, and therefore that it was better that the British public's hopes not be raised beyond the means of fulfilling them.

## Modern talismans

Miracle drugs enable hope. In 1947 a well-known journalist, Chapman Pincher from the *Daily Express*, quoted a physician as saying, 'I have 25 patients now for whom streptomycin is the only hope. It would not save them all, but some might pull through.'[71] This quote shows that even in recent decades it has been common for individuals to ascribe miraculous powers to drugs and medical procedures, a cultural form touching on life and death issues. Moreover, in the period of seeming immunity from infection brought about by the antibiotic revolution, 'miraculous' drugs played a key role in many people's thinking about these subjects. It appears that there is a need that is at least partially satisfied through individuals' attachment of magical powers to specific medicinal substances or procedures. We can see this in terms of the attempt to avoid loss, here the ultimate loss, death, by holding on to a fantasy that streptomycin might save them. The miracle drug may thus fulfil, for some patients and members of their families, a crucial function of psychological defence, by allowing them to imagine a happy ending. The intensity of some people's demand for the drug, even in the face of official assertions that it could not rationally be expected to have any effect, is understandable as a response to a personal crisis. There is no other hope, no alternative treatment; all the energy is invested in the streptomycin solution to the problem. The drug has a talismanic quality and has attributed to it magical or heightened powers, beyond what the official reports say.

The object of magical thinking is somehow set apart as a special phenomenon. In contrast with traditional magical cases wherein this specialness might arise by virtue of an association with ancient wisdom, miracle drugs are distinguished by being new and modern. The Medical Research Council continually played on its expert knowledge of 'the latest' American reports, on the assumption that the most recent would be the best. This quality of novelty immerses wonder drugs, ironically enough, in some very strong traditions, namely the stereotyped ways we have of talking about innovation, ways that exaggerate the importance of differences between new and old.[72] Miracle drugs in this respect are similar to patent medicines in being described as revolutionary and unique. There are, for example, many precedents for recent claims that one or another aspect of Viagra's social impact is 'unprecedented'. The romanticisation of novelty surely contributes to why penicillin, a product of fermentation, looms much larger in popular culture than do the sulphonamides, products of chemical synthesis techniques that were fairly routine at the time of innovation. Considered as a media phenomenon, streptomycin followed closely in the mould, so to speak, of penicillin. For anyone outside a pharmaceutical manufacturing concern, there was nothing remarkable about the method of production of streptomycin in particular, but the whole notion of antibiotics was still very novel. What was special about streptomycin was its ability to treat conditions in which penicillin and sulphonamides had proved ineffective, including tuberculosis. Wonder drugs attain their distinctiveness partly through saving lives in cases of conditions that have been heretofore incurable; as the public becomes accustomed to seeing effective treatments emerge for an ever-widening range of diseases, we might perhaps expect the public's fascination to be displaced onto other objects.

Miracle drugs are a symbol of modernity, or perhaps more recently, postmodernity.[73] The Director of Britain's National Institute for Medical Research argued that the development of streptomycin production would necessarily involve training of a type that was 'essential to modern chemical industry'.[74] Wonder drugs once exemplified a forward-looking culture: by the end of the Second World War it was commonly presumed that even more effective new drugs were just around the corner, and that it was only a matter of time until they were discovered. This association with modernisation is not, and never has been, regarded in a uniformly positive light. A basic point often forgotten or caricatured in the historical literature is that there was inevitably resistance to wonder drugs, of the societal rather than the bacterial kind. We should recall that for years, streptomycin and the other chemotherapies of tuberculosis continued to be regarded by many practitioners as adjuncts to sanatorium treatment and collapse therapy, even though industrial officials apparently argued for production sponsorship on the basis that the drug might, if proved effective, actually replace prolonged hospital treatment. Over-prescription of antibiotics has long symbolised the flaws of modern medicine, in the eyes of both rationalisers and holists.[75] The recurring warnings in recent years, to the effect that the end of the antibiotic era is upon us, are a sign of faith under siege. Some popular writers appear surprised that there has turned out to be a dark side to the progress of medicine, while others trumpet the widespread emergence of antibiotic-resistant bacteria as a sign that orthodox medicine has failed us and that we must now turn to some other saviour. A spokesman for thalidomide victims writes bitterly, 'We remind the world of dreams shattered and mothers, families and friends forever scarred by the "wonder drug" of the past, now returned to use';[76] scathing quotation marks express his sense that the promise held out by science and by the pharmaceutical companies has been betrayed.

Miracle drugs, through their association with health and the saving of life, accrue a special moral status in comparison with other modern technological objects that may be either consumerist or warlike. Medical care is perhaps the most apt illustration of the 'active moralistic collectivism' that David Marquand posits as characteristic of the period in British history from the end of the war to the mid-1950s.[77] In March 1947, a few months after passage of the National Health Service Act, Dr Barnett Stross, a backbench Labour MP, asked the Parliamentary Secretary for Health, regarding the production and distribution of streptomycin,

> Is my hon. Friend aware that our civilisation will be judged by the care we take of our sick, and, therefore, by this type of work, rather than by the possession of motor cars, refrigerators, or how many of us chew gum?[78]

What is particularly interesting about miracle drugs is that the talismanic attachment is made to an object specifically and strongly associated with science.[79] And this sets up a tension, in that we may see the miracle drug as a symbol of faith in non-faith. The discoverers and managers of these drugs walk a fine line. On the one hand they need their product to be seen positively and they accrue status from being seen as the geese that lay the golden eggs. But on the other hand, public enthusiasm is seen as a dangerously uncontrollable force, and is deprecated as irrational, even superstitious.[80] The case of traditional religious miracles displays a similar tension between elites upholding stringent criteria of miraculous status and lay people or ordinary priests whom the hierarchy views as overly flexible, if not credulous. But the latter case lacks the miracle drug's dependence on elites who may be unsympathetic to *any* belief that transcends rationality and hard scientific evidence.

The symbolism attached to a drug may be explicitly faith-based. Some reformers, inside and outside the medical profession, have invoked spiritual ideals in concert with the treatment of the whole patient, in contrast with a supposedly mechanistic prescription for antibiotics. But other believers did not consider faith healing an alternative to antibiotic treatment; rather, for them, antibiotics *were* a gift from God. Late in 1946, an unmarried woman in County Down, Northern Ireland, began her letter to Waksman:

> I am only one of the hundreds of thousands of people who must have blessed your name for your wonderful discovery of streptomycin. I have been an invalid for seven years through paralysis in the lower limbs – the doctors call it spastic paraphlegia [sic] – I am otherwise a perfectly healthy person aged 50, but cannot walk without the aid of two crutches. Terrific nerve pains in legs and feet – giving almost constant pain. My doctor thinks that injections

of streptomycin will be very helpful to me – in fact that I may be cured. What do you think, Doctor Waksman?[81]

She ended her request, 'Thanking you in anticipation and may God bless you always'.[82] The history of tuberculosis written by physician Frank Ryan quotes, without comment, another letter that came to Waksman from Charleston, South Carolina:

> So you see, because you laboured and discovered the drug streptomycin, and because of the prayers of all the good people who heard of our baby's illness, our son is with us, today, healthy, happy, and a normal boy in every way. Yours is God given work.[83]

With the threat of uncontrollable public responses continually in the background, pharmaceutical manufacturers and anyone else with direct responsibility for the drugs tend to avoid, indeed to disown, any claim that their product is a miracle drug. A carefully framed denial can stir up the desired buzz of interest while shielding pharmaceutical manufacturers from charges that they have unfairly raised the hopes of the public – and regulatory intervention has increased the importance of this factor since the 1930s. Media pundits can afford to be more free-wheeling, but even in the 1940s the words 'wonder' or 'miracle' often appeared in quotes. Rumour is an important element of talk about wonder drugs. 'Already the names of even newer chemotherapeutic remedies are mentioned. One hears of claviformin, for example, also called patulin, and of helvelic acid'.[84] Some display of caution about the miracle drug is *de rigueur* for the sake of the commentator's credibility. It was often said that streptomycin was 'not a cure-all', as a preface to making optimistic remarks about its properties. Chapman Pincher wrote, 'I must stress that no cures are claimed. Recovered patients must stay healthy for four more years before the possibility of relapse can be discounted. But the cautiously worded report of the trials credits streptomycin with the dramatic relief of several types of obstinate tubercular disease'.[85] William Feldman said during his series of Harben Lectures in London,

> My colleagues and I view the present status and future possibilities of chemotherapy in clinical tuberculosis with hopeful enthusiasm, being ever mindful of the fact that neither streptomycin nor any of the other known substances that have proved effective in experimental animals can fully qualify as the long awaited curative drug.[86]

If the miracle drug fails, the disillusionment that follows can be harsh. Gods who disappoint are rapidly transformed into devils. Witness the bitterness of some people's denunciation of AZT, or the rather different case of angry letters to the discoverers of streptomycin, Waksman and Albert Schatz, blaming them for the hearing loss that was a 'side effect' of the drug.[87]

The degree of lay and medical enthusiasm for wonder drugs may fluctuate widely over time. It is well established in the literature that some new drugs follow a similar pattern of acceptability. Highly favourable publicity appears, there is a rush in the market, and then adverse events receive prominent publicity, with the result that demand levels off, or sometimes falls, eventually stabilising as the market matures. Demand is of course the outcome of a wide range of economic, political and cultural factors in addition to medical evidence, as for example Michael Worboys has described in comparing the adoption of pneumonia treatments in the USA and Britain.[88] The diffusion of medicines encompasses factors (such as marketing, oligopoly, and force of habit) that rationalist 'therapeutic reformers', as Harry Marks has dubbed them, have often seen as corrupting influences on prescribing decisions that in an ideal world should, they believe, be based solely on therapeutic efficacy.[89] Numerous scholars have insisted that the problems in producing objective knowledge are even more difficult in the case of clinical medicine than in the scientific fields examined in the classic case studies in sociology of science. But whereas the discipline of Science and Technology Studies has tended to assert that knowledge in general and particular cases is socially constructed, one need not subscribe to an ideal of value-free science in order to lay charges of bias, as John Abraham has reminded us. He quotes Barry Barnes, 'By recourse to its own normal practice, scientific work can itself be criticised and, if one insists on putting it so, revealed as ideologically determined'.[90] The story above of the toxicity scare juxtaposes the bureaucracy's public statements, driven by a logic of managing demand, and private statements that give credence to independent scientific evidence.

## Conclusion

The stories of discovery of wonder drugs have often played on the element of serendipity, and this has surely contributed to their talismanic specialness. *Penicillium notatum* was often likened (not quite accurately, but this is beside the point) to an ordinary bread mould, or the mould on oranges. To transform an apparently commonplace substance into a life-saving drug, was that not astonishing? The rotten cantaloupe found in a market in Peoria, from which was isolated a high-yielding strain of *Penicillium*, achieved a legendary status. The story of spores of *Penicillium* mould drifting in through an open window in Fleming's laboratory at St Mary's has been retold many times. Likewise with streptomycin, the story was told that a farmer living near Rutgers University brought a sick chicken to Waksman's lab for examination, and that the swab from the chicken's throat yielded the streptomycin-producing strain of *Actinomyces griseus*. And these well-worn anecdotes bring me to my concluding theme, mythology in historiography. Donald McGraw has pointed out the repetitious nature of the existing accounts of antibiotics.[91] Our basic understanding of the history of the antibiotics has remained largely unchallenged for decades – with the notable exception of Wai Chen's interpretation of penicillin as a 'weedkiller' that interested Fleming only for its application to the growing of clean bacterial cultures at St Mary's vaccine laboratory[92] – while writers pursue ever more esoteric – I use the word advisedly – details of the historical record. Antiquarianism in the history of medicine is of course a familiar phenomenon, and set in that context, the lack of novelty in these accounts is no great defect; the retelling of familiar stories serves a ritual function. But if our accounts of the wonder drugs are myths that illustrate idealised characteristics of science, then errors in these accounts, left to stand unchallenged, would be seen to undermine the scientific enterprise itself. The science journalist David Wilson devoted practically a whole book to correcting popular misconceptions about the discovery and development of penicillin, and the bacteriologist Ronald Hare argued convincingly that the open window story could not have been true, while Schatz insisted that the chicken in New Jersey was healthy.[93] While they are certainly justified in seeking accuracy, we are bound to ask why it matters so much. Surely we can see at least some such writers as defending a faith in scientific objectivity by purging the historical record of any accretion of mythical elements. Of course a myth, by its very nature and function, tends to defy the efforts of non-believers to make factual corrections to it. Our efforts as historians to place events in perspective will usually have but modest effects on belief systems of any kind.

## Acknowledgements

This paper is based on research partially funded by the Wellcome Trust. I am grateful for feedback from Toine Pieters, Marijke

Gijswijt-Hofstra, other participants of the symposium, the anonymous referees, and Tim Boon.

### Notes

1. www.ussc.alltheweb.com lists 4200 documents containing 'miracle+drug', (visited 11 June 2000); www.ussc.alltheweb.com lists 6725 documents containing 'wonder+drug', (visited 11 June 2000).
2. M. Gijswijt-Hofstra, H. Marland and H. de Waardt (eds), *Illness and Healing Alternatives in Western Europe* (London: Routledge, 1997).
3. B. Smith, 'Gullible's Travails: Tuberculosis and Quackery 1890–1930', *Journal of Contemporary History*, 20 (1985), 735–56, quotation at 740.
4. R. B. Mullin, *Miracles and the Modern Religious Imagination* (New Haven and London: Yale University Press, 1996).
5. D. Eveleigh and C. Schaffner, 'Reflections on the Fiftieth Anniversary of the Discovery of Streptomycin', *Society for Industrial Microbiology News*, 44 (1994), 177–84. See also, for example, H. A. Lechevalier, 'The Search for Antibiotics at Rutgers University', in J. Parascandola (ed), *The History of Antibiotics* (Madison, WI: American Institute of the History of Pharmacy, 1980); M. Wainwright, *Miracle Cure: The Story of Penicillin and the Golden* Age of Antibiotics (Oxford: Blackwell, 1990); *idem*, 'Streptomycin: Discovery and Resultant Controversy', *History and Philosophy of the Life Sciences*, 13 (1991), 97–124; A. Schatz, 'The true story of the discovery of streptomycin', *Actinomycetes* (Udine, Italy), 4 (1993), 27–39; S. A. Waksman, *The Conquest of Tuberculosis* (London: Cambridge University Press, 1964).
6. Waksman, *op. cit.* (note 5), 164–5.
7. L. Bryder, *Below the Magic Mountain: A Social History of Tuberculosis in Twentieth-Century Britain* (Oxford and New York: Clarendon Press, 1988), 255.
8. D. Masters, *Miracle Drug: The Inner Story of Penicillin*, (London: Eyre and Spottiswoode, 1946); H. Bottcher, *Miracle Drugs: A History of Antibiotics* (translation from the German edition of 1959), (London: William Heinemann Ltd, 1963), interestingly retitled *Wonder Drugs* for the American market (Philadelphia, PA: Lippincott, 1964); Wainwright (1990) *op. cit.* (note 5).
9. Closest in spirit to the present paper is D. Cantor, 'Cortisone and the Politics of Drama, 1949–55', in J. V. Pickstone (ed.), *Medical Innovations in Historical Perspective* (New York: St. Martin's, 1992). This literature is large and diverse. See, for example, M. Bliss, *The Discovery of Insulin* (Toronto: McLelland & Stewart, 1982); G. M.

Hobby, *Penicillin: Meeting the Challenge* (New Haven: Yale University Press, 1985); R. Hare, *The Birth of Penicillin and the Disarming of Microbes* (London: Allen and Unwin, 1971); D. P. Adams, '*The Greatest Good to the Greatest Number': Penicillin Rationing on the American Home Front, 1940–1945* (New York: Peter Lang, 1991); H. Marks, 'Cortisone, 1949: A Year in the Political Life of a Drug', *Bulletin of the History of Medicine* 66 (1992), 419–39; T. Pieters, 'Interferon and its First Clinical Trial: Looking Behind the Scenes', *Medical History,* 37 (1993), 270–95.

10. A recent Witness Seminar held at the Wellcome Institute for the History of Medicine brought to light much information on the under researched topic of the antibiotics that were developed after penicillin. See E. M. Tansey and L. A. Reynolds (eds), *Post Penicillin Antibiotics: From Acceptance to Resistance? Wellcome Witnesses to Twentieth Century Medicine,* vol. 6. (London: The Wellcome Trust, 2000).

11. For an elaboration of this argument, see D. Edgerton, 'From Innovation to Use: Ten Eclectic Theses on the Historiography of Technology', *History and Technology* 16 (1999), 111–36. Notable exceptions within the literature on drugs in the 'miracle' category include Cantor, *op. cit.* (note 9) and Adams, *op. cit.* (note 9).

12. N. Rogers, 'Women and Sectarian Medicine', in R. D. Apple (ed), *Women, Health and Medicine in America* (New Brunswick, NJ: Rutgers University Press, 1992); R. Juette, G. B. Risse and J. Woodward (eds), *Culture, Knowledge, and Healing. Historical Perspectives on Homeopathic Medicine in Europe and North America* (Sheffield: European Association for the History of Medicine and Health Publications, 1998).

13. Smith has called attention to quacks' remedies as 'godsends... in a peculiarly Protestant world'. Smith, *op. cit.* (note 3), 740.

14. Masters, *op. cit.* (note 8), 7.

15. Medical Research Council, *Report of the Medical Research Council for the Years 1945–48,* Cmd 7846, *Parliamentary Papers* xviii (1948–9), 1–283, quotation at 22.

16. H. H. Gerrans to E. Mellanby, 25 January 1946, Public Record Office (PRO), Kew, Medical Research Council Files FD1/3258.

17. E. Mellanby to H. H. Gerrans, 22 February 1946, PRO, FD1/3258.

18. E. Mellanby to H. W. Florey, 12 March 1946, PRO, FD1/6751.

19. E. Mellanby to J. Mackintosh, 6 May 1946, PRO, FD1/3258.

20. H. M. Keith, 'Use of chemotherapy in a case of tuberculous meningitis', *Proceedings of the Staff Meetings of the Mayo Clinic,* 19 (1944), 36–7.

21. Registrar-General, *Statistical Review for England and Wales* (London: HMSO, 1946).
22. Anonymous, 'Four British Firms to Make Streptomycin', *The Times*, (21 September 1946), filed in PRO, FD1/6764; Anonymous, 'Streptomycin', *British Medical Journal*, ii (21 September 1946), 431; Anonymous, 'Home Production of Streptomycin', *Lancet*, ii (28 September 1946), 475.
23. See R. Williams-Thompson, *Was I Really Necessary?* (London: World's Press News Publishing Co. Ltd, 1951), especially 75–7; also PRO, Ministry of Supply Files AVIA49/44.
24. E. Mellanby to C. L. Pattison, 26 September 1946, PRO, FD1/6760.
25. PRO, MRC Files FD1/6760-3.
26. For descriptive accounts of the black markets in goods more mundane than penicillin, see E. Smithies, *Crime in Wartime: A Social History of Crime in World War Two* (London: Allen and Unwin, 1982); idem, *The Black Economy in England Since 1914* (Dublin: Gill and Macmillan, 1984); and D. Hughes, 'The spivs', in M. Sissons and P. French (eds), *Age of Austerity* (London: Penguin, 1964), 86–105.
27. See T. R. Henry, 'Control of Streptomycin Throws Suspicion on Black Market Drug', *Washington Star* (16 April 1946), PRO, FD1/6751.
28. Our Special Correspondent, 'Imitation Penicillin in Berlin: Black market arrests', *The Times* (22 April 1946).
29. G. Greene, *The Third Man and the Fallen Idol* (London: Penguin, 1976; original, London: Heinemann, 1950). Raymond Greene, the author's brother, was a physician. For a fascinating account of the creation of the film, see M. Shelden, *Graham Greene: The Man Within* (London: Minerva, 1995), 316–33.
30. G. Greene, *op. cit.* (note 29), 104.
31. C. S. Keefer, 'Official Statement Concerning Streptomycin', *Journal of the American Medical Association*, 131 (4 May 1946), 31.
32. F. Marchbank memo, 28 October 1946, PRO, Ministry of Health Files MH58/636. The vast majority of the PRO's surviving records of streptomycin enquiries are in MRC files (note 25).
33. W. H. Feldman, 'The Chemotherapy of Tuberculosis, Including the Use of Streptomycin', *Journal of the Royal Institute of Public Health and Hygiene*, 9 (1946), 267–88, 297–324, 343–63.
34. [Couzens] memo to F.H.K. Green, 12 October 1946, PRO, FD1/6760.
35. *Ibid.*

36. *Ibid.*
37. S. A. Waksman, *The Literature on Streptomycin 1944–1952* (New Brunswick, NJ: Rutgers University Press, first edn 1948, rev edn 1952). This source cannot be considered exhaustive, and it contains more than a few errors of text and indexing, but it is very suggestive of the weight of research opinion. See R. D. Barnard, 'Streptomyces Fermentation Derivatives in Acute Leukaemia', *Lancet*, i (26 May 1951), 1157–9. Early in 1949, Barnard reported that he began giving acute leukaemic patients a crude by-product of the fermentation of *Streptomyces griseus*. It appears from his paper that the original purpose of this approach had been to provide the patients with vitamin B12, and that remission of leukaemia was only later attributed to an antibiotic component of this by-product.
38. A. L. Thomson memo on phone conversation with Sir W. Dalrymple-Champneys, 5 November 1946, PRO, FD1/6764.
39. P. D'Arcy Hart to A. L. Thomson, 6 November 1946, FD1/6760; J. Drummond to A. L. Thomson, 8 November 1946, PRO, FD1/6760.
40. C. H. Andrewes to E. Mellanby, 18 December 1946, PRO, FD1/1378.
41. A. L. Thomson memo, *op. cit.* (note 38).
42. Harding annotation on A. P. Ryan to Harding, 12 November 1946, PRO, MH58/636.
43. *Hansard*, House of Commons Debates, vol. 435, Oral Answers, col. 2225, 3 April 1947.
44. Anonymous, 'Car Races Rare Drug to Boy', *Daily Express*, c.2 November 1946, and F. H. K. Green to F. Droogmans, 20 November 1946, PRO, FD1/6760.
45. F. H. K. Green to A. L. Thomson, 5 November 1946, PRO, FD1/6760.
46. *Ibid.*
47. H. C. Hinshaw, W. H. Feldman, and K. H. Pfuetze, 'Treatment of Tuberculosis with Streptomycin: A Summary of Observations on One Hundred Cases', *Journal of the American Medical Association*, 132 (30 November 1946), 778–82, quotation at 779.
48. *Ibid.*
49. H. Cairns, E. S. Duthie, and H. V. Smith, 'Intrathecal Streptomycin in Meningitis: Clinical Trial in Tuberculous, Coliform and Other Infections', *Lancet*, ii (3 August 1946), 153–5, quotation at 153.
50. A. L. Thomson to J. G. Wilson, 29 May 1946, PRO, FD1/6760.
51. A. L. Thomson to R. C. Matson, 23 July 1946, PRO, FD1/6760. Emphasis added.

52. Anonymous, 'Streptomycin', 8 October 1946, PRO, FD1/6760. Emphases added.
53. F. H. K. Green to T. H. G. Shore, 24 October 1946, PRO, FD1/6760.
54. [H. Raistrick and & T. B. Keep], 'Streptomycin', PRO, FD1/6759 and MH58/636.
55. Anonymous, 'Streptomycin: The Present Position', *British Medical Journal*, ii (14 December 1946), 906.
56. D. G. Madigan, P. N. Swift and G. Brownlee, 'Clinical and Pharmacological Aspects of the Toxicity of Streptomycin', *Lancet*, i (4 January 1947), 9–11, quotation at 11.
57. Anonymous, 'Streptomycin', *The Times* (23 January 1947).
58. Memo, 'Dr. Henry Welsch [sic]', 28 January 1947, Papers of Professor Selman A. Waksman, Alexandra Library Special Collections, Rutgers University, New Brunswick, NJ, Box 2 Main Series, File 'Streptomycin (British Corres.)'.
59. Telegram, [A.] King, British Commonwealth Scientific Office to [H. L.] Verry, Department of Scientific and Industrial Research, 30 January 1947, PRO, FD1/6769.
60. Telegram, [H. L.] Verry to [A.] King, 8 February 1947, PRO, FD1/6769.
61. F. H. K. Green to Under-Secretary of State, Foreign Office, 16 April 1947, PRO, FD1/6769.
62. A. L. Thomson to E. M. R. Russell-Smith, 5 February 1947, PRO, FD1/6769.
63. J. Drummond to S. A. Waksman, 4 February 1947, Waksman Papers (note 58), 'Streptomycin (British correspondence)'.
64. H. C. Hinshaw to S. A. Waksman, 12 February 1947, Waksman Papers (note 58), 'Streptomycin (British correspondence)'.
65. Anonymous, 'Streptomycin in Tuberculosis', *Lancet*, i (25 January 1947), 144–5.
66. *Ibid.*
67. Anonymous, 'Distribution of Streptomycin', *Lancet*, i (14 June 1947), 833. See, for example, 'Quick Response to Appeal for Drug', *The Times* (28 May 1947).
68. C. Hill to F. H. K. Greene [sic], 16 May 1947, PRO, FD1/6769.
69. Ministry of Health, 'Streptomycin in Tuberculous Meningitis: Ministry Report', *Lancet*, ii (5 August 1950), 230–1, quotation at 230.
70. *Ibid.*
71. C. Pincher, 'Treasury Holds Back the Dollar Drug: 25 Children are Left to Die', *Daily Express*, c.9 July 1948, PRO, FD1/6765.

72. See Edgerton, *op. cit.* (note 11).
73. See R. Bud, 'Penicillin and the New Elizabethans', *British Journal for the History of Science*, 31 (1998), 305–33.
74. C. Harington to J. E. Lennard-Jones, 26 March 1946, PRO, FD1/6751.
75. See J. C. Whorton, 'Antibiotic Abandon', in Parascandola *op. cit.* (note 5).
76. R. Warren, 'Living in a world with Thalidomide: a new reality' (TVAC Position Paper on the return of Thalidomide), (Thalidomide Victims Association of Canada: www.thalidomide.ca/position.html, 1998, visited 13 June 2000).
77. D. Marquand, 'Moralists and Hedonists', in D. Marquand and A. Seldon (eds), *The Ideas that Shaped Postwar Britain* (London: Fontana Press, 1996), 21.
78. *Hansard*, House of Commons Debates, vol. 435, Oral Answers, col. 578, 20 March 1947.
79. For a similar case, see R. D. Apple, *Vitamania: Vitamins in American Culture* (New Brunswick, NJ: Rutgers University Press, 1996).
80. Cantor, *op. cit.* (note 9).
81. J. S. M____ to Dr Waksman, 30 December 1946, Waksman Papers (note 58), 'Streptomycin Letters I'.
82. *Ibid.*
83. F. Ryan, *The Greatest Story Never Told: The Human Story of the Search for the Cure for Tuberculosis and the New Global Threat*, first edn. (Bromsgrove, Worcestershire: Swift Publishers, 1992), 296.
84. M. Goldsmith, *The Road to Penicillin: A History of Chemotherapy* (London: Lindsay Drummond Ltd, 1946), 166.
85. C. Pincher, 'This Drug is Too Good to Hold Up', *Daily Express*, *c.*29 December 1947, PRO, FD1/6761.
86. Feldman, *op. cit.* (note 33), 360.
87. See I. Crab, *The Importance of Disappointment* (London: Routledge, 1994), 102; Ryan, *op. cit.* (note 83); Wainwright (1990), *op. cit.* (note 5), 138.
88. M. Worboys, 'Treatments for Pneumonia in Britain 1910–1940,' in I. Löwy (ed.), *Medicine and Change: Historical and Sociological Studies of Medical Innovation* (London and Montrouge: John Libbey Eurotext, 1993), 317–36.
89. H. M. Marks, *The Progress of Experiment: Science and Therapeutic Reform in the United States, 1900–1990* (Cambridge: Cambridge University Press, 1997).
90. J. Abraham, *Science, Politics and the Pharmaceutical Industry: Controversy and Bias in Drug Regulation* (London: University College

London Press, 1995), 28, citing B. Barnes, *Scientific Knowledge and Sociological Theory* (London: Routledge and Kegan Paul, 1974), 138.
91. D. J. McGraw, 'The History of Antibiotics: A Critical Bibliography', *Bulletin of Bibliography*, 43 (1986), 103–7; *idem*, 'On Leaving the Mine: Historiographic Resource Exhaustion in Antibiotics History', *Dynamis*, 11 (1991), 415–36.
92. W. Chen, 'The Laboratory as Business: Sir Almroth Wright's Vaccine Programme and the Construction of Penicillin', in A. Cunningham and P. Williams (eds), *The Laboratory Revolution in Medicine* (Cambridge: Cambridge University Press, 1992).
93. D. Wilson, *Penicillin in Perspective* (London: Faber & Faber, 1976); Hare, *op. cit.* (note 9); Schatz, *op. cit.* (note 5), 30.

# 11

## About media, audiences and marketing medicines: The interferons

### Toine Pieters

Every so often, during the past 25 years, scientific claims of therapeutic accomplishment in the treatment of cancer have entered the public domain in Britain and the Netherlands. The biographies of these experimental therapies seem to have a familiar pattern in common: implied claims for a cancer cure based on preliminary tests, exaggerated coverage in the media, high public expectations, widespread disappointment and loss of interest when the claims failed to materialise in large scale trials, researchers and administrators forced on the defensive, and finally there seems hardly any reason for continuation of research or for clinical application.

A similar sequence of events unrolled in the course of 1978 following public statements by scientists who claimed to have achieved promising results with the biological substance interferon in preliminary trials on cancer patients. As might be anticipated, the media gave enthusiastic coverage to the implied claims for a cancer cure which laid the foundation for a global interferon hype. The euphoria surrounding interferon as a 'miracle cure' for cancer was short-lived and faded when interferon's performance in large scale cancer trials was disappointing and when it became clear that interferon that it often produced adverse effects in patients.[1]

However similar the course of events in the case of interferon to those of other so-called cancer cures, the most common dead-end scenario of potential cancer remedies did not materialise. Despite having failed to live up to its public promise as a therapeutic breakthrough, interferon succeeded in finding a niche in clinical practice. Today, thousands of patients suffering from certain types of cancer and a number of virus diseases are routinely treated with interferon. This raises the following question, what gave interferon's biography a different turn from most other therapeutic promises in the treatment of cancer?

In an attempt to offer some insights into the processes by which new remedies are evaluated and put into practice, I shall explore the complex events by which the therapeutic value and clinical use of interferon as a new type of cancer drug was shaped between 1978 and 1997. I shall pay special attention to the ways in which the major actors (individual and collective), ranging from doctors, laboratory researchers, patients, journalists, and regulators, to drug company executives, left their mark and influenced the ways in which the interferons were accepted and disseminated.

## Interferon, scientists and the media

In August 1978, the American Cancer Society (ACS) publicly announced that it would spend $2 million on clinical studies with interferon to investigate its value in treating advanced cancer. This was the largest grant the ACS had ever committed to a single project. The fact was obviously not lost on the media, as the press release triggered a wave of interferon-related publicity with headlines such as 'Interferon: The cancer drug we have ignored' or 'New cancer weapon?' and 'Interferon: No miracles without more molecules'.[2] With additional interest shown by radio and television networks, this brought interferon out of the relative seclusion of the laboratory into the limelight of public attention, as we shall see in the next section.

The portrait conveyed most often and most vividly in the mass media showed interferon as a somewhat mysterious, clinically unharnessed, non-toxic natural body substance, claimed to be the hottest, though long ignored, line of biomedical research currently being followed. The idea generated by the media was that if only enough of this extremely scarce and expensive naturally-occurring protein could be made available, a kind of miracle cure for everything from cancer to the common cold was at hand. The double framing of interferon, as a natural solution to a dread disease and as the product of 'cutting-edge' biomedical research, was reinforced by the illustrations used in the media. A case in point was a photograph in *Newsweek* with the legend 'searching for the natural key to interferon' showing scientists in laboratory coats staring hopefully at a sophisticated laboratory set-up composed of a tangle of wires, tubes, retorts and graduated cylinders filled with fluids, seeing things that only they were supposed to recognise.[3] The public image of interferon as a promising product of laboratory-supported scientific medicine was not dissimilar to the associations and legitimisations presented by interferon researchers to their scientific audiences – linking state-of-the-art basic research with achieving future cures at the bedside.[4]

## About media, audiences and marketing medicines

Despite the sobering facts that underlay the bold headlines, the frequent associations of interferon with terms like 'medical breakthrough', 'cancer', 'wonder drug' and 'panacea', built the foundation for a global interferon mania. In addition, the fact that interferon was both costly and extremely hard to come by, and the knowledge that no other biological substance could match interferon's extraordinary biological activity, all encouraged the popular belief that interferon must be highly effective. Most of these descriptions in the media were directly or indirectly inspired by optimistic statements by interferon researchers, though they did their best to pepper their public declarations with 'if', 'could', and 'might'. The claims by genetic engineering firms and leading molecular biologists about the imminent possibility of making available, in large quantities and at modest cost, substances such as interferon that were expensive or difficult to make, intensified public interest.[5]

The race to clone the interferon gene was fascinating in its own right; not because it was one of the first medically significant human genes to be cloned, nor because it proved that genetic engineering had passed, as the *Wall Street Journal* put it, 'from science-fiction fantasy to fact'.[6] Rather, it was the metaphor of a race, in combination with both the promises of a new and wondrous production technology and of a billion-dollar miracle molecule, that made interferon so fascinating for the general public.[7]

The euphoria reached a peak after Biogen and the Schering-Plough Corporation announced at a joint skilfully orchestrated press conference at the Park Plaza Hotel in Boston on 19 January 1980 that through the use of genetic engineering the molecular biologist, Charles Weissmann, and his team were the first to succeed in getting bacteria to produce human interferon in biologically active form. While admitting that there were still a lot of questions to be answered, such as the extent to which the rDNA-made interferon was different from natural interferon, Nobel Prize winner Walter Gilbert, a Harvard professor and chairman of the board of Biogen, predicted that within one or two years the mass production of interferon for use in clinical trials would be feasible.[8]

During the next days and months the story appeared on the front pages of most American newspapers and magazines, and others around the world – in France, Great Britain, and the Netherlands – ran major pieces on it.[9] The event was described by Nicholas Wade in Science in terms of a 'cloning gold rush' that turned molecular biology into big business – with biotechnology stocks rising to record levels in the international stock markets. Popular magazines talked about genetic engineering as the solution to the problem of producing a 'priceless miracle drug'.[10] Cancer centres in America and Europe were inundated with requests for interferon. Countless desperate patients and their families were begging hospitals, doctors, research centres and drug companies to provide them with the new wonder drug.

The interferon mania only added to the media interest: 'Wonder drug hope of Miss Anneli; Amazing case book of the wonder drug doctor', 'Dad's wonder drug plea' and 'Drug brings hope for tumour boy Daniel'.[11] Personification of scientific medicine and disease - projecting the inherent benevolence of medical science on individual scientists, doctors and patients – was a powerful rhetorical tool that journalists routinely used but which helped to maintain and intensify the interferon furore. Imagery replaced content in most cases. Journalists eagerly reproduced the analogy popular among interferon researchers: comparing interferon's move from the laboratory into the clinic with the long, obstacle-filled road that penicillin travelled from Fleming's laboratory to the pharmacist's shelf.[12]

All segments of society had a part in the hype. As Sandra Panem aptly portrayed the situation:

> scientists who genuinely believed that they were on the right track and that money solicited at the expense of candour would be wisely used; investors and the public who wanted interferon to be a wonder drug and did not choose to ask whether the claims might be overstated; and those representatives of the media who reported anecdotes with unbridled enthusiasm.[13]

Until the Biogen announcement, the dramatic portrayal of interferon seemed to work to the advantage of all, and enormous amounts of energy and money were poured into efforts related to interferon in times of otherwise sharp financial cutbacks. However by the spring of 1980 the interferon wonder began to show signs of decay. Confronted by the stormy public reactions, doctors, researchers and the medical authorities began to regard the media frenzy as disturbing and problematic.

Every patient suffering from cancer or a severe virus disease wanted to have access to a drug that was in short supply and had yet to be tested. A lot of distress was involved. In their face-to-face contact with patients, doctors found themselves besieged by demands for a drug that they could not supply, and frustrated by hopes of a cure they could not deliver.[14] At centres where interferon was being tested everyone wanted to be in the trial and doctors had a hard time explaining that nobody could or would be favoured in their selection of trial candidates. In order to determine whether interferon had any 'real' efficacy they had to work in accordance with stringent testing protocols that implied that only patients meeting the highly specific trial requirements would be allowed to participate. In addition, the doctors involved in testing interferon feared that the high hopes of 'the chosen' could affect the scientific validity of clinical trials - their test subjects' own enthusiasm for interferon and their feelings after its administration might work against what was defined as 'objective benefit'.

Despite the fact that the excitement and motives of its own members had played an obvious part in the interferon mania, the medical profession swiftly left the media to carry the blame. Once defined as a threat to the practice of medicine and professional autonomy, physicians on both sides of the Atlantic started making public appeals for a moratorium on publicity about interferon. They were openly supported by the interferon community in their efforts to blame the journalists for raising patients' hopes through irresponsible reporting.[15] The primary concern of those working with interferon was that the continued media frenzy, which had initially worked to the advantage of interferon research, might in the end rebound to the discredit of interferon research itself.[16]

At the same time, medical research organisations, like the British Medical Research Council (MRC) and the Imperial Cancer Research Fund (ICRF), and health administrators, saw the public demands for interferon as a challenge to their authority to evaluate, register and supply drugs.[17] There were worries that private funding bodies and manufacturers would yield to public pressures to provide interferon outside the formal testing channels and, even worse, that a black market for interferon might develop.[18] The authorities realised that it was hard to explain to a patient with cancer that there might be a more effective treatment in the pipeline, but that it could not be generally available for some years, until licensing procedures were completed, by which time he or she might be dead.[19]

Distribution of unlicensed interferon outside the approved medical trials was not only believed to undermine the drug evaluation process, but also the whole state-regulated drug testing practice – established in the 1960s to maintain certain quality and safety standards.[20] With the prospect of improving supplies it seemed even more difficult to resist the public's disinclination to wait and make sure that all available material would be channelled into the official trajectory of the controlled clinical studies that were required for the proper evaluation and licensing of new drugs.[21] Confronted with the desperate efforts of countless families and friends of cancer sufferers to obtain supplies of interferon at any price, the British Government and the major funding bodies for cancer research in the UK decided to issue a joint press notice in May 1980, cautioning against over-optimism and attempts at by-passing the formal drug evaluation route.[22]

In The Netherlands, however, things never reached the stage where the health authorities felt that they had to intervene. There was no influential tabloid journalism and hardly any Dutch companies or institutions had a stake in the development of interferon; there was therefore little breeding-ground for hype. The only prominent Dutch interferon researcher, Huub Schellekens, again and again publicly cautioned against over-excitement.[23]

It can be no accident that, while doctors and authorities were struggling to cope with what they regarded as mass hysteria about interferon, preliminary, unexciting results of the interferon clinical trials sponsored by the American Cancer Society were announced at the annual meeting of the American Association for Cancer Research.[24] The information made available cooled expectations by suggesting that interferon was no more active than other chemotherapeutic agents in treating breast cancer and multiple myeloma. Moreover, contrary to what was hoped for (in particular by outsiders who were sold on interferon as a non-toxic agent), adverse effects were reported similar to those of other cancer medications; the patient who responded best was said to suffer the most serious adverse effects, such as abnormal liver function and even cardiac toxicity, and therapy had to be interrupted.[25] These results placed interferon in perspective, just like any of the many substances being tested for anti-tumour activity.

The redefinition of interferon as a potentially harmful experimental treatment with uncertain therapeutic benefits proved effective in undermining its public image as a wonder drug and put a lid on 'the unquenchable desire for interferon by cancer victims'.[26] The media immediately picked up the message with headlines such as 'Interferon: studies put cancer use in doubt', 'Is it a wonder cure for cancer or the most expensive flop in history?'[27] Unqualified optimism quickly shifted to the other extreme by casting doubt on interferon's potential.

## Beyond interferon

As might be expected, the people working on interferon tried as hard as they could to account for the disappointments in order to safeguard funding. Interferon researchers conveyed the impression that with more questions than answers they were just beginning to explore the potential of interferon. The diversity of interferons with distinct and complementary activities seemed to grow every day, although clinical testing of the first interferon preparations produced with recombinant DNA (rDNA) technology had yet to start. The consensus view was that, although interferon as a single agent might turn out to be useful in treating viral infections, it might ultimately prove most valuable as part of the increasingly popular 'multi-modality' approach in cancer treatment. Interferons could then be used as biological enhancers – helping to increasing the host's own response against the tumour – in combination with the three main cancer therapies of surgery, chemotherapy, and radiation.[28]

By creating an image of interferon as a prototype of a promising, new, but still poorly understood area of cancer therapy known as immunotherapy – one that was going to play a significant role in future cancer practices – interferon promoters succeeded in establishing a more permanent base for support. The overall message was, as a science reporter of the *Washington Post* aptly expressed it in his headline, 'Beyond Interferon'.[29] Cancer treatment centres that aspired to maintain an image of being at the cutting edge of the field of clinical oncology could not afford not to study an experimental therapy that was closely linked with the latest developments in tumour biology and molecular biology.[30] Only the relative scarcity and impurity of interferon preparations withheld them from pursuing interferon research more actively. They waited for the more pure and homogeneous interferons produced from rDNA to become more widely available.

The apparently unremitting optimism within scientific quarters contrasted with the growing scepticism about interferon's potential among senior executives in pharmaceutical companies. Of the 20 or more firms that had announced their intention of investing in interferon development back in 1979, a growing number ceased work on interferon over the period of one year, namely during 1983. They had either lost out in the 'cloning race' or management had negatively assessed interferon's potential both as a therapeutic drug, and as a means to attract capital investment from the stock markets.[31]

•

In the boardrooms of the three 'interferon champions' that had most heavily invested in the substance – the Burroughs Wellcome Company and most notably Hoffmann-La Roche and Schering-Plough – interferon's lacklustre clinical performance in treating tumours as well as virus infections was reason for growing concern.[32] The company officials responsible for investment in interferon had a hard time defending the costly interferon research and development (R & D) programmes. However, they succeeded in convincing the sceptics in management that although interferon might not be a 'magic bullet' in itself, it had enormous potential as a prototype of a new generation of custom-designed biosynthetic drugs that were expected to generate a therapeutic revolution. The promise of scientific and therapeutic innovation appealed most to senior drug company executives, who were less worried about today's profits than about tomorrow's prospects. With patents on most of their top prescription medicines expiring by 1990 and with few potential 'blockbuster' products in the pipeline, drug companies had come to recognise that a new wave of innovation was needed to position themselves for long-term survival.[33]

However, those responsible for the interferon-related R & D programmes were not able to get round the iron business rule of profit generation. The pressure for return on investments in interferon research and development forced the interferon advocates within the companies to adapt their R & D strategies. In line with government-supported research programmes, the pharmaceutical industry focused on interferon as a prototype of a new generation of tailor-made recombinant biologicals to be used as therapeutics in a new kind of disease management: immunotherapy within a multi-modality treatment framework. Apparently the drug companies recognised the strategic and commercial importance of taking advantage of the more general move across medicine towards combination therapy.[34]

However, the regulatory authorities found the combined-modality approach difficult to assess, as their evaluative practice and standards were still governed by a single-agent therapeutic philosophy. For interferon to be considered legally as a new therapeutic drug, it had to be evaluated officially as a single agent. This implied that before licensing procedures could be taken into consideration, the companies had to look for a disease, rare though it might be, that justified a need for interferon.[35]

•

*About media, audiences and marketing medicines*

## Promoting the use of interferon

In the search for suitable diseases as candidates for interferon as a treatment, the drug companies actively supported clinical trials to evaluate the effects of interferon in as wide a variety of diseases as possible. They offered clinical investigators worldwide large quantities, free-of-charge, of their interferon products. Interferons were tested in hepatitis B, various lymphomas, breast cancer, prostatic cancer, multiple sclerosis, *Herpes* keratitis, malaria, AIDS, and many other cancer and virus-related diseases.[36] By the end of 1983 the large-scale testing efforts finally seemed to show signs of paying off. Drug company officials swung into action as soon as the news broke in the fall of 1983 that Jordan Gutterman's research group in the M.D. Anderson Hospital and Tumour Institute in Houston (Texas, USA) had achieved a higher than 80 per cent trial response to 'natural' alfa interferon therapy in patients with a rare form of chronic leukaemia known as 'hairy-cell leukaemia'.[37]

The knowledge that there was hardly any effective treatment for this form of cancer, with estimated mortality rates of about 15 per cent per year, sufficed for those looking for a suitable disease indication.[38] They seemed to take it for granted that among clinical oncologists scepticism prevailed about the overwhelming efficacy claim by Gutterman, who had earned himself a name for over optimistic interpretation of interferon trial data.[39] The companies' first priority was to demonstrate that the dramatic clinical effect could be reproduced by other clinical researchers. Following extensive clinical testing they ultimately succeeded. Consequently licence applications were sent for evaluation to drug regulatory agencies such as the FDA, the British Committee on Safety of Medicines, and the Dutch College ter Beoordeling van Geneesmiddelen.[40]

In 1986, once the FDA, swiftly followed by the British and Dutch regulatory agencies, had licensed Hoffmann La Roche's and Schering-Plough's recombinant alfa interferon products for the treatment of hairy cell leukaemia, the marketing branches of the companies were fully activated as a means to establishing a growing need for interferon.[41] The way in which the companies presented interferon by means of a combination of visuals and narrative to doctors, decision-makers and journalists in the specialist press drew on the same range of images that had influenced the public perception of interferon through the mass media: framing interferon both as a naturally occurring substance in the body and as a state-of-the-art product of modern science and technology.

In 1986 the Dutch interferon researcher Huub Schellekens predicted that interferon would be used more widely within ten years than might be expected on the basis of the approved list of indications, because of the psychology of interferon as a potential 'multi-drug' from the common cold to cancer.[42] Schering-Plough and Roche of course fully endorsed this perceived mechanism and were keen to turn it into a self-fulfilling prophesy. With the relentless support of the drug industry and patients in desperate need of a cure, and through the combination of scientific drive and professional ambition, clinical oncologists and infectious disease specialists in particular continued to change the designs of trials. They tried different combinations (e.g. with cytotoxic drugs or various biological response modifiers) and different routes and durations of administration.[43] In doing so they ultimately tinkered towards success. Fuelled by a potent combination of scientific drive, professional ambition, marketing efforts and a lot of hard work between bench and bedside, interferon was transformed from an orphan-drug into a billion-dollar molecule.

## Conclusions

An important institutional link in the network of relationships that developed around interferon is the role played by the media. I have shown how the media stressed and added certain aspects and thereby contributed to the continual process of reshaping the meaning of interferon. Interferon stories in the media are characterised by one major script, which centres on the theme of 'breakthrough'. Initially the media highlighted the dramatic curative potential of interferon against the dread disease cancer. They framed interferon as a somewhat mysterious and scarce non-toxic body substance, which exerted its anti-tumour effects in a natural way, and at the same time as the latest promising product of laboratory-supported scientific medicine. Subsequently, attention shifted to interferon as the most promising demonstration of a revolutionary production technology, genetic engineering. I described how, by inflating the imaginative combination of two wondrous products of modern science and medicine, the media helped to trigger an international interferon mania. However, I want to stress that, except for a general tendency to reinforce and overstate interferon's promise, the media coverage of interferon was for the greater part a mirror of the expectations, legitimisations and opinions circulating within the biomedical and public realm. A case in point is the difference in reporting between Britain and the Netherlands.

The active, intermediary role of the media is also well illustrated by the turn in the nature of reporting during the early-1980s. Following the dissemination of information in Britain and the USA, specially designed to lower public expectations, the nature of the stories in the press rapidly shifted from medical zealotry in promoting interferon's benefits to the other end of the spectrum: disillusionment about a failed promise.

I then showed how, confronted with the quick erosion of public support, the interferon promotors developed alternative strategies to legitimise work on interferon. Instead of the presumed non-toxic nature of interferon, its perceived unique capacity as a biological agent acting through the immune system was used to attract attention. Moreover, interferon was presented as having an important advantage over conventional therapies: it linked the clinics to advanced laboratory research in tumour biology, molecular biology and immunology. I dubbed the rhetorical strategy that proved effective in establishing a more permanent base for support 'beyond interferon': picturing interferon as a first step towards constituting a medicine of tomorrow.

However, in order to become accepted, interferon needed a therapeutic profile and treatment concept that could be integrated or combined with existing therapeutic practices. In positioning interferon as a helpful and natural *adjunct*, compatible with, and supportive of, existing treatment practices, the pharmaceutical industry succeeded in having interferon relatively quickly absorbed by the medical infrastructure, requiring increasingly large amounts of money for its use. As a consequence, opposition to interferon therapy currently revolves less around questions of need than around questions of cost or economic feasibility that increasingly dominate the political agenda of 'marketplace' medicine in Britain and the Netherlands.[44] However, as the chapter on economic aspects of interferon in the 1997 book, *The Clinical Applications of the Interferons*, shows, economic and commercial considerations are easily linked to medical discourse and are therefore difficult to separate from medical arguments that show the need for interferon treatment.[45]

## Notes

1. For extensive accounts of the early development of interferon, see T. Pieters, 'Interferon and its First Clinical Trial: Looking behind the Scenes', *Medical History*, 37 (1993), 270–95; T. Pieters, 'History of the Development of the Interferons: From Test-tube to Patient', in R. Stuart-Harris and R. Penny (eds.) *The Clinical Applications of Interferons* (London: Chapman & Hall, 1997), 1–19.
2. 'New Cancer Weapon?', Newsweek, (18 September 1978), 90–1; J. Hixson, 'Interferon: The Cancer Drug We Have Ignored', *New York Magazine*, (4 September 1978), 59-64; K. White, 'Interferon: No Miracles Without More Molecules', *Medical Tribune*, (18 October 1978).
3. *Newsweek, op. cit.* (note 2).
4. Discussing the interleukine-2 hype of the mid 1980s, Ilana Löwy noted similar connections between the public and the scientific realm. I. Löwy, *Between Bench and Bedside* (Cambridge, MA: Harvard University Press, 1996), 158.
5. Early in September 1978 the public announcement of the cloning of the first medically significant human gene to make human insulin hit the headlines, was said to open up a new and most exciting era in biology, and only added to the public interest for interferon. V. Cohn, 'Scientists in California Create Gene to Make Human Insulin', *The Washington Post*, (7 September 1978).
6. H. Lancaster, 'Potent Protein; Medical Researchers Say the Drug Interferon Holds Great Promise', *The Wall Street Journal*, (6 December 1979).
7. This is nicely illustrated by a cover story of *Newsweek* magazine entitled 'DNA's New Miracles'; "By turning bacteria into living factories scientists can cure disease and create new forms of life"; *Newsweek*, (17 March 1980).
8. N. Wade, 'Cloning Gold Rush Turns Basic Biology into Big Business', *Science*, 208 (1980), 688–92; S. Andreopoulos, 'Sounding Board: Gene Cloning by Press Conference', *New England Journal of Medicine*, 302 (1980), 743–6.
9. 'Medical Breakthrough Reported', *Los Angeles Times*, 21 January 1980; 'L'interferon: Enjeu d'une Competition Mondiale Scientifique et Industrielle', *Le Monde*, (6 February 1980); 'Cancer Treatment Available Soon', *Guardian*, (20 March 1980); The Big If-interferon', *The Listener*, 29 February 1980; 'Interferon Duurste Stof ter Wereld', *Telegraaf*, (29 mei 1980); 'The Making of a Miracle Drug', *Newsweek*, (28 January 1980); interview with K. Cantell, (4 May

1992), Helsinki; interview with J. Sonnabend, (13 November 1993), New York.
10. Wade, *op. cit.* (note 8); Anonymous, 'At only $100 Million a Gram, This 'Miracle' has a Future', *Science Digest*, (April 1980).
11. '"Wonder" Drug Hope of Miss Anneli', *Sunday Mirror*, (1 June 1980); 'Dad's Wonder Drug Plea', *Sunday Mirror*, (8 June 1980); and 'Drug Brings Hope for Tumour Boy Daniel', *Daily Telegraph*, (12 April 1980).
12. K. Cantell, 'Why is Interferon not in Clinical Use Today?', in I. Gresser (ed.) *Interferon* (London: Academic Press, 1979), 2–28, 3.
13. S. Panem, *The Interferon Crusade* (Washington, DC: Brookings Institution, 1984), 99.
14. Anonymous, 'Publicity on Interferon has Caused Great Distress', *The Times*, (10 June 1980).
15. Editorial, 'What not to Say about Interferon', *Nature*, 285 (1980), 603–4.
16. M. Edelhart, *Interferon: The New Hope for Cancer* (Reading, MA: Addison-Wesley Publishing Company, 1981), 1–9; Anonymous, 'Interferon: The Hopes and the Reality', *BMA News Review*, (September 1980), 18–22.
17. Letter from the Department of Education and Science to Sir John Eden, MP, 12 June 1980, MRC Archives File No. S806/5.
18. A flourishing black market rapidly developed in often dubious interferon samples, fuelled by those rich, famous and desperate enough to try anything like the dying film hero, John Wayne, and the dying, exiled, Shah of Iran.
19. Letter from MRC to ICRF, 23 June 1980, MRC Archives File No. D1009/40.
20. MRC internal note, 23 June 1980, MRC Archives File No. D1009/40
21. Interview with J. Petricciani, 6 November 1993, Cambridge, MA; interview with D. Tyrrell, 21 May 1990, Salisbury, Hampshire, UK.
22. MRC internal note, 27 June 1980, MRC Archives File No. D1009/40; Press notice, 13 May 1980, MRC Archives File No. D1009/40.
23. F. Conggrijp, 'Interferon is Duurste Stof ter Wereld', *Telegraaf*, 29 mei 1980; E. Boer, 'Interferon – Wordt Huid Verkocht voor de Beer is Geschoten?', *NRC-Handelsblad*, 14 mei 1980; 'Anti-virusmiddel Stap Dichterbij', *Volkskrant*, (16 mei 1980).
24. Anonymous, 'Interferon Results "Promising", ACS will Commit Additional $3.4 Million', *The Cancer Letter*, (22 February 1980).
25. Anonymous, 'Interferon Results Cool Expectations', *The Cancer*

*Letter*, (6 June 1980).
26. M. Edelhart, *Interferon: The New Hope for Cancer* (Reading, MA: Addison-Wesley Publishing Company, 1981), 6.
27. H. M. Schmeck, 'Interferon: Studies Put Cancer Use in Doubt', *New York Times*, 27 May 1980; Anonymous, 'Is it a Wonder Cure for Cancer or the Most Expensive Flop in History?', *Daily Star*, (19 June 1980).
28. S. Krown, 'Prospects for the Treatment of Cancer with Interferon', in J. Burchenal and H. Oettgen (eds), *Cancer: Achievements, Challenges, and Prospects for the 1980s* (New York: Grune & Stratton, 1981), 367–79; R. Johnson, 'Interferon: Cloudy but Intriguing Future', *Journal of the American Medical Association*, 245 (1981), 109–16; P. Newmark, 'Interferon: Decline and Stall', *Nature*, 291 (1981), 105–6; M. Sun, 'Interferon: No Magic Bullet Against Cancer', *Science*, 212 (1981), 141–2.
29. C. Fenyvesi, 'Beyond Interferon', *The Washington Post*, (14 June 1981), 28.
30. Interview with Ernest Borden, 12 October 1992, Wisconsin.
31. T. Powledge, 'Interferon on Trial', *Biotechnology*, (March 1984), 214–28.
32. In 1983 Hoffmann-La Roche and Schering-Plough reportedly allocated 15 percent of their research budgets – more than $40 million each – to interferon; Powledge, *op. cit.* (note 31); Interview with N. Finter (Wellcome), 25 May 1990, Beckenham, Kent, UK; interview with L. Gauci (Hoffmann-La Roche), 18 June 1990 in Basle.
33. Powledge, *op. cit.* (note 31); A. Wycke, 'Molecules and Markets', *The Economist*, (7 February 1987); Gauci, *op. cit.* (note 32); and, interview with J. Warbeer (Schering-Plough), 24 June 1988, Brussels.
34. Petriccianni, *op.cit.* (note 21); and Gauci, *op.cit.* (note 32).
35. *Op. cit.* (note 34). For similar cases of drugs looking for diseases, see R. Vos, *Drugs Looking for Diseases. Innovative Drug research and the Development of the Beta Blockers and the Calcium Antagonists* (Amsterdam: Kluwer Academic Publishers, 1991); N. Oudshoorn, *Beyond the Natural Body: Archeology of Sex Hormones* (New York: Routledge, 1994).
36. 'Interferon May Help AIDS Victims', *New Scientist*, (3 November 1983); 'Interferon Tested on Sclerosis', *The New York Times*, (21 November, 1981); and, N. Finter and R. K. Oldham (eds), *Interferon, In Vivo and Clinical Studies*, vol. 4, (Amsterdam: Elsevier, 1985); 'Update on Interferon', *News Service American Cancer Society*,

dated 11 February 1983, NCI Archives File No. DC8301-006691; and, 'Intron A', press information video tape produced by Schering-Plough in 1986 on the occasion of the market introduction of their interferon product.

37. J. Quesada, E. Hersh and J. Gutterman, 'Hairy Cell Leukemia: Induction of Remission with Alpha Interferon', *Blood*, 62 (1983), 207a.

38. J. Quesada, J. Reuben, J. Manning et al, 'Alfa Interferon for Induction of Remission in Hairy Cell Leukemia', *New England Journal of Medicine*, 310 (1984), 15–18;. Petriccianni, *op. cit.* (note 21); Gauci, *op. cit.* (note 32).

39. Powledge, *op. cit.* (note 31), 227.

40. 'Anticancer Interferon Available Soon', *Hospital Doctor*, (22 September 1983). In contrast to interferon products that were still in the investigational stage and limited in their clinical use (phase I, II, III testing), licensed products that would be available for general commercial distribution and use by the medical profession must meet a variety of extra regulatory requirements, at least in the United States, as prescribed by the Good Manufacturing Practice (GMP) provisions and the General Provisions for Licensed Biologicals (GPLB) Code of Federal Regulations; J. Petricciani, E. Esber, H. Hopps *et al*, 'Manufacture and Safety of Interferons in Clinical Research' in P. Came and W. Carter (eds), *Interferons and their Applications* (Berlin: Springer-Verlag, 1984), 357–70, 359.

41. Interview with T. Pike (Hoffmann-La Roche), 22 June 1990, Basle.

42. See interview with Schellekens included on 'Intron A', press information video tape produced by Schering-Plough in 1986 on the occasion of the market introduction of their interferon product.

43. C. Pinsky (ed.), 'Biological Response Modifiers', *Seminars in Oncology*, 13 (1986), 131–227; D. Parkinson (ed.), 'The Expanding Role of Interferon-Alfa in the Treatment of Cancer', *Seminars in Oncology*, 21 (1994), 1–37; Stuart-Harris and Penny, *op. cit.* (note 1).

44. Anonymous, 'In Parliament: Beta Interferon', *Bulletin of Medical Ethics*, (March 1998), 2.

45. A. Shiell and G. Salkeld, 'The Economic Aspects of Interferon', in Stuart-Harris and Penny, *op. cit.* (note 1).

# 12

## The billion dollar molecule:
## Taxol in historical and theoretical perspective[1]

*Vivien Walsh and Jordan Goodman*

One of the few organic compounds which, like benzene and aspirin, is recognisable by name to the average citizen.[2]

Taxol is an anti-cancer drug available in clinics throughout the world for the treatment of ovarian and breast cancer. Approval for some other types of cancer has either been granted or is pending, depending on the country concerned, while clinical trials for other uses continue worldwide. Taxol is the best-selling anti-cancer drug in history, world sales having reached $1.2 billion in 1998,[3] the first time an anti-cancer drug has had sales as high as a billion dollars. Taxol is made and sold by Bristol-Myers Squibb, the world's largest supplier of anti-cancer drugs and fourth largest pharmaceutical company.[4] In most countries the company essentially sets the price of the drug, and taxol is its second largest pharmaceutical earner, contributing around ten per cent to its total drug sales.

To make sure that the world knows that taxol is the property of Bristol-Myers Squibb, the name Taxol® was registered as a trademark on 26 May 1992 and the name paclitaxel was created for all uses that did not refer explicitly to that company's product. This was despite the fact that for the first thirty years its research and development was carried out in the public sector, largely funded and managed by the US Government. Taxol became the property of Bristol-Myers Squibb in the first place when the firm entered into a series of Co-operative Research And Development Agreements (hereafter CRADAs) in 1991 with various agencies of the US Government to develop taxol commercially.

This paper is about medical–biological objects, and the process by which they emerge through practice to become innovations. We explore narratives other than the dominant story of taxol, oft-repeated in both the scientific and popular press: those other narratives that might have been enacted but in fact were not. We examine the tension between public knowledge and private property, in the appropriation as private property of a drug that had been developed in the public sector practically to the point of commercial production. We analyse the way in which the drug taxol has changed its identity, its status as property and even its name, since it first came to the attention of western science in the 1960s. Over the following 30 years taxol kept being made and remade, and at each stage of this process it had different people speaking for it, claiming it as theirs, taking possession of it, and giving it a different name. Finally we consider taxol's co-existence with its source, *Taxus brevifolia*, the Pacific yew tree in whose bark it was first found, and the changing identity and status as property of the tree as they co-evolved with those of taxol.

## The cultural biography of an object

In exploring the way in which taxol has changed its identity, its status as property and its name, we may be said to be writing its biography. Igor Kopytoff, in writing about the process of commoditisation, argues that objects, like people, have biographies:

> ....an eventful biography of a thing becomes the story of the various singularisations of it, of classifications and reclassifications in an uncertain world of categories whose importance shifts with every minor change in context. As with persons, the drama here lies in the uncertainties of valuation and of identity.[5]

Contingency, or non-essentialism, is central to Kopytoff's ideas about the biography of objects,[6] and his approach appealed to us because this is an important feature of the story of taxol, too. In the social studies of science appeals to take account of, and incorporate, contingency have been made by a variety of authors, and from several disciplinary perspectives, including Steve Shapin,[7] Donald MacKenzie,[8] Paul David,[9] David Noble[10] and Donna Haraway.[11] However, the only other attempt to apply Kopytoff's ideas to pharmaceuticals, as far as we know, has followed life cycles within prescribed stages rather than revealing events as contingent.[12] This paper explores two of the paths that were taken as the stories of taxol unfolded in the USA and France, revealing the dominant narrative of taxol as contingent: things might have been otherwise.

Any conceptual framework within which the evolution of taxol is to be revealed must recognise the contingency of the actors, but the model of personal biography does not quite accommodate taxol's peculiar state of co-existence with its source, *Taxus brevifolia*, nor its ability to appear in different roles in different milieux at the same time and to have different identities over time. We have chosen to combine biography with the approach of actor-network theory, in which the distinction between objects and humans is not given, but made and remade; and which offers the research and narrative strategy of following the object wherever it leads, thus allowing a relationally-based biography to be constructed.[13] Instead of settling on one trajectory in time, or dissecting the object and its situation into different categories or compartments, Latour suggests that the 'fragile thread' of the object's associations, or the transformations of the various actors involved in the story, are simply followed through the various networks of which they are a part.[14] 'Following the actors' also has resonances with George Marcus's 'multi-sited ethnography' in the field of anthropology.[15]

The recognition of the inherent instability and contingency of the actors and their networks, which are constantly regrouping and forming new objects and new networks, is a central tenet of actor-network theory. This ability to deal with transformation and change is one of its advantages. A network in this approach is not a predictable series of linkages of well defined, stable elements; instead the components can at any moment redefine their identity and their mutual relationships in a new way, and bring new elements into the network. 'An actor network is simultaneously an *actor* whose activity is networking heterogeneous elements, and a *network* that is able to redefine and transform what it is made of'(emphasis added).[16] Other useful notions specific to actor-network theory include 'enrolment',[17] or the process by which an actor enlists other participants into the network, so that the other actors are convinced that they will be able to realise all their separate aims by the achievement of a common goal, with which all their interests become bound up; 'translation', in which the goals of the project are presented to the new actors to be enrolled in such a way that they will be seen as equivalent to their own various specific aims; and 'obligatory passage points' which are the 'unavoidable conduits through which they (the actors) must pass in order to articulate both their identity and their raison d'être'.[18]

Actor–network theory allows things as well as humans to be actors, but, as Callon and Law say 'by themselves, things don't act. Indeed ...there are no things "by themselves" ...instead there are relations, relations which (sometimes) make things'.[19] All the interests of the other actors, people and things, techniques, instruments and so on, are inscribed on the object. The object becomes like an archive, a text of all the actors and events that have gone before.

Marilyn Strathern makes a similar point when she says that, of their own accord,

> things fetishize people's past decisions.... The thing itself will identify what people have to be mobilised... You do not necessarily want to reopen all the negotiations. You do not reinvent the conventions of commerce with strangers each time you handle money. It is there in the banknote.[20]

Biography in Kopytoff's terms is based on the changing meanings given to an object by successive users, but he does not make reference to the network of which the object is a part. The actor-network approach, on the other hand, does not make property and ownership endogenous attributes of the network, nor does it analyse them in its terms, although successions of identities achieved when a series of inscriptions is made on an object might constitute an example of what John Law calls 'relational materiality'.[21] Kopytoff does introduce the notions of property, ownership and property rights, but these are seen primarily as enabling, in the sense of delivering meaning. Without reference to the network, it might seem that the succession of meanings is random, rather than cumulative. But if a network perspective is introduced, without property and ownership being introduced as endogenous attributes of the network, the object's position within the network remains unproblematic.

Marilyn Strathern writes from an anthropological perspective, which shows how centralising ideas about property can make a useful contribution to actor-network approaches.[22] Placing property and ownership as a product and essential feature of the network has potentially profound effects for network translations, and has distinct advantages for understanding how networks may be cut, and how the actor-network of *Taxus brevifolia* was indeed cut on two occasions during the stories we unfold. The story of taxol helps to illuminate connections between objects, networks and property. By following taxol, we can identify the interests different actors have had in it, and the decisions that have been made, or not made, as these are inscribed on the object. Its identity at any point in time is determined by and inseparable from the network of practitioners who are associated with it. It is, therefore, not possible to speak of taxol as a final object, but only an object in the process of emergence. To define its characteristics at any time requires capturing it during this process. In what follows we explore the way in which taxol changed its identity and its status as property in the course of appropriation firstly by the state, claiming to represent 'the public', and then by private industry. We return now to the moment when the object that was to be called taxol was about to be revealed for the first time to Western science and medicine.

### What's in a name?

Taxol is not just an anti-cancer drug: it is also a molecule found in the bark and some other parts of the Taxus species, commonly known as the yew. It is most concentrated in the Pacific Yew or *Taxus brevifolia*, found in the temperate rainforest of the Pacific Northwest, from Northern California to British Columbia. Taxol and *Taxus brevifolia* co-evolved over millennia, but both remained hidden from modern Western science and medicine until relatively recently. They were revealed as part of an inter-agency agreement between the National Cancer Institute (NCI) and the US Department of Agriculture (USDA), to collect plants worldwide and screen them as potential anti-cancer agents. The agreement lasted from 1960 to 1981, during which time some 115,000 extracts from 15,000 plant species had been tested for activity (still only representing an estimated six per cent of the world's plant species). Taxol is so far the only plant product screened as part of that programme to have reached the clinic.

USDA botanist Arthur Barclay and a small team collected samples from *Taxus brevifolia* in Washington State in 1962. The strategy was to sample everything. At this point the 'name' given to the collection of *Taxus brevifolia* was the USDA number B-1645, with separate accession numbers for the different samples: PR-4959 for the twigs, needles and fruit, and PR-4960 for the reddish stembark. The samples were dried and sent to the extraction laboratory under contract to the NCI, from which crude plant extracts were made and sent to other NCI sub-contractors to test for potential anti-cancer activity. In 1964 the extract of PR-4960 showed cytotoxic activity, on which basis it was sent to Monroe Wall and colleagues at the Research Triangle Institute, North Carolina, also working under contract to the NCI, who undertook the task of isolating the compound responsible for the observed activity. The crude plant extract, a crimson liquid, was given a name in accordance with NCI protocol: NSC670549. Meanwhile, the USDA focused its attention on the source, *Taxus brevifolia*, gathering not only its bark but also information about the tree and its habitat. Bob Perdue, in charge of the plant programme at USDA, regularly reminded his collaborators that the objectives of the plant screening programme were not only to get plant products to the clinic as anti-cancer drugs, but to get those plants to crop status. He was therefore concerned to investigate *Taxus* species that could be cultivated as an alternative to wild *Taxus brevifolia*.

Wall's laboratory began separating fractions of the extract, the most active being that labelled F021. In 1966 they isolated a white crystalline substance – indicating that it was a pure compound – which they now designated K172 (NCI nomenclature gives pure compounds a 'K' prefix). A chemists' label was also attached to K172: the molecular formula $C_{23}H_{26}O_7$, which was tentatively proposed to indicate the proportions of the atoms making up the molecule. In 1967, Wall decided on the name taxol for the crystals isolated from the active extracts of *Taxus brevifolia* stembark. The first published reference to the name 'taxol' was in a paper published in 1969,[23] the year the NCI officially adopted taxol as its molecule by giving it a new 'name': NSC125973. By 1970 Wall and Wani had revised the molecular formula for taxol as $C_{47}H_{51}NO_{14}$, and proposed a structure that would describe the arrangement in space of this combination of atoms, published in 1971, which we have reproduced as Figure 12.1. It had the taxane ring structure common to taxane alkaloids (natural products from the *Taxus* species) but also a side chain essential to its activity. Figure 12.1 is a representation of taxol of a kind that conveys meaning to chemists in particular: as a result of their experience and tacit knowledge they can deduce information about its likely reactivity with other chemicals, how it might be made in the laboratory (and with what problems) and even whether it is likely to be toxic or looks like a molecule with potential for further investigation as a drug. By representing taxol in this way, the chemists in some senses made it theirs, requiring translation to explain to non-chemists what the diagram signified.

So, in the manner of a relay race, *Taxus brevifolia* passed its bark to Arthur Barclay and the USDA in 1962, who passed it to Monroe Wall in 1964 via other sub-contractors; Wall, in turn, passed the molecule to the NCI in 1971 to be put through further analysis. The change in title to the object was signified by changes in its 'name': B-1645, PR-4959 & PR-4960, NSC 670549, F021, K172, $C_{23}H_{26}O_7$, NSC 125973, $C_{47}H_{51}NO_{14}$, and the structural formula shown in Figure 12.1. Taxol had changed from what was, to humans in industrial societies, an unknown, unidentified substance that had some purpose for the protection or survival of either *Taxus brevifolia* as a species or the individual yew tree, through these various stages, to an NCI designated compound with a name; a crystalline structure; various physical and chemical properties; a new chemical formula;

*The billion dollar molecule*

*Figure 12.1*
*A chemist's two-dimensional representation of the three dimensional structure of taxol: ceci n'est pas une molécule*

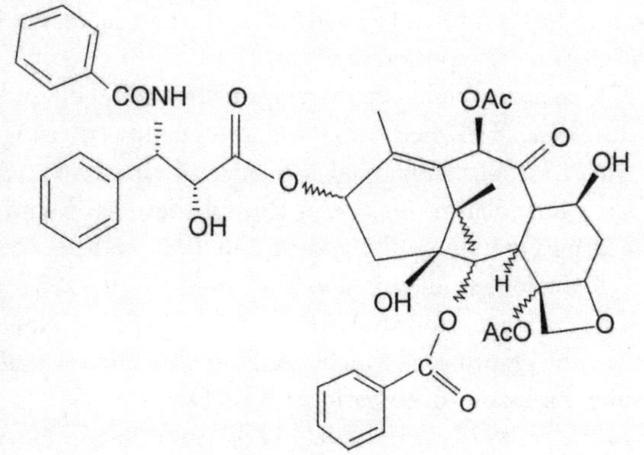

> We have labelled Figure 12.1 'Ceci n'est pas une molécule' after the surrealist paintings 'Ceci n'est pas une pomme' and 'Ceci n'est pas une pipe' by Magritte. He was making the point that his pictures were representations of an apple and a pipe, rather than a real apple or a real pipe. However, anyone who knew either of Magritte's representations would be able to recognise a real apple or pipe from them. In the case of the molecular diagram, however, it bears no obvious relation, certainly not visually, to the white crystals which are known as 'pure taxol'. This kind of representation is a theoretical conceptualisation of atoms, molecules and structure, which acts as a shorthand to chemists, but is meaningless to anyone who has not been 'initiated'. And even with the necessary chemical knowledge, it would not be possible to recognise the crystals as taxol as a result of seeing the diagram.

and a (chemical) architect's diagram representing the three dimensional arrangement of the atoms in space. Meanwhile the USDA was promoting another identity for taxol, that of a natural product residing in the bark of a living organism, and the implications of that, such as the desirability of knowing more about *Taxus brevifolia*, other *Taxus* species, and the occurrence of taxol; and of investigating cultivation.

•

## From molecule to drug

But the stories are not over yet. In 1971 the molecule was handed over to another part of the NCI's Cancer Chemotherapy National Service Center (CCNSC) to begin its process through the NCI's decision network: from assays with mouse tumours to the filing of an application to begin human trials in 1982, the first successful results of which began to be reported in 1988.

By 1978 taxol had shown activity against two difficult and slow-growing tumours, B16 melanoma and the mammary xenograft, a primary breast tumour implanted into specially bred mice. After a delay while a formulation for use in clinical trials was found, taxol became a Drug Development Candidate in 1980 and passed to the next stage, toxicology studies in laboratory animals. In 1982 it passed on to a further stage, approval for an Investigational New Drug Application, the granting of which would initiate clinical trials, and a new 'name' for taxol: Investigational New Drug.

Meanwhile, in 1977, samples had been sent to Susan Horwitz, a molecular pharmacologist at the Albert Einstein College of Medicine in New York, who was investigating the mechanism of biological activity of natural products with antitumour activity. She and her colleagues made the remarkable observation that taxol had a unique mechanism of action: its cytotoxic effects were caused by the molecule's ability to stabilise and inhibit the disassembly of the cell's microtubules, leading to the arrest of cell division. Cell biologists became very excited as they realised they had a new research tool with which to study cell dynamics, because the actions of microtubules remained suspended in the presence of taxol. At the same time, taxol's unique structure and mechanism of action offered the possibility of opening up a whole new area of cancer chemotherapy, based on other molecules with similar structures and mechanism of action. The NCI was flooded with requests for samples, and nearly 3,000 articles were published between 1980 and 1992.

While this was happening, the interaction between the NCI and the USDA, which focused attention on taxol as both a potential anticancer drug and as a natural product in a living organism, came to an end. The NCI had acted as the spokesperson of taxol as a potential anticancer drug, ensuring that this identity was revealed by the work of its sub-contractors and grant-holders, while the USDA, through its own network of sub-contracts and agency contacts, had supplied the bark from *Taxus brevifolia* and collected information about the tree and about the presence of taxol in other species of the

*Taxus* genus. Each participant had their own agenda, but continual negotiations and discussions ensured that they all worked for a common objective. When the inter-agency agreement was terminated by senior officials at the NCI in 1981, taxol was cut adrift from its identity as a natural product. The search for information about taxol across the *Taxus* genus was abandoned, and no further information was sought about the yew's habitat, the variety of *Taxus* species, how many Pacific yews there were, whether taxol could be obtained from renewable parts and/or from other species, or whether cultivation was a realistic option. Furthermore, the NCI had to make its own arrangements for the collection of bark.

## Contingent story

In France, however, both identities of taxol were kept in view. Pierre Potier, head of the Institut de Chimie des Substances Naturelles (ICSN) of the Centre National de la Recherche Scientifique (CNRS), was interested in natural products as potential anticancer agents and had been working on the synthesis of other antimitotic compounds when he read about Susan Horwitz's discovery of taxol's unique mechanism and the excitement it generated. He decided to look at taxol himself, curious about possible alternative sources. ICSN was situated in a park (also owned by CNRS) full of *Taxus baccata*, but, as he knew from Wall and Wani's 1971 publication, taxol was present in this species only in minute quantities. Potier thought it possible that he might find another substance in *Taxus baccata* needles that might act as a precursor for a semisynthetic route to taxol and new compounds related to taxol that might also have anticancer properties.

In 1980 ICSN signed a collaborative agreement with the chemical and pharmaceutical firm Rhône-Poulenc, to explore the chemistry of taxoids, to build structure-activity relationships, and to seek new and patentable anticancer compounds. Potier and colleagues extracted 10-deacetyl baccatin III (10-DAB), which was present in substantial concentrations and easy to isolate, with a yield much higher than that of taxol from dried bark. These results were reported in 1981. The significance of this paper for the future of taxol was that it used a renewable resource as its starting material, although that would not become an issue until later.

10-DAB had the familiar taxane ring structure, but it lacked the side chain found in taxol. Potier's group knew from Wall and Wani's work that both were essential for taxol's antitumour activity. The side chain, they thought, could be made synthetically and attached to

10-DAB to produce taxol. Meanwhile another CNRS research unit, that of Andrew Greene at Grenoble, had been working on other biologically active natural products. Pierre Potier proposed a collaborative project in which his group would isolate 10-DAB and work on any problems posed by the molecule's shape for attaching the side chain, while Greene's group would synthesise the side chain, and together they would combine both parts to form taxol. In 1985 the Grenoble group synthesised the side chain in the same orientation as it appeared in naturally occurring taxol. The next task was for the two groups to attach the side chain in exactly the right place (the thirteenth carbon atom, $C_{13}$), a non-trivial task since there were four carbon atoms where the side chain might have been attached and the desired one was the most difficult to get at. Taxol was finally prepared semisynthetically in 1988, and a patent was taken out in the name of CNRS by Rhône-Poulenc.[24]

## Clinical trials

Meanwhile, back in the USA, Phase I clinical trials of taxol had begun in April 1984 and a year later – the year in which Greene's group synthesised the taxol side chain – taxol passed through to Phase II clinical trials, which consumed a considerable amount of taxol. At this point the source of taxol, *Taxus brevifolia*, began to make itself felt as an actor in the US story again, as collecting and processing more bark became a matter of urgency. The National Forests were closed to logging and collecting over long periods of time, owing to acute fire risk, while sometimes the bark was of such poor quality that the yield of taxol was only a fraction of that anticipated. The forest, the sole source of taxol, demonstrated the extent to which it could not be tamed, could not be relied upon to deliver its supplies. Several Phase II trials, including that on breast cancer, chosen as a result of taxol's activity on the mammary xenograft, were suspended owing to lack of taxol.

In 1988, William McGuire at the Johns Hopkins Oncology Center reported that taxol had remarkable activity against ovarian cancer, the second largest killer of women and the least amenable to chemotherapy. Gordon Cragg of the NCI Natural Products branch reported: 'there is intense interest in taxol. People are begging for it.'[25] Bids for an unprecedented amount of bark were announced. At the same time, a growing concern about the plight of the Pacific Northwest's old growth forests raised environmental consciousness about *Taxus brevifolia*, and it became clear that environmental considerations would probably permit only one or two more large collections of dried bark.

Meanwhile, Taxol was competing for funds with other compounds in pre-clinical and clinical investigation and money was beginning to get very tight. Matthew Suffness, head of the Natural Products Branch of the NCI and generally viewed as taxol's 'product champion', reported in 1986 that the cost of working up the bark into taxol would be $1.5 million.[26] There was not enough money, for example, for research on alternative methods of producing taxol. The reports from clinical trials were thus both exciting and frightening. If taxol were to prove to be effective against the major cancers of the time, the demand for the drug in clinical use would be phenomenal. Whatever the population of *Taxus brevifolia* it was finite and being depleted. Cancer was not.

The lack of the information that the USDA might have collected, had it continued to be part of the network of actors playing out the taxol story, had now become a serious problem. The supply of enough bark and the extraction and purification of taxol for trials pushed the NCI to its limits, although it had continued to ignore the turn towards cultivated species that the program heads at USDA had proposed as early as the late-1960s. Neither did it consider exploring any other alternative routes. That bark had become an obligatory passage point, or locked in as the source of taxol, meant not just that alternative solutions to making taxol had receded; in addition, as demand for bark grew so did the mortality of *Taxus brevifolia*, since stripping bark kills the tree; and approval for clinical use would be made on the strict requirement that taxol was made from the bark using Good Manufacturing Practice, as approved in the New Drug Application. Taxol made in any other way would have to go through a new round of clinical trials and a new process of approval by the Food and Drug Administration (FDA).

Matthew Suffness expressed his anxiety about supplies of taxol to John Douros,[27] his former boss at the Natural Products Branch, who had gone to work at Bristol-Myers. The NCI's Taxol Working Group discussed collaboration with a pharmaceutical company. It was inevitable that a pharmaceutical company would be involved in the commercialisation of any drug developed at the NCI, given American cultural attitudes that generally favoured market forces, business enterprise and a minimum of government intervention or public spending. But it was not yet certain what role such a company would have.

Finally, in 1988, the Taxol Working Group, in discussing the supply issue seriously, considered alternatives to bark collection.[28] Some favoured mass propagation. Others proposed collaboration with a biotechnology company to develop a process using genetic engineering or tissue culture methods. Total synthesis was ruled out, on the grounds that too many chemical steps would be needed for it to provide a commercially viable process. Surprisingly, no mention at all was made of semi-synthesis, that is preparation from an intermediate extracted from a species of *Taxus*, and indeed Matthew Suffness seems to have explicitly ruled it out,[29] although Potier and Greene's semisynthetic route to taxol was about to be published,[30] and Suffness had been aware of the work leading up to it from 1981.[31] Therefore, semi-synthesis from renewable parts of yew was a route that might have been taken by the NCI, but was not.

By September 1988 the Taxol Working Group learned that the sum needed to complete the extraction and purification of taxol from collections of bark already made or scheduled was now $2 million, but only one-tenth this amount was available, and some of it had already been committed to another promising product (bryostatin). By this time, of the several possible ways in which the NCI might have solved its dilemma, it was clear that it had decided to cut its association with taxol and deliver it, plus the data and revelations it had generated (and its problems) to a pharmaceutical company. The main part of the Working Group's discussion was now how to get a pharmaceutical company to collaborate, and the nature of such a collaboration, not whether such a collaboration was in everyone's best interests.

## Privatisation

The mechanism chosen for the handover to a firm was a Cooperative Research and Development Agreement (CRADA), an instrument designed to facilitate the transfer of commercially exploitable knowledge from federal agencies to private industry, under the terms of the Federal Transfer of Technology Act (1986). The Federal Register of 1st August 1989 announced that a pharmaceutical company was sought to develop taxol to marketable status 'to meet the needs of the public and with the best terms for the government'. By the deadline only four companies had submitted proposals, Bristol-Myers,[32] Rhône-Poulenc,[33] Unimed[34] and Xechem.[35] Cancer is the West's second major disease but oncology is only of minor interest to pharmaceutical companies: anticancer drugs in 1990 accounted for less than 3 per cent of the world's drug market, compared with 17 per cent for cardiovascular drugs.[36] Bristol-Myers Squibb produces most of the world's anticancer drugs, and already had a special relationship with the NCI because of the high profile of anticancer drugs in their portfolio. Rhône-Poulenc had been developing taxotère in collaboration with Potier and Greene, but did not have a presence in the oncology field like Bristol-Myers Squibb, and besides was not US-owned.[37]

There appears to have been a clear preference for Bristol-Myers Squibb as the CRADA partner, even before the final proposals were received. In the memo covering the final stage of the selection process, Dale Shoemaker of the NCI Regulatory Affairs Branch asked the Taxol CRADA Review Committee to 'review the proposals and let me know if you still feel Bristol-Myers should be selected for the Taxol CRADA'.[38] Within a few days the decision was taken. In January 1991 the CRADA was signed by the NCI and Bristol-Myers Squibb, giving the company exclusive access to all the data needed to file for clinical approval. Two further CRADAs were signed in mid-June 1991 by Bristol-Myers Squibb with the USDA and the Department of the Interior, to provide exclusive access to *Taxus brevifolia* on federal land. The molecule had finally arrived at a pharmaceutical company, 25 years after its isolation in Monroe Wall's laboratory in North Carolina. It was in the final stages of leaving the NCI and public ownership to become private property.

The FDA approved taxol for use in the treatment of refractory ovarian cancer in December 1992, and Bristol-Myers Squibb was granted five years exclusive marketing rights to the drug under the terms of the Waxman-Hatch Act (1984), passed to give intellectual property rights to products that had no patent. Taxol, being both a natural product and in the public domain for 25 years by this time, could not be patented. In the meantime, the delayed breast cancer trial due to take place in 1985, had finally got underway in January 1990. The results were outstanding: and taxol was found to be active against a cancer that affects a much larger population than ovarian cancer – some 200 000 in the USA alone. Taxol duly received FDA clearance for use against metastatic breast cancer in 1994. But the consumption of taxol promised to be more than ten times as great as the calculations based on ovarian cancer results had suggested. Bristol-Myers Squibb had acquired the rights to commercialise taxol, and exclusive access to the public sector intellectual and material property needed to do so, but with them came an even greater supply problem than expected.

### Controversy

In 1991, and again in 1993, taxol became a hot political issue in the United States as the participants in its biography were questioned and cross-examined in two Congressional hearings. The issue that taxol raised for the politics of the nation was whether the arrangements between the public and the private sector were in the public's best interest. The first hearing (29 July 1991) focused on the exclusive agreements between Bristol-Myers Squibb and the three Federal Agencies, and the granting of a monopoly to one firm.[39] Congressman Ron Wyden (Democrat – Oregon) from the chair stated that the CRADA did not protect the public interest, did not assure a reasonable level of commercial fair play, did not assure responsible management of a limited natural resource, and did not stimulate the transition to an alternative supply.

The second hearing (25 January 1993) was more generally on the pricing of drugs co-developed by Federal laboratories and private companies, with special reference to taxol. Drugs developed with Federal funding were priced at a considerably higher level than those developed without. It was argued that Bristol-Myers Squibb had not discovered taxol, nor had it paid for or carried out clinical trials: that is, it had not taken the risks normally used to justify high prices and profits. Consumer groups argued that the public was paying twice for taxol, once as taxpayers and once as consumers. However, the Congressional hearings did not ask the question 'did it have to turn out this way?' but 'since we have this system, is this the best way of managing it?'

*Taxus brevifolia* too had become a political phenomenon in the early 1990s. The Environmental Defence Fund, a Washington-based activist group seeking legal and economic solutions to environmental problems, had petitioned the Department of the Interior to list *Taxus brevifolia* as a threatened species in 1990. They took care to enfold biomedical practice with species protection, by enlisting in support of the petition Bill McGuire, the head of the ovarian cancer trial, and Susan Horwitz, the biologist who discovered taxol's unique mechanism of action. Despite this strategy, the media hyped the story up into one of 'cancer wars': the interests of cancer patients vs. the protection of the environment. The Fish and Wildlife Service turned down the petition in January 1991, but *Taxus brevifolia* got its own act, the Pacific Yew Act (1991) and it too was subjected to its own Congressional hearing (4 March 1991).

*Taxus brevifolia*, like taxol, changed its identity over time, from a 'trash' tree that was burned on slash piles because it was of no commercial value in logging operations, to the most valuable species in the forest. It became an important symbol of the fate of the American temperate rainforest, and the planet's ecosystem in general.

*Taxus brevifolia* became an icon of resistance to what many believed was the imminent disappearance of an entire eco-system. It also reminded people how little they knew about the forests, how they worked, and particularly what hidden human benefits there were waiting to be discovered: that is, it gave a concrete meaning to the word 'biodiversity'.

So Taxol wound its way through the drug development program, a tortuous path with many setbacks, its attributes as an anticancer agent emerging more clearly, but its identity as such an object still in the making. It became a Drug Development Candidate, an Investigational New Drug, a New Drug approved by the FDA, and a commodity on the market, sold by a drug firm. It had other identities, too, since it had also become an important research tool for cell biologists, and for chemists one of the most complex natural products they had ever seen, challenging them to try and make it in the laboratory. At some stage it became an image on a computer screen, which showed the arrangement of atoms in three dimensions and could be reacted in virtual reality with proteins to predict its likely biological and toxic effects. But for a time its owners lost sight of another identity it had, as a natural product obtained from a living organism, and this contributed to its becoming the subject of a series of political controversies.

## Cutting the network

No sooner had the tree hit the headlines and appeared on prime time television than it disappeared again from the public conscience. At the beginning of 1993, Bristol-Myers Squibb announced that it was effectively pulling out of the Pacific Northwest ancient forests and sourcing its raw materials and operations as far away as possible from this political hot spot, in the Himalayas, Milan, Germany and Ireland. It was ending its contract with the bulk supplier of taxol, who obtained the active chemical from the bark. It was moving to a supplier that used a semisynthetic process instead of an extractive process, and moving from the Pacific yew as raw material to the European and Himalayan yew. Although the NCI had greeted the French semi-synthesis with less than overwhelming enthusiasm as a solution to the supply problem,[40] NCI funding for taxol chemistry projects in American universities began to take off soon after it was reported, so that by 1992 some 30 groups were working on the synthesis of taxol,[41] and Bob Holton at Florida State University patented semisynthetic routes to taxol in 1990 and 1991,[42] which he licensed to Bristol-Myers Squibb.

Ownership is a phenomenon that limits the size of networks or even cuts them, which is what occurred when the USDA lost its share in the ownership of taxol, and again what happened in the aftermath of Bristol-Myers Squibb's becoming the 'owner' of taxol and moving out of the forest. Almost overnight, the networks built around the voices of *Taxus brevifolia* began to disintegrate, as the voices themselves became silent. With one action, Bristol-Myers Squibb cut all the networks that had sustained *Taxus brevifolia* as a political actor. To get some idea of the size and scope of the taxol network we can look at those who had taken part in an NCI sponsored workshop on taxol and *Taxus* in Bethesda, MD (where the main offices of the NCI were located) in June 1990. The areas of expertise represented by the 194 participants included agronomics, chemistry, clinical studies, tissue culture, genetic engineering, mechanism of action and resistance, venture capital, licensing, and regulatory affairs. About a quarter of the audience came from the corporate sector, including pharmaceutical firms, biotechnology companies, bulk chemical producers, small-scale loggers and major timber companies.

Some of those present from the Pacific region, concerned about the fate of *Taxus brevifolia*, had later formed the Native Yew Conservation Council in order to draft a conservation plan for the tree as a national strategic resource in the fight against cancer. When Bristol-Myers Squibb pulled out of the forest, the Native Yew Conservation Council ceased to meet and even some of its members' informal and social links were cut. A plant species, which had been transformed from being waste to being precious, was transformed back again.

But none of the events, the actions and reactions of those who participated in the drama, was inevitable. Taxol threw the spotlight on to *Taxus brevifolia*, not because of some natural or inevitable connection, but because the decisions taken by key actors along the historical path from the 1960s led to such an outcome. It could have been quite different. If decisions had been taken in the late 1960s and 1970s to seek cultivars as the raw material for taxol production, then newspapers would not have been carrying stories about *Taxus brevifolia*, no Congressional hearing would have been held, and no special yew conferences would have been organised and attended. If the NCI had followed the path pursued in the 1980s by natural product chemists in France on semi-synthesis, there would have been no NCI-sponsored workshop on taxol and *Taxus* and no creation of the Native Yew Conservation Council, the tree's most public voice. If the commercialisation had been carried out differently,

Congressional hearings might not have been held and controversies in the public domain might not have taken place.

As it was, taxol became an obligatory passage point for NCI administrators and scientists seeking to justify the state definition and management of 'the war against cancer' and how to fight it, to legitimise the plant screening program (which had not otherwise resulted in any clinically useful drugs), and to succeed in their careers. Meanwhile *Taxus brevifolia* and the forest became obligatory passage points in the supply of taxol in the USA. Finally, Bristol-Myers Squibb after the signing of the CRADA, made itself an obligatory passage point to those who wanted taxol for the treatment of cancer or for research.

## Property

Property or ownership is one of the attributes of an object, and changes in ownership are a form of translation that can appear by enrolling new actors or cutting the network. Thus taxol passed from being the 'property' of *Taxus brevifolia*, to being briefly the property of the US Department of Agriculture and then became the property of the National Cancer Institute, a Government agency claiming to act on behalf of 'the public', so that in theory the public owned taxol. Finally, it became the property of Bristol-Myers Squibb, and thus private property, no longer in the public domain.

In most pre-industrial societies, no-one owned the trees in the forest, and no-one had any concept of the substance that is now called taxol. When taxol was 'owned' by *Taxus brevifolia*, the tree was there for anyone to use as they saw fit – symbolically in ceremonies to represent death, or elsewhere to represent everlasting life; to make bows or furniture; or for medical treatments. The 'public' had more freedom to use the yew than it had when ownership became officially vested in 'the public' through the state. Once taxol belonged to the NCI and *Taxus brevifolia* to the Department of the Interior (Bureau of Land Management) and the Department of Agriculture (Forest Service), members of the public could not in practice exercise any ownership rights over either taxol or *Taxus brevifolia*.

When taxol belonged to the NCI, other actors were sub-contracted to work on it, including chemists, biologists and clinicians, and in varying degrees they assumed certain 'ownership' rights within the conventions of science and the boundaries imposed by the NCI. Thus Monroe Wall and his colleagues named the compound 'taxol' and the NCI and USDA immediately began to use the name Wall *et al* had chosen, as did other scientists. Chemists and others spoke as though the name 'belonged' to Wall, just as new reactions and theories tend to be named after the scientist who first proposed them. The structural formula was described as his. Similarly the practice of science put Susan Horwitz's name on taxol's mechanism of action and Andrew Greene's, Pierre Potier's and Bob Holton's on the semi-synthesis of taxol, although the dominant narrative usually refers to the work of Holton rather than Potier and Greene.

But, though science assigns the achievements to the scientists mentioned, intellectual property in a legal sense is quite a different matter altogether. The right to exploit discoveries, that is make money from them, depends on patents, trademarks, licenses and CRADAs. Taxol had not been patented as a product by Bristol-Myers Squibb, Wall, or anyone else, but despite the widespread belief in the scientific community and elsewhere that the name 'taxol' was either in the public domain or in some senses 'belonged' to Monroe Wall, Bristol-Myers Squibb were able to make it their own by trademarking it in 1992. As a result, the firm was able to rewrite history. Their account of Wall and Wani's work refers to the isolation of 'paclitaxel', more than 20 years before the word had been invented.[43] In the medical database MEDLINE the word 'paclitaxel' generates references to about 600 abstracts of work on taxol between the first publication of the name 'taxol' (1969) and the date of registration of Taxol® (1992), even though the word 'paclitaxel' is in none of the publications.

Under trademark law, Bristol-Myers Squibb is prepared to enforce their rights to own the name taxol by taking legal action against those who challenge their property rights by producing a similar product themselves, or even those who use its name without the ®. In this endeavour, the firm has enlisted the support of state agencies, just as state agencies earlier enrolled the firm in the enterprise of manufacturing and distributing taxol. That is, countries have been threatened with trade sanctions[44] if they permit any firm other than Bristol-Myers Squibb to market generic taxol in that country, even though it would be entirely legal, since taxol is unpatented.

The journal, *Nature*, in an editorial in 1995,[45] urged the company to relinquish the trademark on the grounds that 'taxol' had been used by the research community for at least two decades. Bristol-Myers Squibb's lawyers made it clear that journals should not use the name taxol to refer to the substance derived from the Pacific yew, but only to the anticancer drug sold by Bristol-Myers Squibb Co.[46] As

Rosemary Coombe points out, trademark law has become a powerful vehicle for the suppression of unwelcome speech or social commentary.[47]

Bristol-Myers Squibb took out a successful lawsuit against the small Québécois firm Corporation Biolyse Pharmacopée Internationale, which made taxol from the needles and branch tips of the fast-growing *Taxus canadensis*,[48] accusing them of misleading the medical profession by passing off their preparation as that of Bristol-Myers Squibb.[49] In 1998, 30 years of work by the National Cancer Institute – and all the public sector researchers whom the NCI financed and coordinated – were dismissed in a few words by Bristol-Myers Squibb: 'Taxol was developed in the early-1960s and languished for almost 30 years because nobody could make it', said by Bruce Ross, who had been the firm's chief negotiator with the NCI in setting the price of taxol in 1992.[50]

## Conclusion

In order to write the biography of taxol, we have followed it as it wound its way through the procedures of science and the decision networks of state agencies and into the political arena, finally being appropriated by a pharmaceutical company. We have explored some of the networks as they were constructed during the process of enlisting different actors into the performance of the taxol drama – and the way they were cut when the USDA's collaboration with the NCI was terminated and again when Bristol-Myers Squibb pulled out of the forest. We have examined ways in which taxol changed its identity, and the different layers of meaning that may be given to 'property', as taxol passed successively through different hands. We followed the stories, incorporating their different identities of taxol, as they unfolded differently in France and in the USA. It is the American taxol story on which emphasis and publicity is focused, and in that sense it is the unfolding of events in France – in which the natural product and the anti-cancer drug were both key identities of taxol, and in which controversies neither over the environment nor over intellectual property rights appear to have been engendered – which shows the contingent narrative, the story that might have been the dominant tale but in fact was not.

## Notes

**Key to primary material**
**FRD** Papers in the Natural Products Branch, National Cancer Institute
**GCB** Papers in the Grants and Contracts Operations Branch, National Cancer Institute
**NPB** Papers in the Natural Products Branch, National Cancer Institute

1. The narrative in this chapter is based on a large number of sources, published, unpublished and oral, too numerous to cite individually. Full references can be found in J. Goodman and V. Walsh, *The Tree, the Molecule and Cancer: The story of taxol* (Cambridge: Cambridge University Press, 2001). From the late-1960s to the early-1990s taxol was the chemical name for one product found in the bark of *Taxus brevifolia*. Then it was trade marked and became a brand name for Bristol-Myers Squibb's drug. At the same time the word paclitaxel was invented for the molecule (all uses except Bristol-Myers Squibb's drug). Similarly Taxotere was a semisynthetic molecule which was made by a chemical reaction with a substance obtained from *Taxus baccata*. When it, too, was trademarked and became Rhône-Poulenc's brand, another name was invented for all other uses of the molecule.
2. K. C. Nicolaou, W-M. Dai and R. K. Guy, 'The chemistry and biology of taxol', *Angewandte Chemie International Edition*, xxxiii (1994), 15–44, especially 15.
3. 'Bristol-Myers Squibb reports record fourth quarter and annual sales (1998)', www.prnewswire.com, visited 20 January 1999.
4. Based on prescription drug sales in Tracey Barker, 'Merck accelerates, Glaxo falters', *Scrip Magazine*, (January 1999), 39.
5. Igor Kopytoff, 'The cultural biography of things: Commoditisation as a process', in Arun Appadurai (ed), *The Social Life of Things: Commodities in Cultural Perspective* (Cambridge: Cambridge University Press, 1986), 64–91.
6. Art historians have used an approach based on biographies of things in recounting the histories of art objects. In 1995, the Association of Art Historians had 'Objects, histories and interpretations' as the theme of their annual conference in London. Debbora Battaglia argued this point in her paper 'Do objects have individual histories: a critical examination from postcolonial New Guinea'.
7. Steven Shapin, 'History of science and its sociological

reconstructions', *History of Science*, 20 (1982), 157–211.
8. Donald MacKenzie, 'Marx and the machine', *Technology and Culture*, 25 (1984), 473–502.
9. Paul David, 'Clio and the economics of QWERTY', *American Economic Review*, 75 (1985), 332–7.
10. David F. Noble, 'Social choice in machine design: the case of the automatically controlled machine tools, and a challenge for labor', *Politics and Society*, 8 (1978), 313–47.
11. Donna Haraway, 'Universal donors in a vampire culture – it's all in the family: Biological kinship categories in the twentieth century United States' in William Cronon (ed), *Uncommon Ground* (New York: W. W. Norton, 1996), 321–66.
12. S. van der Geest, S. R. White and A. Hardon, 'The anthropology of pharmaceuticals: A biographical approach', *Annual Review of Anthropology*, 25 (1996), 153–78.
13. See, for example, Bruno Latour, *Science in Action* (Cambridge, MA: Harvard University Press, 1987).
14. Bruno Latour, *We Have Never Been Modern* (Cambridge, MA: Harvard University Press, 1993), 2–3; idem, *The Pasteurisation of France* (Cambridge, MA: Harvard University Press, 1988), 10.
15. George Marcus, 'Ethnography in/of the world system: The emergence of multi-sited ethnography', *Annual Review of Anthropology 34* (1995), 95–117.
16. Michael Callon, 'Society in the making: the study of technology as a tool for sociological analysis' in W. E. Bijker, T. P. Hughes and T. J. Pinch (eds), *The Social Construction of Technological Systems: New directions in the sociology and history of technology* (Cambridge, MA: MIT Press, 1987), 93.
17. Actor network theory uses the word *intéressement*.
18. V. Singleton and M. Michael, 'Actor networks and ambivalence: General practitioners in the UK cervical screening programme', *Social Studies of Science*, 23 (1993), 227–64.
19. Michel Callon and John Law, 'Agency and the hybrid collectif', *The South Atlantic Quarterly*, 94 (1995), 485.
20. Marilyn Strathern, *Property, Substance and Effect: Anthropological essays on persons and things* (London: Athlone Press, 1999), 194.
21. John Law, *Organising Modernity* (Oxford: Blackwell, 1994), 100–4. Marilyn Strathern *op. cit.* (note 20), 193 makes this point.
22. Marilyn Strathern, 1999, *op. cit.* (note 20). See also Marilyn Strathern, 'Cutting the Network', *Journal of the Royal Anthropological Institute*, 2 (1996), 517–35.
23. R. E. Perdue and J. L. Hartwell, 'The search for plant sources of

anti-cancer drugs', *Morris Arboretum Bulletin*, 20 (1969), 35–53.
24. M. Colin et al, 'Preparation of baccatin III derivatives as antitumour agents', *European Patent Application* EP 336,851, 10 October 1989; French Patent Application 884,513, 6 April 1988.
25. Cragg, notes on conversation with Brian Leland-Jones, 13 April 1988, NPBI/2.
26. Suffness to New, 9 December 1986, NPB(S).
27. Suffness to Douros, 6 July 1988, FRD4.
28. Minutes of the August 1988 meeting, NPBI/3.
29. Suffness to Douros, 6 July 1988 FRD4.
30. Jean-Noël Denis *et al*, 'A highly efficient practical approach to natural taxol', *Journal of the American Chemical Society*, 110 (1988), 5917–19.
31. Correspondence between Suffness and Potier and Suffness and Greene from 1981, GCB1.
32. Bristol-Myers is a US-based multinational drug firm, which merged with Squibb in October 1989.
33. Rhône-Poulenc is a French-based multinational chemical firm with manufacturing and marketing activities in the USA and other countries.
34. Unimed is a small US firm.
35. Xechem is a small US firm bought by Fujisawa, one of Japan's largest pharmaceutical firms, in September 1989.
36. *Scrip Yearbook 1991*, 61 and *Scrip Yearbook 1992*, 73.
37. One of the aims of the Federal Transfer of Technology Act, and of the CRADA, was to discourage the exploitation of the output of research supported by the US government by or to the benefit of foreigners. Rebecca Eisenberg, 'Public research and private development: patents and technology transfer in government sponsored research', *Virginia Law Review*, 82 (1996:), 1663–1727; and personal communication, 25 May 1999.
38. Shoemaker to members, Taxol CRADA review committee, 29 November 1989, NPBII; and Rebecca Eisenberg, *op. cit.* (note 37).
39. In the course of the investigations in the run-up to the hearing, concern was expressed as to whether the competition had been fair. For example, Robert Wittes had been Associate Director of the Cancer Therapy Evaluation Program in the NCI's Division of Cancer Treatment 1983–8; moved to Bristol-Myers to be Senior Vice-President for Cancer Research in November 1988; and returned to the NCI in August 1990 as Chief of the Medicine Branch of the Clinical Oncology Program. No evidence was

produced, however, to suggest that Wittes' revolving door experiences had anything to do with the CRADA or the firm's success.

40. The *Journal of the National Cancer Institute* reported the Potier-Greene synthesis without mentioning their names or giving a reference, see Elaine Blume, 'Investigators seek to increase taxol supply', *Journal of the National Cancer Institute*, 81 (1989), 1122–3.
41. Charles Swindell, 'Taxane diterpene synthesis strategies – A review', *Organic Preparations and Procedures International*, 23 (1991), 465–543.
42. Robert Holton, 'Method for preparation of taxol using an oxazinone', *European Patent Application* 400,971 (1990), *US Patent* 5,015,744 (1991); 'Method for preparation of taxol using a ß-lactam', *European Patent Application* 428,376 (1991), US Patent 5,175,315 (1992).
43. Bristol-Myers Squibb, 'The development of Taxol® (paclitaxel)', (March 1997).
44. Ralph Nader, James Love and Robert Weisman to Vice President Gore, 29 July 1997 (www.cptech.org/pharm/goreonsa/html, visited 16 February 1999).
45. Anonymous, 'Names for hi-jacking', *Nature*, 373 (2 February 1995), 370.
46. Stephen Chesnoff, 'The use of Taxol as a trademark' *Nature*, 374 (16 March 1995), 208; Madeleine Jacobs, 'What's in a name? (editorial)', *Chemical and Engineering News*, (21 October 1996), 5.
47. Rosemary J Coombe, *The Cultural Life of Intellectual Properties: Authorship, Appropriation and the Law* (Durham, NC: Duke University Press, 1998), 72.
48. Gilles Gagné, 'Biolyse pourrait s'emparer du marché de Taxol grâce à l'If du Canada', *Le Soleil (Québec)* (13 November 1993).
49. Affidavit of Christine Poon, President of Bristol-Myers Squibb Canada Inc., Bristol-Myers Squibb (plaintiff) and Corporation Biolyse Pharmacopée Internationale (defendent), Federal Court of Canada, Trial Division, T-946-94, 29 June 1995.
50. Quoted in Li Fellers, 'The medicine market', *The Washington Post Magazine* (31 May 1998), 24.

# 13

### Afterword:
### Who Cares? Remedies, care and cultures of healing in the twentieth century

*Godelieve Van Heteren*

Who cares?

On the brink of yet another biotechnological therapeutic revolution, this time involving genes, biomaterials, chips, data-matching and – profiling, e-commerce, patenting of biological substances, multimillion corporate investments and deadly competition, it is indeed fascinating to reflect on the question: Remedies, who cares? At one level, simple answers can be given. Today, most patients care about effective, quick and painless remedies for their ailments, which restore and prolong good quality life; remedies preferably delivered to them at little personal expense and devoid of side effects. Most Western doctors also care about such remedies in caring for their patients. In addition, they may wish remedies publicly underscore their professional power to heal, and may feel strongly about advancing research and opening new avenues for the development of such remedies.

In turn, biotechnological companies and pharmaceutical industries have their own cares about remedies. Their concerns are mainly inspired by the drive to stay commercially afloat in a market where experts predict that only a handful of global players will survive into the twenty-first century. Consequently, innovative industries care primarily about developing remedies which lead to profit maximisation and market control. Finally, national governments care anxiously about remedies, since for them remedies not infrequently signal danger. For health departments increasingly desperate to control costs, new remedies in particular can be a threat to healthcare budgets. In 1998, in most West European countries, expenditure figures on pharmaceuticals grew officially by 6 to 10 per cent, an annual growth rate way out-of-line with the 'autonomous' growth levels of 2.3 to 3 per cent in health care which most governments consider 'acceptable'.[1] Governments, therefore, fear that new remedies – pharmaceuticals especially – could undermine their already greatly strained budgets.[2]

In the face of all these diverse forms of 'caring' about remedies on the part of patients and providers, producers and cost-controllers, who will care about historical attempts to study remedies as indicators of cultures of healing in the twentieth century? That, I assume, depends. It depends on the extra ammunition that historical analyses can offer to the critique of modern healing practices. It depends on the critical insights which historians bring to bear on the rapid changes in products and procedures of healing which have materialised during this century. In short, it depends on how historians answer the question: What do remedies tell us about the political, social and moral economies of healing in the modern world?

### Assessing healing cultures by their remedies: building blocks for further research

One might expect that by putting 'twentieth century remedies' centre stage, the spotlight would fall on specific dimensions of modern healing cultures: on their material aspects and economics; on the specific requirements of therapeutic research and control that have emerged; on the high levels of technology involved; but equally on the specific beliefs still vested in remedies in a secularised world. The articles presented in this volume, of course, cover just a tiny selection of remedies: opium, homoeopathic remedies, streptomycin, contraceptives, interferon and taxol. And even though the remedies' roles in history are being examined in multifarious ways, by historians who draw on the best of anthropology, the social and political sciences, and ethnography, the contributions are only a beginning of the endeavour to compare cultures of healing. Yet from the articles, important building blocks for larger historical frameworks can be assembled. Five areas for further immediately suggest themselves:

I. Remedies: indicators of changing powers and dependencies- their social dimension

II. Remedies: indicators in healing and health care of the role of economy and patterns of productivity – their economic dimension.

III. Remedies: indicators of material interaction and the 'life of things' in healing and health care – their radical social-philosophical implications

*Afterword*

IV. Remedies and the end of national health care – their health-political perspective

V. Remedies and care – the social-moral dimension of remedies and healing cultures

My discussion of each of these areas begins with a short recommendation in the form of a subheading.

## I. Remedies, changing powers and dependencies

We need further studies of the changing powers and dependencies in twentieth century healing and the specific impact of remedies on the balances of power.

A first observation one can make is how healing relationships have shifted in contents, composition and location over the last two hundred years, attracting an ever greater arsenal of objects to mediate between healer and patient. While James Boswell in the 1760s, upon falling ill, would still simply visit his 'friend Douglas', a surgeon in Pall Mall, 'a kind hearted, plain, sensible man'[3] in his house to be bled or purged, healing relationships have since been rapidly shifted from homes and backrooms to ever more medicalised environments, permeated with technology, upheld by insurance systems and certified by the state. Healing environments have become busy scenes, densely populated with objects for diagnosis, therapy and prevention; entities of diverse origins, involving multiple layers of commercial interest. The changing milieu of healing relations is indicative of broader transformations in social dependencies and power structures. It parallels the crowding of social relationships generally with ever more gadgets and non-human mediators.

Under a healing relationship, traditionally, a connection has been understood between two human beings: somebody who is ill and wishes to be cured, and a(n) (self-)appointed person who provides services of cure and care. By their very nature, healing relationships have always contained elements of power and dependency. At the most basic level, one thinks of the dependencies of a sick person who is forced to confide in someone else to obtain a cure or relief from suffering, granting this person power over his or her life and body. Equally, one can imagine dependencies of the healer on the patronage or cooperation of his/her patients. With the widening network of parties involved: from apothecaries to pharmaceutical companies, from boards of hospital governors to the modern manager, from town councillors to the state, the patterns of dependency and control attached to healing relationships have also grown in complexity.

More than ever, therefore, it has become pertinent for a historian to ascertain which relationships do inform the practices of healing, and which social actors populate the field at any given time. It is significant to establish in which environments modern healing relationships primarily take shape (whether in homes or hospitals, laboratories or industries).

A first stage of examining the role of remedies in healing relationships should involve establishing where remedies become situated in these dynamic social networks. Where does the kidney-dialysis-machinery fit into the picture? What place is given to the artificial lung or to psychopharmacological substances? From which starting conditions do insulin, penicillin, or taxol set out to attain their central place in the processes of healing, and by which routes do they arrive there? Having obtained a clearer perspective on the social location of a remedy, one could proceed to ask: what shifts in powers and dependencies result from their presence in healing relationships? What occurred, for instance, between physicians and diabetics upon the arrival of insulin, what awaits surgeons and patients once telesurgery takes off?

## II. Remedies: indicators in healing and health care of the role of the economy and patterns of productivity

> We urgently need further study of the economics of Western healing as part of a critical historical consideration of twentieth century capitalism and its physical and ideological forms of 'production'. The naive use of economic models as heuristic devices is not sufficient for developing such a critique.

As soon as we focus on the social locations and roles of remedies, our attention is bound to be drawn to the more material sides of the culture of healing. Studying twentieth century remedies, from Salvarsan to gene therapy, obliges us to think about the connections between remedies and the Western economy, commercialism, and industrial and post industrial forms of producing goods, ideas and values.[4]

The economics of healing to date remains an under researched area. Certainly, much social historical work has been devoted to exploring the ways in which, since the Enlightenment, health care has been moulded by public aims and concerns for 'the wealth of the nation', culminating in a wide array of public health services and the development of health insurance arrangements. And in circles of sociologists, social and political economists, political philosophers

## Afterword

and ethicists, there is an unmistakable revival of interest in the transformations which capitalism underwent in the twentieth century. These studies provide sharp critiques of the ways in which twentieth century capitalism restructured our public domains, and of the ideological stances it brought in its wake, including its definitions of 'the good life', individual autonomy, health and disease. But there is a serious need for solid historical studies that examine this changing productivity ethos in healing by addressing, for instance, the spillover of industrial forms of production into the organisation of knowledge and healing practices. If perspectives informed by critical economics figure in medical historical works at all, they often occupy a subordinate position.

However, it is curious to note that while a critical, economically informed historiography of twentieth century medicine is urgently required, many historians of medicine have begun to use as interpretative tools economic notions that they ought to explain more critically. Thus, it is striking to observe how, since the 1980s, models such as 'the medical marketplace' or 'the production cycle' have gained popularity among historians of medicine as conceptual tools through which the fate of healing products and procedures can be traced. Surely, adopting models which have originated in economic or managerial theories may be handy for organising the critical debate about changing cultures of health care. One could indeed use 'the medical market' as a 'heuristic device' (Willem de Blécourt, Chapter 9). And schematic aids like the 'production cycle' can assist one in assessing who is in control of each of the phases of a modern 'production' process. Then why not apply them to 'the production of health'? It would be naive, however, to ignore the significance of the specific moment in time when theoretical tools like the 'medical market' were embraced by historians. Nor is it wise to ignore how our cultural criticism of social processes has become tacitly pervaded with economic categories.

It remains to be seen what critical awareness the application of notions such as 'the medical marketplace' or 'the production cycle' are capable of yielding. Let's look at a few examples in this volume. At one level, Willem de Blécourt's account of the selling tactics of Dutch 'hygienic shops' in the early years of the twentieth century can be read as a story of clever marketing. His article touches on the veiled language and circumventing strategies that had to be used by owners of these shops to attract customers to buy contraceptive devices and abortificants at a time when such products were illegal or taboo.

Lara Marks's article (Chapter 8) concerning the various test environments for the pill for women, can also be analysed as a struggle for distribution and market control, this time through control of the test environments. Although not written explicitly in those terms, Marks illustrates how between 1959 and the late-1960s a large voluntary organisation, the Council for the Investigation of Fertility Control (CIFC), happened to control most early application research on the pill in Britain. Marks tries to explain why this situation existed and suggests that the close affiliation of the CIFC with another party in the market, the Family Planning Association (FPA), was a key factor. The FPA was the main distributor of contraceptives in the United Kingdom during those years.

Similarly, the articles by Stuart Anderson, Frank Huisman and Rein Vos can also be read as pertaining to the 'medical marketplace'. The authors discuss the changing profiles and positions of apothecaries, chemists and druggists in Great Britain and the Netherland respectively, and deal with socio-political and cultural aspects of the distribution of remedies. Huisman (Chapter 2) elaborates the changing professional profile of the Dutch pharmacist following the 1865 Medical Acts. Vos (Chapter 3) describes the world of apothecaries in the Netherlands before their cartel was dismantled in the 1970s under pressure of European legislation. He characterises the post-war Dutch apothecaries as caught up in a major struggle between their commercial and professional interests, a familiar theme in social historiography. Anderson (Chapter 4) presents an elegant study of the changing profile of British chemists since the inter-war period. He distinguishes four periods since the 1920s in which chemists reconfigured their occupational status as distributors of remedies. He relates the perceived changes to shifts in culturally accepted advisory roles, the chemists' accessibility to patients as well as their relationship with physicians, and the changing structures of payment for remedies. An economically reductionist reading of his story would turn it into one about how distributors constantly adapted themselves to the evolving market.

Nonetheless, while almost all the historical accounts in this volume could be selectively read as bearing upon elements of production, marketing, and dissemination of remedies, equally they demonstrate the complexity of cultural factors hidden behind such terms. A cultural-historical examination of production forces – even when drawing heavily on economically oriented heuristic aids – will immediately encounter broader social tensions and cultural frictions. A good example is Kate Fisher's article (Chapter 7) about cultures of contraception in the twentieth century. Through an economic looking glass, this paper could be interpreted as describing the difficulties of marketing and distributing new contraceptives. But such a reading would fail to do justice to the cultural heterogeneity that instantly surfaces. Fisher's interviews with individuals who married in the inter-war years, show the great diversity of public response to attempts by movements such as the Marie Stopes' birth clinics to 'modernise' birth control in Britain and control the market. Fisher's findings challenge the assumptions so often reiterated in arguments about the medicalisation of birth control. Contrary to the monolinear idea that the availability of new contraceptives would automatically lead to their widespread distribution and application, Fisher's research demonstrates how the cultural responses to new contraceptives were much more mixed, with many people continuing to adhere to traditional contraceptive practices.

In sum: the recent introduction of economic intellectual aids in historical studies highlights how economically oriented Western culture (and its self-criticism) has become. The models are useful in focusing attention on important forces and features of a culture's production system. But any application of such models in cultural studies almost immediately also brings home how 'culturally embedded' most economic phenomena continue to be. A more detailed assessment of the role of economics in healing cultures, which a study of remedies could easily inspire, requires a more comprehensive critical framework.

### III. Remedies: indicators of material interactionism and the 'life of things' in healing and health care

> Some authors in this volume have adopted the ethnographic method of 'following a remedy around' in order to 'write the biography of a remedy'. These methodologies underpin radical sociological views of twentieth century healing cultures in which non-human entities are granted an ever greater actor-role in social networks of relationships. More case studies with remedies as main 'protagonists' are needed in order to assess the degree of material interactionism to be found in twentieth century healing cultures.

A number of contributors to this volume have chosen to investigate remedies in terms of 'the biography of a remedy'. This perspective is philosophically significant. Granting 'life' to remedies underscores the deep sense in which material objects have invaded practical consciousness in the twentieth century to the point where cultural critics apply a 'sociological discourse' to things, discuss their 'actor status', and observe 'material interactionism' in many dehumanised, technology-driven, social environments. As Thomas Richard's once phrased it in a masterful study of modern advertising and commodification: Things have come to speak for themselves, 'a language of their own'.[5] In the modern world, healing 'things' have come to standardise human bodies, stabilise practices, help define disease and abnormality.[6,7]

Writing a biography of a remedy implies 'following the object and observing in which strange environments it will lead you' (Jordan Goodman and Vivien Walsh in Chapter 12). Given the great diversity of *curricula vitae* of twentieth century remedies, their 'biographies' are bound to reflect this heterogeneity. Not all the 'biographers' in this volume, however, are equally radical in allowing a remedy to dominate its own life story. Some authors delve into the changing status of a substance, which may not always start out as a remedy, but only eventually obtain this status. These authors try to spell out the circumstances that turn a substance into a remedy, or - similarly - to examine the new social and cultural effects that a substance may acquire once it is established as a remedy. Others investigate the environments in which a remedy is tested and produced, marketed and disseminated. A third group concentrates on finding out more about the ways in which remedies are received. Several articles in this volume testify to the fact that even in the twentieth century, rich sets of tales circulate, revealing the many forms of hope and belief which patients continue to attach to healing products. Such stories also show how faith is not infrequently enhanced by the public statements of researchers and officials, or the public relations machinery of industries. Following a remedy around can show that social actors (from researchers to health department officials) are most influential in shaping 'the profile' of a given substance. Their activities participate in the major moral task of defining which actual conditions should be 'remedied'.

Most authors in this volume adopt a middle ground between viewing remedies as 'passive objects' or viewing them as semi-autonomous 'social actors'. In her nuanced discussion of the shifting cultural status of 'opium' and 'nicotine', Virginia Berridge (Chapter 1), for instance, examines the social construction of the distinction between remedies and narcotics by a variety of human agents. Berridge demonstrates how differently opium and nicotine became culturally defined through a variety of changes in economic, political and social circumstances. Ultimately Berridge is interested in remedies as indicators of specific medico-political regimentation. She therefore focuses most keenly on the socio-political 'localisations' which opium and nicotine attained during their journeys in the world.

Nelly Oudshoorn (Chapter 6) follows her protagonist, 'the pill', through clinical trials and various research environments. She points to the *status aparte* of these 'remedies' as 'substances for healthy people' and explores what consequences the specific characteristics of contraceptives had for the research efforts concentrated on them. Oudshoorn compares two historical cases of contraceptive testing: the research projects in the 1950s and 1960s preceding the introduction of the pill for women, and the tedious research efforts which surrounded the testing of hormone injections for men in the 1980s and 1990s. She notices important changes in clinical research protocol, differences in recruiting men or women as research subjects, and the disparity of medical interest in the testing of these remedies for men and women.

A completely different aspect of a remedies' 'biography' is explored by Alan Yoshioka (Chapter 10) when he points out the extreme fluctuations in socio-cultural evaluation of drugs. Drawing on his extensive research into the socio-economic and policy debates surrounding the introduction of streptomycin into Britain, Yoshioka sets out to explain when and how streptomycin became labelled a 'wonder drug', and why. In analysing the intricacies of the introduction of streptomycin, Yoshioka focuses renewed attention on the influence of hope and faith in promoting remedies at the 'zenith of public trust in doctors and modern medicine'. He highlights the complicated forces – not least the media – and the cultural semantics surrounding substances that reach the status of wonder or miracle drug in modern times. By studying the ups and downs of wonder drugs, Yoshioka argues, it should become possible to trace the most important values in current health culture.

Similarly, Toine Pieters (Chapter 11) follows the trail of his protagonist 'interferon' through the ever more closely related worlds of clinical and biological research, bioindustry, highpowered government agencies and the media, in search of an answer to the question why and how the public fame of interferon oscillated since the late-1970s. After having been a highly promising 'antiviral penicillin', interferon made a come back in the 1970s as a cancer drug, much stimulated by the media, followed, however, by a quick erosion of public support. To explain how interferon survived, Pieters sketches a detailed picture of the alliances that built up around interferon in order to force its reentry onto the drugs market. He shows how research on interferon helped to reconfigure the various relationships between pharmaceutical companies, clinicial researchers, and clinicians. He also portrays how informal oncological practices were regrouped around interferon, how in interferon research notions stemming from immunology, molecular biology and genetic engineering were consolidated and fed into a new bioclinical definition of cancer, and a new therapeutic rationale.

In Pieters' social constructivist account, 'interferon' already figures as a dynamic protagonist. The most radical 'biographers' of remedies in this volume, however, are Jordan Goodman and Vivien Walsh (Chapter 12). They present no less than 'a series of biographies of taxol'. Taxol leads Goodman and Walsh all over the globe: to the forests of Oregon, the focal points of American ecological activists, to chemical laboratories in France, and cell biology laboratories as well as the pharmaceutical research labs of Bristol-Myers Squibb.

In the stories of Pieters, and Goodman and Walsh especially, the fundamental question of material interactionism surfaces: what is the actor status of objects in the ever more dehumanised social networks of relationships? More and more remedies in the twentieth century raise this question. Although still produced by human beings, certain remedies appear to be attaining ever more independent, active roles, once they are introduced to the world.

## IV. Remedies and the end of national health care

> More study is needed about how twentieth century remedies – which participate in global commercial structures – affect national health care systems

In this volume we have seen how, from a cultural viewpoint, remedies function locally, nationally and internationally. Increasingly, as the later chapters show, comparisons between national healing cultures which centre around remedies are almost impossible. In the course of the twentieth century, the production and dissemination of remedies have become more and more internationally organised. And the same forces that produce international remedies also turn patients into international consumers. Prescription and control of remedies, however, are still largely in the hands of national authorities and bound by local conventions and national regimentation. These control mechanisms explain in part why consumption patterns of treatments and remedies can still differ from country to country.[8] As a result, on an almost daily basis we witness tensions created between

*Afterword*

demanding consumers-patients and anxious governments by the increasing 'globalisation' of remedies. The way remedies have come to move in the world in the course of the twentieth century puts ever more pressure on the boundaries between local, national and international health care arrangements. In the late-twentieth century, one only has to refer to the new sales techniques aimed directly at patients via the Internet, to imagine how quickly existing balances may be shifted again. Since remedies participate in global commerce, they are perhaps the largest time bomb within national health care systems. And thus they may radically transform and even abolish any 'national' elements left in cultures of healing today.

## V. Remedies and care

> Historical studies of twentieth century remedies should focus more explicitly on the kinds of cultures of care modern remedies help to shape or sustain.

One major area of cultural historical inquiry could be: the evaluation of how changes in available sets of remedies relate to changes in care. Even with the high public acclaim some therapeutic innovations have received in the twentieth century, it remains worthwhile to assess the types of care and cures these innovations have helped to promote, at whose expense and to what avail? What forms of treatment and care, for instance, did the psychopharmacological substances in the 1950s replace and at what cost? Why have large numbers of patients throughout the twentieth century turned to healing products and procedures outside the mainstream? These are questions with social–ethical implications. They pertain to the issue of defining the goals remedies are supposed to serve: increasing life expectancy, removing human frailty from public view, creating images of the 'infinite body' and technical fix, improving life style? Research in this area should encourage historians to determine more explicitly what new values are attached to health and disease, bodily interventions and manipulations of life with each reconfiguration of a healing practice due to the arrival of a new remedy.

In order to explore the shifts remedies bring about in care, I have found it useful to employ a typology of care which the American political scientist Joan Tronto introduces in her book *Moral Boundaries* (1993).[9] Tronto aims at developing clearer political and social moral understanding of modern life through solid empirical descriptions of the distribution of care and its substantiating values in modern societies. Continuous empirical assessment of relationships of care, she argues, will enhance public awareness of the kinds of dependency and power at work in social relations, and clarify the most significant threads in the modern social fabric. Tronto distinguishes between four categories of 'care', beginning with *caring about*, the general recognition that something/somebody requires care even if one does not act upon it. The chief value attached to this type of caring is attentiveness. Tronto's second category is *taking care of*, assuming responsibility for somebody's needs and finding out how to respond to them, even if one does not actively provide services. Responsibility is the key value here. Thirdly, there is *care giving*, by which Tronto refers to all the activities involved in the direct meeting of needs for care. The main value attached to care giving is competency. Finally, there is *care receiving*, a category which Tronto uses for being sensitive to how the activities undertaken to meet a need are actually received by the subject of care. The key value 'responsiveness', Tronto argues, springs from a basic recognition of human beings' fundamental fragility, and from the ability to register the viewpoint of someone else, without presuming the other is exactly like oneself.

Tronto's schematic delineation of different types of care allows one to distinguish more clearly between different care roles that people in modern societies can adopt. 'Taking care of' in Tronto's definition leans in the direction of management. Care relations of this type are associated with power, public affairs, big responsibilities. By contrast, 'care giving' is more direct, smallscale and frequently associated with the private sphere, where emotions, dependencies and weaknesses become more easily visible. In current practice, 'care giving' relations tend to rest more heavily on women or people of poorer socio-economic backgrounds.

Each of Tronto's categories of care assumes a particular degree of moral distance-closeness to the subject of care. Bearing this in mind, it would be intriguing to examine what the changes in kinds of remedies signify in terms of enhancing particular forms of care over others. In the course of the twentieth century, much direct care giving, for instance, has been replaced by pharmaceutical regimentation.

Likewise, the fact that patients turn to alternative treatments and remedies (such as homeopathy which forms the subject of Marijke Gijswijt-Hofstra's Chapter 5) is frequently defended by references to the 'more direct and humane care' they allegedly receive in these domains.

*Afterword*

## Concluding remarks

The articles collected in this volume leave, not surprisingly, many subjects undiscussed. A critique of commercialism could be further developed on the basis of some of the papers. Similarly, the revolutionary late-twentieth century biotechnological and managerial changes that are reconfiguring remedies once again could be studied in detail, using some of the methods developed in this volume. Pieters and Goodman and Walsh, in particular, do take account of the many changes in production of remedies or the production biases which have occurred since the Second World War and such studies deserve emulation. Also more could be done in assessing patients' attitudes towards remedies. In this volume, the articles discussing miracle drugs and responses to contraceptives offer a first indication as to how one might proceed.

In short, each of the articles provides insights which are rich enough to advance cultural historical research along the lines outlined above. And the authors manage to do so while endowing black-and-white statements – so often found in older theoretical treatises on modernisation and industrialisation, capitalism and technology – with proper shades of grey. So, in answer to the question: 'historical studies of remedies, who cares?' One could say: 'We all do'. Historical studies matter. In a liberalizing, commercialising culture, with strong economic push factors, these historical studies continue to focus our attention on pluralism, cultural heterogeneity and multiple motivations. Although a powerful neocapitalist production ethos has come to surround remedies, cultural studies of remedies can still demonstrate that a multitude of social actors continues to define their various interests in healing relations, and endow them with anxiety and hope, criticism and compliance, fear and faith.

## Notes

1. For further European statistics on pharmaceutical and biotechnological production, see: *European Commission Communication on the Single Market in Pharmaceuticals* (CP98/127E, 2 December 1998); or: 'Benchmarking the Competitiveness of the EU Pharmaceutical Industry', *Europe Economics* (report), (December 1998).
2. G. Van Heteren, 'Europese farmaceuten. Weg of derde weg?', *Medisch Contact*, 54/13 (1999), 472–4.
3. *Boswell's London Journal 1762–1763* (reprint 1950, 1952) (London:

The Reprint Society, 1952), 54.
4. See, for example, Jonathan Liebenau, *Medical Science and Medical Industry: The Formation of the American Pharmaceutical Industry* (Basingstoke: Macmillan in association with the Business History Unit of the University of London, 1987).
5. Thomas Richards, *The Commodity Culture of Victorian England. Advertising and Spectacle, 1851–1914* (London and New York: Verso, 1991), 4.
6. For the roles of objects in modern social networks, see Bruno Latour, *Science in Action: How to follow scientists and engineers through society* (Cambridge, MA: Harvard University Press, 1987). Also B. Conein, N. Dodier, L. Thévenot (eds), *Les Objects dans l'action: De la maison au laboratoire. Collection Raisons Pratiques* (Paris: Editions de l'Ecole des Hautes Etudes en Sciences Sociales, 1993).
7. Dick Willems, *Tools of Care: Explorations into the Semiotics of Medical Technology* (Amsterdam: Thesis Publishers, 1995). See also Marc Berg, Annemarie Mol (eds), *Differences in Medicine. Unraveling Practices, Techniques, and Bodies* (Durham, NC, and London: Duke University Press, 1998).
8. Lynn Payer, *Medicine and Culture. Varieties in Treatment in the United States, England, West Germany, and France* (London: Penguin Books, 1988).
9. J. C. Tronto, *Moral Boundaries: A Political Argument for an Ethic of Care* (New York and London: Routledge, 1993), especially chapters 4 and 5, 101–155.

# Index

## A

abortion, Netherlands, *190–1, 191–2, 195–6*
academic discipline, pharmacy as, Netherlands, *36–8*
Ackerknecht, Erwin, *2*
Action on Smoking and Health (ASH), *25*
actor-network theory, *247–8*
Adams, Dr RE, *16*
addiction
 nicotine, *25–9*
 opiate, *16, 18*
Addiction Research Unit, *265*
advertising
 drug, in US medical journals, unqualified, *65*
 Dutch 'hygienic' products, *184–6, 196*
 tobacco, *21*
Advisory Council on the Misuse of Drugs (ACMD) Part 1 report on *AIDS and Drug Misuse*, *19*
AIDS and methadone, *19*
alkaloids, opiate (incl. opium), *4, 12–20, 29*
allopathy and homoeopathy, *105–6, 109–14*
America *see* US
American Cancer Society and interferon, *230, 234*
Amsterdam
 'deskundigen', *192*
 hygienic articles advertised, *184*
 university/universities
 homoeopathy at Free University, *111*
 Willem Stoeder (professor) at, *37–8, 38–40, 40, 43*
Andrewes CH, *209–10*
Andrews, Jennifer, *89, 90*
antibiotics, *203–27*
anticancer drugs *see* cancer
antihistamine as cold remedy, unqualified advertising in US medical journals, *65*
ASH (Action on Smoking and Health), *25*
Ayres, Wilfred, *81*

## B

Baird, Professor Sir Dugald, *161*
Banners Pure Drug Company, *80*
Barbanel, David, *88, 93*
Barclay, Arthur, *249, 250*
barrier contraception, interwar years, *142–3*
BBC radio appeals for streptomycin, *209–10, 211, 214*
Bearman, Jack, *81–2, 82–3*
Benz, Ronald, *82*
Betting, Hendrik Wefer, *37, 43*
Bevan, Aneurin, *210, 213*
Biogen and interferon gene, *231*
Biolyse Pharmacopée and taxol, *263*
biotechnology, *269*

*Index*

*see also* genetic engineering
Bird, Captain Oliver, *160*
Birmingham, oral contraceptive study, *163–4, 169*
birth control *see* family planning
bleeding, break-through, oral contraceptives, *167–9, 169–70*
'Blue Cross' hygienic articles, *185*
*BMJ* and streptomycin, *206, 210, 212, 213*
*Book for Men, 193*
*Book for Women, 189, 194*
Boots (the chemist), *76*
Brain, Sir Russell, and CIFC trials, *161*
Brain Committee and drug misuse, *17–18*
breast cancer, taxol, *252, 254, 257*
Bristol-Myers-Squibb and taxol, *245, 256–7, 258, 259–61, 262*
*British Medical Journal* (*BMJ*) and streptomycin, *206, 210, 212, 213*
Brommet, Jakob, *188*
bryostatin, *256*
Burroughs Wellcome and interferon, *236*

## C

C list, *47*
    hygienic articles and, *193*
cancer
    drugs treating
        interferon, *229, 230, 230–4, 235*
        taxols *see* taxol
    lung, smoking and, *21*
    prostate, male contraceptive agents used in, *135*
cap, cervical, *142, 143*
    rejection/discontent, *148, 152*
    safety (efficacy), *147*
    care and remedies, *279–80*
Cave, John, *92*
Central Health Council (Netherlands), *114, 115*
Centre National de la Recherche Scientifique (CNRS), taxol studies, *253*
cervical cap *see* cap
Charles, Enid, *144, 148*
Charles, Sir John, *21*
Chemist and Druggist Certificate, *75*
chewing gum, nicotine, *27*
Chief Medical Officer, Sir John Charles, *21*
children and smoking, *21–2*
China, opium situation, *14*
cigarette smoking *see* tobacco
cloning of interferon gene, *230–1*
cocaine, *14, 15, 18*
    as 'dangerous drug', *16*
Cohen IS, *114*
cold remedy, unqualified advertising in US medical journals, 65
commercialism and Dutch pharmacy, *62–6*
Committee on Safety of Medicines (CSM) on smoking, *24*
    and nicotine replacement therapy, *27*
condoms (sheaths)
    Dutch hygienic shops selling, *194*
    inter-war Britain, *143, 151, 153*
contraception, *5–7, 123–82*
    in Britain, *5–6, 141–82*
        interwar years, *6, 141–57, 275*
        oral contraceptive

studies, *128, 130, 159–82*
in Netherlands, hygienic shops selling products for, *189–91*
abortion and, *190–1, 191–2*
Co-operative Research and Development Agreements (CRADAs) and taxol, *245, 256–7*
Council for the Investigation of Fertility Control (CIFC), *6, 159–82, 274*
Cragg, Gordon, *254*
Crime and Disorder Bill, *29–30*
Crisp, Ronald, *86–7*
Cytrel, *23*

## D

10-DAB, *253–4*
Dalrymple-Champneys, Sir Weldon, *210*
'dangerous drugs', opiates as, *15–20*
Dangerous Drugs Act (1920), *16, 17*
Daube, Mike, *25*
Dawkins, Sylvia, *142–3*
10-deacetyl baccatin III, *253–4*
Deaconesses' hospital (Utrecht), homeopathy, *110*
dependency in 20th C. healing, *271–2*
dependency on nicotine, *25–6, 27*
see also Drug Dependence units
'deskundingen', *191–2, 196–7*
diaphragms (contraceptive), *143*
Dickman, Alan, *83*
disease, early-20th C. ideas on fighting, *2*
doctors/physicians (incl. general practitioners), Great Britain, *86–8, 90–3*
lesser accessibility (1989-95), *90–1*
patient barriers to visiting, *78–9*
pharmacist relationships post-NHS introduction, *86–8, 90, 92*
pre-NHS, *82–3*
prescriptions from see prescriptions
smoking cessation, *22*
doctors/physicians (incl. general practitioners), Netherlands pharmacist relationships with, *41–3*
Dodds, Sir Charles, *161*
Doll, Dr Richard, *21*
Donkers and Dutch drugstores see drugstores
Douros, John, *255*
Droog EAM, *108*
drug abuse (illicit drugs), *4, 12–20, 29*
Drug Dependence units, *18*
druggists, Dutch, *64*
pharmacists in competition with, *41, 46–8*
pharmacists involved with activities of, *61–2*
self-medication and, *64*
drugstores (and Donkers proposal), *58–9, 66*
responses to Donkers proposal, *59–66*
political nature of debate, *62*
Drummond, Sir Jack, *213*
Dutch Society for the Advancement of Pharmacy see Pharmaceutical Society

# E

economics of healing/health care, *272–5*
education and training in pharmacy
  Great Britain, *75–6*
  Netherlands, *36–8*
Education Law (1876), Dutch, *36, 37, 41, 61*
enemas, administering, *43*
Enovid, *132, 133*
Eykman JF, *41*

# F

family planning (birth control) in Britain, interwar years and the working classes, *6, 141–57*
  methods, *142–50*
family planning (birth control) clinics
  inter-war years, *141–57*
  oral contraceptive studies, *163–4*
Family Planning Association (Great Britain)
  approved list of oral contraceptives, *173–4*
  in trials of oral contraceptives, *160, 161, 162, 163, 164, 165*
Family Planning Association (Puerto Rico) in oral contraceptive trials, *128*
FDA *see* Food and Drug Administration
Feldman, William, *205, 218*
females *see* women
Feyerabend, Colin, *26*
Fisher, Evelyn, *146*
Florence, Lella Secor, *144, 147, 147–8, 152*
Food and Drug Administration (FDA), approval by
  oral contraceptives, *132–6, 170*
  taxol, *255, 259*
Foundation of United Dutch Pharmacies, *58–9*
France, taxol studies, *253–4, 259*
Free Hospital for Women, oral contraceptive studies, *125*
Frogatt, Sir Peter, *26, 28*

# G

galenic remedies, Netherlands, *41*
Gelder, Herman Van, *45*
General Dutch Pharmaceutical Student's Society, *66*
general practitioners *see* doctors; primary care
genetic engineering, interferon gene cloned via, *230–1*
Germany, opium industry, *15*
Gilbert, Joyce, *80*
Gilbert, Walter, *231*
Gladstone, William Ewart, *13*
Goodman, Grace, *80, 84*
Gorman, Mr, *84–5*
Green Cross, *185*
Greene, Andrew, *254, 256, 257, 262*
Greene, Graham, *The Third Man*, *207*
Groningen, hygienic shop, *188*
Groningen university professor
  Johan F Eykman, *41*
  Pieter Cornelis Plugee, *37*
Gruber AJ, *103*
Gunning, Jan Willem, *37–8, 40–1, 49–50*

# H

Hague (The), hygienic shops in, *184–5*

## Index

abortion and, *191, 195–6*
  Sanitas chain, *188*
Hague Convention of 1912 (and meetings at The Hague from 1911-12), *14, 15*
Hahnemann, Samuel, *99, 100–1, 105, 106, 112, 113*
hairy-cell leukaemia, interferon in, *237*
Hambro, Sir Charles, *208*
*Handelingen* (of Society of Homoeopathic Practitioners in the Netherlands), *103, 104, 105, 107, 113*
Hardy's (Thomas) Bob Loveday, *12*
Hare, Ronald, *220*
Haverhoek R, *109*
health care
  Dutch system, *57, 60*
  ending of national systems of, *278*
Health Education Authority, Ann McNeill of, *28*
Herman, John, *89–90*
heroin, *17, 18*
Heyermans, *64*
Hill, Dr A, *162–3*
Hill, Sir Austin Bradford, *21*
Himes, Norman and Vera, *144*
HIV and methadone, *19*
Hoffman-La Roche and interferon, *236, 237, 238*
Hofman, Jan, *50*
Holton, Bob, *259, 262*
Homan, Christine, *86*
Homan, Peter, *88, 90, 92–3*
homeopathy *see* homoeopathy
*Homoeopathisch Bibiotheek* (Homoeopathic Library), *109*
*Homoeopathisch maandblad*, *103, 104, 105, 106, 108, 109*
*Homoeopathisch tijdschrift*, *104, 116*

homoeopathy, Dutch, *5, 99–121*
  19th C., *101–4*
  20th C., early, *104–17*
    allopathy and, *105–6, 109–14*
  purity issues, *101, 104–9*
*Honorary Code for Pharmacists*, *66*
hormonal contraceptives (incl. preparations - the pill), clinical testing, *6, 123–40, 159–82, 274, 277*
  approval for marketing and testing, *132–6*
  Britain, *6, 149–52, 159–82*
    aims of larger trials, *167–72*
    dose considerations, *167–9, 170*
    formulations, *170*
    methods for administering, 171
    organising larger trials, *163–5*
    preliminary trials, *161–3*
    recruiting volunteers for larger trials, *165–6*
  health/safety risks, *133–4, 136, 162*
Horowitz, Susan, *252, 258, 262*
Hunter RB, *24*
*Hygiene for Women*, *197–8*
'hygienic' shops/establishments, Dutch, *7, 183–202, 273*
  advertisements, *184–6, 196*
  contraceptives, *189–91*
  meanings, *196–8*
  medicines, *193–5*
  Sanitas chain/name, *188–9, 192, 194, 195*
  sources of information, *186–7*

# Index

## I

ICRF and interferon, 233
illicit drugs, 4, 12-20, 29
immunotherapy in cancer, 235
Imperial Cancer Research Fund and interferon, 233
Independent Scientific Committee on Smoking and Health (ISCSH), 23–5, 26, 27, 30
India, opium, 14
Institut de Chimie des Substances Naturelles (ICSN), taxol studies, 253
interferons, 7, 229–43, 277–8
   media and scientists and, 231–6, 238–9
   promoting use of, 237–8

## J

Jackson, Dr Margaret, 161, 162
*JAMA* (*Journal of the American Medical Association*), Mayo Clinic's streptomycin study, 210, 213
Joseph, Sir Keith, 23
*Journal of the American Medical Association* (*JAMA*), Mayo Clinic's streptomycin study, 210, 213

## K

Kallenbach family
   CG Kallenbach, 102
   FWO Kallenbach (son of CG), 102, 106–7, 107, 111, 112, 113, 117
Kawasan 25350, 194
Kendall, Alan, 79–80
Knowles, Geoffrey, 85, 89, 92
Kuyper, Abraham, 110, 113

## L

*Lancet* and streptomycin, 206, 210, 212, 213–14
Law on Higher Education (1876), Dutch, 36, 37, 41, 61
Law on Physicians (1878), Dutch, 36
leeches, administering, 43
Leiden University
   Eduard Alexander Van der Burg (professor) at, 37, 41
   homoeopathy at, 110
   homoeopathic candidate for pharmacological chair, 113
*Leipziger Populäre Zeitschrift für Homöopathie*, Dutch edition (*Homoeopathisch tijdschrift*), 104, 116
leukaemia
   hairy-cell, interferon use, 237
   streptomycin in, 208–9
LHRH vaccine in prostate cancer, 136
Linstead, Sir Hugh, 86
list C *see* C list
Lloyds (the chemist), 76
London School of Hygiene and Tropical Medicine (1950s) and smoking, 21
lung cancer and smoking, 21
lynestrenol (Lyndiol), 129–30

## M

McGuire, William (Bill), 254, 258
McNeill, Ann, 28
males *see* men
Martens HAAJ, 69
Maskew, Jack, 80
material interactionism, 275–8
Mayo Clinic's streptomycin study,

210, 213
media
    interferon and, *231–6, 238–9*
    male contraceptive pill and, *129–31*
    streptomycin and, *206, 207, 209–10, 211*
Medical Act (1818), *102*
Medical Act (1865 - Thorbecke's Medical Laws), *35–50, 60–1*
    homoeopathy and, *103*
    hygienic articles and, *186*
    Stb. 60 article 9 (transitional provision), *42–3*
    Stb. 61 article 1, *47*
    Stb. 61 article 4, *44*
    Stb. 61 article 6, *44*
    Stb. 61 article 30, *47*
Medical Advisory Committee of Council for the Investigation of Fertility Control, *161*
Medical Research Council (MRC)
    interferon and, *233*
    streptomycin and, *206, 208, 209, 211, 212, 213, 214, 215*
Medical State Inspection, *44, 45, 46, 47*
Medicines Act (1958), Dutch (=Medicines Supply Act), *63–4, 64, 65, 66, 71*
Medicines Act (1968), UK, *23, 24, 81*
melanoma, taxol, *252*
Mellanby, Sir Edward, *205, 206*
Membership of Pharmaceutical Society, *75*
men
    contraception for
        Dutch hygienic shops and, *190*
        inter-war Britain, *150–3, 154*
    oral contraceptive studies, *126, 129–31, 135–6, 136*
    hygienic articles, *187, 190, 193*
meningitis, tuberculous, streptomycin in, *206, 208, 210–11, 212, 213, 213–14*
mental institution, oral contraceptive studies, *126–7*
methadone, *18–20*
Mieg J, *108, 113, 114*
Ministry of Health and streptomycin, *205–6, 210, 211, 213, 214*
'miracle' drugs, *7, 203, 214–19*
    as modern talismans, *214–19*
Misuse of Drugs Act (1971), *24*
*Monthly against Quackery*, hygienic articles and, *187*
    venereal disease, *193*
Morality Act (1911), *191*
morphine, *13, 14, 15*
Motké HP, *59, 60*
MRC *see* Medical Research Council
Mulder, Gerrit Jan, *37*
Munting DK, *107–8, 112, 113*
Murray, Clive, *87, 91*

# N

Naks, Jerzy, *88, 91*
narcotics (opium and opiates), *4, 12–20, 29*
National Cancer Institute (NCI)
    plant collection and drug screening, *249*
    taxol and, *250, 252, 254, 255, 255–6, 256, 257, 259, 260, 260–1, 261, 263*
National health care systems, ending, *278*

## Index

National Health Insurance Act (1911), 78, 79
National Health Service *see* NHS
National Insurance, 78
National Pharmaceutical Association, 88
Native Yew Conservation Council, 260
NCI *see* National Cancer Institute
*Nederlandsche homoeopathisch artsenijboek*, 115
Nederlandsche Maatschappij ter bevordering der Pharmacie *see* Pharmaceutical Society
Neo-Malthusian League and hygienic articles, 190, 191, 197
New Smoking Material, 23
news media *see* media
NHS
    contraception service, 175
    pharmacy after founding, 77, 83–93, 94
        patient–pharmacist relationship, 84–5
    pharmacy before, 77, 77–83, 93–4
        doctor–pharmacist relationships, 82–3
        patient–pharmacist relationship, 81–2
        ready availability of pharmacists, 79–81
nicotine, 21–9
    addiction, 25–9
    blood assay, 26
    manipulating content in cigarettes, 26–7
*Nicotine, Smoking and the Low Tar Programme*, 26
nicotine replacement therapy, 27, 28
Noorderpost, hygienic articles, 187, 188, 192

### O

oestrogen dosage, British trials of the pill, 169
Oosterhuis RAB, 116, 117
opium (and opiate alkaloids), 4, 12–20, 29
oral contraceptives *see* hormonal contraceptives
*Organon*, 100, 101
Organon (drug company), contraceptive pill, 128, 132
Otosclerosis and streptomycin, 207
Oudenrijn, homoeopathic hospital, 110
ovarian cancer, taxol, 254, 257, 258
over-the-counter products, Great Britain, 87
    nicotine products, 27
Owen, David, 23
Oxford's Radcliffe Infirmary, streptomycin study, 211

### P

Pacific yew *see Taxus* spp.
paclitaxel, 262
    *see also* taxol
Parke-Davis, contraceptive pill and, 128, 133
Parkes, Dr Alan, 161
Patel, Majula, 91
Paulsen, Alvin, 129–30
penicillin, 205, 215, 220
    in *The Third Man*, 207
*Penicillium notatum*, 219–20
Pereira, Jonathan, 12
Pharmaceutical Chemist (PhC) Diploma, 75–6
Pharmaceutical Society, Dutch (Royal Dutch Society for the

# Index

Advancement of Pharmacy;
Nederlandsche Maatschappij ter
bevordering der Pharmacie;
NMP), *35*
   annual reports of 1866/1867,
*40*
   commercialism and, *65*
   Foundation of United Dutch
Pharmacies and role of, *58*
   Gunning addressing General
Assembly (1887), *49–50*
   public image concerns, *37*
   sickness funds/welfare services
and, *66, 68–9*
   state's role with pharmacies
and, *38*
   supervision of pharmacists'
trade and, *45*
   weekly magazine *see*
Pharmaceutical Weekly
Journal
Pharmaceutical Society, Great
Britain, Membership of, *75*
Pharmaceutical Weekly Journal
(*Pharmaceutisch weekblad*)
   on commercialism, *66*
   editor in chief (Van Itallie),
*43, 47–8, 50*
   foundation, *40*
   Hofman's article at 50th
anniversary of, *50*
   Stoeder's articles in, *39*
*Pharmaceutisch weekblad see*
Pharmaceutical Weekly Journal
pharmacists (and pharmacy),
British, *5, 75–97*
   1920-95, *75–97*
      'ask your pharmacist'
campaign, *88–9*
      doctor relationships with
*see* doctors
      NHS and *see* NHS

      patient relationships
with, *88–90, 91–2*
      practice in community,
*76–7*
      re-emergence from 1982,
*88*
      training, *75–6*
   opium and, *16, 17*
pharmacists (and pharmacy),
Dutch, *5, 35–74*
   1865-c.1950, *35–55*
      competence, *40–1*
      druggists and *see*
druggists
      education and training,
*36–8*
      evolution of professional
identity, *60–2*
      physician relationships
with, *41–3*
      science and trade and,
*48–50*
      supervision of their trade,
*43–5*
   1950s onwards, *57–74*
      drugstores *see* drugstores
      welfare services (sickness
fund) and, *57, 62, 66–9*
pharmacopoeia, Dutch,
homoeopathic supplement,
*104–5, 108, 114–16*
Pharmacy Acts (Britain), *12, 13*
physicians *see* doctors
Physicians Law (1878), Dutch, *36*
pill, the *see* hormonal contraceptives
Pincher, Chapman, on
streptomycin, *214, 218*
Pincus, Geoffrey, *124–8, 133*
Pinkhof H, *196*
plants, collection and screening for
anticancer properties, *249*
Platz, Hugo, *116*

## Index

Plugge, Pieter Cornelis, *37*
Potier, Pierre, *253, 254, 256, 257, 262*
powers, changing, in 20th C. healing, *271–2*
prescriptions after NHS introduction
  *see also* pharmacists
  charges, *85–6, 91*
  errors on doctor's part, *93*
  impact, *85–6*
  number written, *83*
primary care, smoking cessation, *22*
  *see also* doctors
productivity, patterns of, in healing/health care, *272–5*
progesterone (in oral contraceptive studies), *125*
  approval by FDA, *132, 133*
progestins/progestogens (=modified progesterone/progesterone derivatives) in oral contraceptives, *126–7, 128*
  approval as drug, *133*
  dosage, British trials, *167–9*
prostate cancer, male contraceptive agents used in, *135*
*psora* theory, *100–1*
psychotics, oral contraceptive studies, *126–7*
Puerto Rico, oral contraceptive studies, *126, 127–8, 169*
Pyke, Margaret, *161*

## Q

quackery and quack remedies, *48*
  *see also* Monthly against Quackery; Society Against Quackery

## R

Radcliffe Infirmary (Oxford),
  streptomycin study, *211*
  radio appeals for streptomycin, *209–10, 211, 214*
Raw, Martin, *22*
registered trademark, TaxolR[O], *245, 262–3*
Rhône-Poulenc, taxol patent, *254*
Roberts, Elizabeth, *78*
Roche (Hoffman-La Roche) and interferon, *236, 237, 238*
Rock, John, *125–6, 127*
Rolleston Committee, *16*
Rosenberg, Charles, *2*
Ross, Bruce, *263*
Royal College of Physicians (RCP)
  on smoking, *24*
  1962 report, *21, 25*
  1971 report, *23, 25*
Royal Commission on Opium, *14*
Royal Dutch Society for the Advancement of Pharmacy *see* Pharmaceutical Society
rubber goods, Sanitas, *194*
Russell, Michael, *26, 28*

## S

Salipyrin Riedel, prescribing, *61*
Sanitas chain of hygienic shops, *188–9, 192, 194, 195*
Sanitas pills, *187*
scabies theory, *100–1*
Schatz, Albert, *204, 219, 220*
Scheele, Carl Wilhelm, *40*
Schering-Plough Corporation and interferon, *231, 236, 237, 238*
Schwabe, Willmar, *109, 110, 116, 117*
  Dutch edition
    (*Homoeopathisch tijdschrift*) of *Leipziger Populäre Zeitschrift für Homöopathie*, *104, 116*
science, pharmacist as man of

## Index

(Netherlands), *48–50*
Searle, oral contraceptives
    British study, *161, 162, 172*
    marketing approval, *132, 133*
self-medication and Dutch
  druggists, *64*
sequential oral contraceptive pill, *170*
sexually-transmitted (venereal)
  disease in men, remedies, *193–4*
Shanghai Opium Commission, *14, 15*
sheaths *see* condoms
Shoemaker, Dale, *257*
sickness funds system, Dutch, *57, 62, 66–9*
Sieffert, Dr G, *110*
*similia similibus curentur*, *99, 107, 113, 117*
Simpson, David, *25*
smoking *see* tobacco
social dependency in 20th C. healing, *271–2*
Society Against Quackery (Society for the Repression of Quackery), *45, 46, 48*
    hygienic shops and, *195*
Society for the Advancement of Homoeopathy in the Netherlands (Vereeniging tot Bevordering van de Homoeopathie in Nederland), *106, 109–10*
    founding, *102–3*
    and homoeopathic supplement to pharmacopoeia, *114, 115*
    membership requirements, *112–13*
    monthly journal (*Homoeopathisch maandblad*), *103, 104, 105, 106, 108, 109*

Society for the Suppression of the Opium Trade, *14*
Society of Apothecaries, *76*
Society of Champions of Homoeopathy, *102–3*
Society of Homoeopathic Practitioners in the Netherlands (Vereeniging van Homoepathische Geneesheeren in Nederland), *102–3, 105, 111–12*
    founding, *102–3*
    proceedings of (*Handelingen*), *103, 104, 105, 107, 113*
spermicides and spermicidal products
    British trials, *163*
    Dutch hygienic shops, *190*
Spivack, Edith, *92*
sponges (as contraceptives), *142, 143*
Stakman, Dr, *185*
Stocks, Percy, *21*
Stoeder, Willem, *37–8, 38–40, 40, 43*
Stokvis BJ, *111*
Stopes, Dr, hygienic articles of, *185*
Stopes, Marie, and her birth control clinics, *141, 142, 143, 144, 146, 148, 149, 150*
streptomycin, *7, 203–27, 277*
    lay images, *205–14*
Stross, Dr Barnett, *217*
substance abuse (illicit drugs), *4*
Suffness, Matthew, *255, 256*
sulphonamides, *215, 216*
Supreme Court of Netherlands, *44, 48*
Swyer, Dr Gerald, *161, 162*
symbolism of 'miracle', *214–19*
Syntex, oral contraceptive marketing approval, *132, 133*

# T

talismans, 'miracle' drugs as, 214–19
tar in cigarettes, manipulating content, 23, 26–7
taxol, 8, 245–67
   clinical trials, 254–6
   controversies/politics, 257–9
   discovery/early studies, 248–53
   ownership/property, 260, 261–3
   privatisation, 256–7
*Taxus* spp. (yew), 250, 251, 252–3
   *baccata*, 2
   *brevifolia* (Pacific yew tree), 240, 246, 249, 252, 254, 255, 258–9
      environmental/ecological concerns, 258–9, 260
   *canadensis*, 263
thalidomide, 216
Thau, Dr Rosemary, 135–6
The Hague *see* Hague
*The Third Man*, 207
Thomson, Sir Landsborough, 209, 211–12
Thorbecke JR, Medical Laws *see* Medical Act
Tobacco Products Research Trust, 26
tobacco smoking, 21–9, 29, 30
   alternative products/product modification, 23, 26–7
trademark, TaxolR[O], 245, 262–3
training *see* education
tuberculosis, streptomycin in, 206, 208, 210–11, 212, 213, 213–14, 218
Tyler, Dr Edward, 128

# U

United States *see* US
university education in pharmacy, Netherlands, 36–8
US (America)
   advertising in medical journals, unqualified, 65
   FDA of *see* Food and Drug Administration
   nicotine and addiction in, 29–30
   opium/opiates and, 14–15, 17
   oral contraceptive studies in/by people from, 124–8, 129–30, 132–6, 160, 170
   streptomycin in
      shipments to Britain, 206–7
      toxicity concerns, 213
   taxol in, 245–67
US Department of Agriculture (USDA)
   plant collection and drug screening, 249
   taxol and, 250, 251, 252, 255
Utrecht, homeopathy in/near to, 110
Utrecht university, Hendrik Wefer Bettink, 37, 43

# V

Van den Wal GH, 114
Van der Burg, Eduard Alexander, 37, 41
Van der Harst PL, 110, 112
Van der Stempel ML, 114, 116, 117
Van der Wielen P, 114
Van Dijk F, 110

Van Itallie, Leopold, *43, 47–8, 50*
Van Nunen JAJ, *59*
Van Roijen family, *117*
  JIAB Van Roijen (son of SJ), *108–9*
  SJ Van Roijen, *103, 111, 114*
venereal disease in men, remedies, *193–4*
Vereeniging tot Bevordering van de Homoeopathie in Nederland *see* Society for the Advancement of Homoeopathy
Vereeniging van Homeopathische Geneesheeren in Nederland *see* Society of Homoeopathic Practitioners in the Netherlands
Vereeniging van Voorstanders der Homoeopathie, *102–3*
von Bakody, Professor Theodor, *103, 107, 113*
von Bönninghausen, Baron CMF, *102*
Voorhoeve, Johannes (of Dillenburg), *106, 112*
Voorhoeve family (of the Hague), *117*
  Carl Theodor Voorhoeve (son of NAJ), *110, 115*
  NAJ Voorhoeve, *103, 106, 107, 112, 113, 117*

# W

Waites, Geoffrey, *136*
Waksman, Selman, *204, 209, 213, 217–18, 219*
Wald, Nicholas, *26, 28*
Wall, Monroe, *249, 250, 261–2*
Warner, John Harley, *2*
Waxman–Hatch Act, *257*
*Weekblad van het regt*, *42*
Weissmann, Charles, *231*
welfare services (sickness fund) and Dutch pharmacists, *57, 62, 66–9*
White Cross, *185*
WHO (World Health Organization), heroin and, *17*
Wilberforce, William, *13*
withdrawal method (birth control), *147–8, 149–50, 152*
women (females), Dutch, and hygienic articles, *107–8, 187, 194–5*
  contraceptives, *189, 190*
women (females), Great Britain contraception
  oral methods *see* hormonal contraceptives
  responsibilities vs those of men in interwar years, *150–2*
  as customers of pharmacists, *77*
  as pharmacists, *76–7*
'wonder' drugs *see* 'miracle' drugs
Worcester State Hospital, oral contraceptive studies, *126–7*
working classes, birth control *see* family planning
World Health Organization, heroin and, *17*
Wouters JT, *113, 113–14, 114, 115–16, 117*
Wright, Helena, and her birth control clinic, *161, 162*
Wu, Fred, *130*
Wyden, Ron, *258*

# Y

yew *see Taxus*

# Z

*zuiverheid*, *104*

# The Republic of Science
The Emergence of Popper's Social View of Science 1935-1945

Ian C. Jarvie

Amsterdam/Atlanta, GA 2001. 263 pp. (Series in the Philosophy of Karl R. Popper and Critical Rationalism 15)
ISBN: 90-420-1515-2            EUR 48.-/US-$ 45.-

This book offers a careful re-reading of Popper's classic falsificationist demarcation of science, stressing its institutional aspects. Popper's social thinking about science, individuals, institutions, and rationality is tracked through The Poverty of Historicism and The Open Society and Its Enemies as he criticises and improves his earlier work. New links are established between the works of the 1935-1945 period, revealing them as a source for criticism of the institutions and governance of science.

Contents: Preface. Chapter 1 Introduction: Science as an Institution. Chapter 2 Popper's 1935 Proto-constitution for the Republic of Science. Chapter 3 Problems in a Science of Social Institutions. Chapter 4 An Enriched View of Institutions. Chapter 5 Science and Society as Learning Institutions. Chapter 6 Conclusion: The Republic of Science. Sources and References. Index of Names. Index of Subjects.

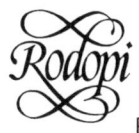
Editions Rodopi B.V.
USA/Canada: One Rockefeller Plaza, Ste. 1420, New York, NY 10020,
Tel. (212) 265-6360,
Call toll-free (U.S. only) 1-800-225-3998, Fax (212) 265-6402
All other countries: Tijnmuiden 7, 1046 AK Amsterdam, The Netherlands.
Tel. ++ 31 (0)20 611 48 21, Fax ++ 31 (0)20 447 29 79
Orders-queries@rodopi.nl                    www.rodopi.nl

# Realismus Disziplin Interdisziplinarität

Hrsg. von Dariusz Aleksandrowicz und Hans Günther Ruß.

Amsterdam/Atlanta, GA 2001. 354 pp.
(Schriftenreihe zur Philosophie Karl R. Poppers und des kritischen Rationalismus 14)
ISBN: 90-420-1535-7                EUR 64,-/US-$ 60.-

Vom Blickpunkt der Wissenschaftslehre des Kritischen Rationalismus aus erscheint der Gedanke, es solle über die Grenzen der Disziplinen hinweg theoretisiert und geforscht werden, als keine atemberaubende Erfindung. Das Wort "Interdisziplinarität" ist nicht eindeutig, was man aber sinnvollerweise darunter verstehen kann, betrachtet der kritische Rationalismus als eine Konsequenz des (metaphysischen) Realismus. Deswegen weist das Thema "Realismus" auf den Kontext hin, in dem das Problem der Interdisziplinarität gestellt werden kann. Das kommt in den Beiträgen des ersten Teils des Sammelbandes zum Ausdruck. Die im zweiten Teil versammelten Abhandlungen betreffen Fragen, die sich aus der "disziplinenübergreifenden" Anwendung der kritisch-rationalen Ansätze auf spezielle Probleme ergeben.

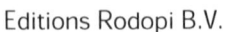

Editions Rodopi B.V.
USA/Canada: One Rockefeller Plaza, Ste. 1420, New York, NY 10020,
Tel. (212) 265-6360,
Call toll-free (U.S. only) 1-800-225-3998, Fax (212) 265-6402
All other countries: Tijnmuiden 7, 1046 AK Amsterdam, The Netherlands.
Tel. ++ 31 (0)20 611 48 21, Fax ++ 31 (0)20 447 29 79
Orders-queries@rodopi.nl                www.rodopi.nl

# National Stereotypes in Perspective
Americans in France, Frenchmen in America

Ed. by William L. Chew, III

Amsterdam/New York, NY 2001. X,433 pp.
(Studia Imagologica 9)
ISBN: 90-420-1365-6     EUR 82,-/US-$ 77.-

Since the late 18th century, when they first entered into an alliance during the American Revolution, the French and Americans have had a long and sometimes stormy relationship based on a complex mix of mutual admiration, cultural criticism, and sometimes downright disgust for the "other." The relatively new interdisciplinary field of imagology, or image studies, allows us to place the dynamics of such a relationship into perspective by grounding its analysis firmly in the study of national stereotypes, in the process providing new insights into the mentality of the observer. For if anything, image studies demonstrate again and again that national character is not—as assumed uncritically for centuries—an innate essence of the "other", but rather a self-serving functional construct of the observer.

For the table of contents please refer to our website

*Rodopi* Editions Rodopi B.V.
USA/Canada: One Rockefeller Plaza, Ste. 1420, New York, NY 10020,
Tel. (212) 265-6360, Call toll-free (U.S. only) 1-800-225-3998, Fax (212) 265-6402
All other countries: Tijnmuiden 7, 1046 AK Amsterdam, The Netherlands.
Tel. ++ 31 (0)20 611 48 21, Fax ++ 31 (0)20 447 29 79
Orders-queries@rodopi.nl                     www.rodopi.nl

# Essays on the Song Cycle and on Defining the Field

Essays on the Song Cycle and on Defining the Field. Proceedings of the Second International Conference on Word and Music Studies at Ann Arbor, MI, 1999.

Edited by Walter Bernhart and Werner Wolf in collaboration with David Mosley Amsterdam/Atlanta, GA 2001. XII,253 pp. (Word and Music Studies 3)

ISBN: 90-420-1575-6                       EUR 57.-/US-$ 53.-
ISBN: 90-420-1565-9                       EUR 23.-/US-$ 21.-

This volume assembles twelve interdisciplinary essays that were originally presented at the Second International Conference on Word and Music Studies at Ann Arbor, MI, in 1999, a conference organized by the International Association for Word and Music Studies (WMA).

The contributions to this volume focus on two centres of interest. The first deals with general issues of literature and music relations from culturalist, historical, reception-aesthetic and cognitive points of view. It covers issues such as conceptual problems in devising transdisciplinary histories of both arts, cultural functions of opera as a means of reflecting postcolonial national identity, the problem of verbalizing musical experience in nineteenth-century aesthetics and of understanding reception processes triggered by musicalized fiction.

The second centre of interest deals with a specific genre of vocal music as an obvious area of word and music interaction, namely the song cycle. As a musico-literary genre, the song cycle not only permits explorations of relations between text and music in individual songs but also raises the question if, and to what extent words and/or music contribute to creating a larger unity beyond the limits of single songs. Elucidating both of these issues with stimulating diversity the essays in this section highlight classic nineteenth- and twentieth-century song cycles by Franz Schubert, Robert Schumann, Hugo Wolf, Richard Strauss and Benjamin Britten and also include the discussion of a modern successor of the song cycle, the concept album as part of today's popular culture.

*Rodopi*

Editions Rodopi B.V.
USA/Canada: One Rockefeller Plaza, Ste. 1420, New York, NY 10020,
Tel. (212) 265-6360, Call toll-free (U.S. only) 1-800-225-3998, Fax (212) 265-6402
All other countries: Tijnmuiden 7, 1046 AK Amsterdam, The Netherlands.
Tel. ++ 31 (0)20 611 48 21, Fax ++ 31 (0)20 447 29 79
Orders-queries@rodopi.nl                                    www.rodopi.nl

# Marteaus Europa oder der Roman, bevor er Literatur wurde

Eine Untersuchung des deutschen und englischen Buchangebots der Jahre 1710 bis 1720.

Olaf Simons

Amsterdam/Atlanta, GA 2001. 765 pp. (Internationale Forschungen zur Allgemeinen und Vergleichenden Literaturwissenschaft 52)
ISBN: 90-420-1226-9                             EUR 136,-/US $127.50

Bewähren sich vor 1720 noch die Wissenschaften der Nationen als der ursprüngliche Gegenstand der Literaturkritik, so ändert sich dies im Lauf des Jahrhunderts: Die Literaturbesprechung wendet sich Romanen, Dramen und Gedichten zu und etabliert am Ende die Literaturgeschichten, die uns noch heute beschäftigen.

Die Literaturbetrachtung gewinnt mit den poetischen und fiktionalen Schriften einen Gegenstand, mit dem sie sich bis in den Schulunterricht ausbreiten kann. Gleichzeitig verändert sie den Markt, dem sie sich zuwendet. Im Blick auf das Romanangebot des frühen 18. Jahrhunderts wird dies deutlich: Einen skandalösen, aktuellen, ungemein europäischen Markt nehmen die Leser in Leipzig wie in London vor 1720 wahr, wenn sie den Romanmarkt berühren - einen Markt, der sich gegenwärtig als historischer und politischer unter kaum erträglichen Manieren den privatesten Nutzungen anbot.

Die vorliegende Untersuchung unterstellt, daß die Literaturbetrachtung diesen Markt - an seiner Reform interessiert - von Anfang an disqualifizierte. Ein breites Aufgebot an Zeitzeugnissen, unter denen sie das Angebot überblickt, stellt sie dazu den späteren Literaturgeschichtsschreibungen gegenüber. Romane, die wir gewohnt sind, getrennten nationalen Literaturen und Epochen zuzuordnen, werden dabei als Produktionen eines größeren europäischen Marktes greifbar.

 Editions Rodopi B.V.
USA/Canada: One Rockefeller Plaza, Ste. 1420, New York, NY 10020,
Tel. (212) 265-6360, Toll-free (U.S. only) 1-800-225-3998, Fax (212) 265-6402
All other countries: Tijnmuiden 7, 1046 AK Amsterdam, The Netherlands.
Tel. ++ 31 (0)20 611 48 21, Fax ++ 31 (0)20 447 29 79

Orders-queries@rodopi.nl                             www.rodopi.nl

# Schuld Und Sühne?
Kriegserlebnis und Kriegsdeutung in deutschen Medien der Nachkriegszeit (1945-1961) Internationale Konferenz vom 01 - 04.09.1999 in Berlin.

Hrsg. von Ursula Heukenkamp

Amsterdam/Atlanta, GA 2001. 403 pp.
(Amsterdamer Beiträge zur neueren Germanistik 50.1)
ISBN: 90-420-1425-3        Bound EUR 75,-/US $70.-
ISBN: 90-420-1415-6        Paper EUR 27,-/US $26.-

Inhalt
Vorbemerkung
Band I: FIGURATIONEN VON KRIEG UND KAMPF (textkritische Beiträge)
   1. Kriegserzählungen.
   2. Schlachtbeschreibung Stalingrad
   3. "Der jugendliche Geist" – Jugend im Krieg.
   4. Folgen ohne Ursachen – Heimkehr
   5. Kriegserinnerung – keine Memoiren

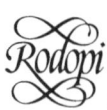
**Editions Rodopi B.V.**
USA/Canada: One Rockefeller Plaza, Ste. 1420, New York, NY 10020,
Tel. (212)265-6360, Toll-free (U.S. only) 1-800-225-3998, Fax (212) 265-6402
All other countries: Tijnmuiden 7, 1046 AK Amsterdam, The Netherlands.
Tel. ++ 31 (0)20 611 48 21, Fax ++ 31 (0)20 447 29 79

Orders-queries@rodopi.nl             www.rodopi.nl

# Schuld Und Sühne?
Kriegserlebnis und Kriegsdeutung in deutschen Medien der Nachkriegszeit (1945-1961) Internationale Konferenz vom 01 - 04.09.1999 in Berlin.

Hrsg. von Ursula Heukenkamp

Amsterdam/Atlanta, GA 2001. 405-827 pp.
(Amsterdamer Beiträge zur neueren Germanistik 50.2)
ISBN: 90-420-1445-8       Bound EUR 80,-/US $74.-
ISBN: 90-420-1435-0       Paper EUR 30,-/US $28.-
Bde 1-2 ISBN: 90-420-1445-5

Inhalt
Vorbemerkung
Band II: KRITIK DER ERINNERUNG
   1. Erinnerungspolitik und Institutionalisierung
   2. Deutschlandbilder
   3. West-östiche Kriegsbilder

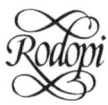
**Editions Rodopi B.V.**
USA/Canada: One Rockefeller Plaza, Ste. 1420, New York, NY 10020,
Tel. (212)265-6360, Toll-free (U.S. only) 1-800-225-3998, Fax (212) 265-6402
All other countries: Tijnmuiden 7, 1046 AK Amsterdam, The Netherlands.
Tel. ++ 31 (0)20 611 48 21, Fax ++ 31 (0)20 447 29 79

Orders-queries@rodopi.nl            www.rodopi.nl

# Theoretical Interpretations of the Holocaust

Ed. by Dan Stone

Amsterdam/Atlanta, GA 2001. IX,239 pp.
(Value Inquiry Book Services 108)
ISBN: 90-420-1505-5          EUR 45.-/US-$ 42.50

This book aims to show the many resources at our disposal for grappling with the Holocaust as the darkest occurrence of the twentieth century. These wide-ranging studies on philosophy, history, and literature address the way the Holocaust had led to the reconceptualization of the humanities. The scholarly approaches of Pierre Klossowki, Georges Bataille, and Maurice Blanchot are examined critically, and the volume explores such poignant topics as violence, evil, and monuments.

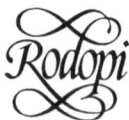

**Editions Rodopi B.V.**
*USA/Canada:* One Rockefeller Plaza, Ste. 1420, New York, NY 10020,
Tel. (212) 265-6360, *Call toll-free* (U.S.only) 1-800-225-3998,
Fax (212) 265-6402
*All Other Countries:* Tijnmuiden 7, 1046 AK Amsterdam, The Netherlands.
Tel. ++ 31 (0)20 6114821, Fax ++ 31 (0)20 4472979
**orders-queries@rodopi.nl**          www.rodopi.nl

# The Model Man
A Life of Edward William Bok, 1863-1930

Hans Krabbendam
Amsterdam/Atlanta, GA 2001. IX,262 + 16 ill. pp. (Amsterdam Monographs in American Studies 9)
ISBN: 90-420-1495-4          EUR 50,-/US-$ 47.-

Edward William Bok was the most famous Dutch-American in early twentieth-century America thanks to his thirty-year editorship of the *Ladies' Home Journal*, the most prestigious women's magazine of the day. This first complete coverage of Edward Bok's life places him against his ethnic background and portrays him as the spokesman for and the molder of the American middle class between 1890 and 1930. He acted as a mediator between a Victorian and a modern society, reconciling consumerism with idealism. As a Dutch immigrant he became a model for successful adaptation to a new country and modern times. He used his national reputation to restore America's internationalism in the 1920s. His life story is relevant to those interested in the history of immigration, journalism, the rise of big business, the women's movement, and the Progressive Movement.

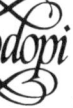
Editions Rodopi B.V.
USA/Canada: One Rockefeller Plaza, Ste. 1420, New York, NY 10020,
Tel. (212) 265-6360, Call toll-free (U.S. only) 1-800-225-3998, Fax (212) 265-6402
All other countries: Tijnmuiden 7, 1046 AK Amsterdam, The Netherlands.
Tel. ++ 31 (0)20 611 48 21, Fax ++ 31 (0)20 447 29 79
Orders-queries@rodopi.nl          www.rodopi.nl

# What is the Meaning of Human Life?

Raymond Angelo Belliotti

Amsterdam/Atlanta, GA 2001. VIII,176 pp.
(Value Inquiry Book Series 109)
ISBN: 90-420-1296-X                EUR 34,-/US-$ 32.-

This book examines core concerns of human life. What is the relationship between a meaningful life and theism? Why are some human beings radically adrift, without radical foundations, and struggling with hopelessness? Is the cosmos meaningless? Is human life akin to the ancient Myth of Sisyphus? What is the role of struggle and suffering in creating meaning? How do we discover or create value? Is happiness overrated as a goal of life? How, if at all, can we learn to die meaningfully?

Contents:
Foreword by Jan Narveson
Preface
ONE Meaning and Theism
TWO Nihilism, Schopenhauer, and Nietzsche
THREE The Myth of Sisyphus
FOUR The Meaning of Life
FIVE Value
SIX Why Happiness is Overrated
SEVEN Death
Notes
Bibliography
About the Author
Index

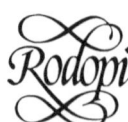
Editions Rodopi B.V.
USA/Canada: One Rockefeller Plaza, Ste. 1420, New York, NY 10020,
Tel. (212) 265-6360,
Call toll-free (U.S. only) 1-800-225-3998, Fax (212) 265-6402
All other countries: Tijnmuiden 7, 1046 AK Amsterdam, The Netherlands.
Tel. ++ 31 (0)20 611 48 21, Fax ++ 31 (0)20 447 29 79
Orders-queries@rodopi.nl                         www.rodopi.nl

# After the GDR
New Perspectives on the Old GDR and Young *Länder*

Edited by Laurence McFalls and Lothar Probst.

Amsterdam/Atlanta, GA 2001. IV,310 pp.
(German Monitor 54)
ISBN: 90-420-1336-2          Bound EUR 73,-/US-$ 68.-
ISBN: 90-420-1326-5          Paper EUR 30,-/US-$ 28.-

This volume represents the efforts of fifteen scholars from Europe and North America to work through the complex and sometimes compromising past and the current struggles that together define eastern German identity, society, and politics ten years after unification. Their papers offer an exemplary illustration of the variety of disciplinary methods and new source materials on which established and younger scholars can draw today to further differentiated understanding of the old GDR and the young *Länder*. In a volume that will interest students of German history, cultural studies and comparative politics, the authors show how utopian ideals quickly degenerated into a dictatorship that provoked the everyday resistance at all levels of society that ultimately brought the regime to its demise. They also suggest how the GDR might live on in memory to shape the emerging varieties of postcommunist politics in the young states of the Federal Republic and how the GDR experience might inspire new practices and concepts for German society as a whole. Most importantly, the papers here testify to the multidisciplinary vitality of a field whose original object of enquiry disappeared over a decade ago.

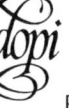
Editions Rodopi B.V.
USA/Canada: One Rockefeller Plaza, Ste. 1420, New York, NY 10020,
Tel. (212) 265-6360,
Call toll-free (U.S. only) 1-800-225-3998, Fax (212) 265-6402
All other countries: Tijnmuiden 7, 1046 AK Amsterdam, The Netherlands.
Tel. ++ 31 (0)20 611 48 21, Fax ++ 31 (0)20 447 29 79
Orders-queries@rodopi.nl                              www.rodopi.nl

# WOMEN AND MODERN MEDICINE

*Edited by Anne Hardy and Lawrence Conrad*

Amsterdam/Atlanta, GA 2001. V,293 pp.
(Clio Medica 61 /
The Wellcome Series in the History of Medicine)
ISBN: 90-420-0871-X      Bound EUR 68,-/US-$ 63.50
ISBN: 90-420-0861-X      Paper EUR 27.-/US-$ 25.-

Modernising scientific medicine emerged in the nineteenth century as an increasingly powerful agent of change in a context of complex social developments. Womens' lives and expectations in particular underwent a transformation in the years after 1870 as education, employment opportunities and political involvement extended their personal and gender horizons. For women, medicine came to offer not just treatment in the event of illness but the possibilities of participation in medical practise, of shaping social policies and political understandings, and of altering the biological imperatives of their bodies. The essays in this collection explore various ways in which women responded to these challenges and opportunities and sought to use the power of modernising Western medicine to further their individual and gender interests.

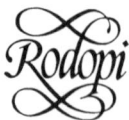

**Editions Rodopi B.V.**
*USA/Canada:* One Rockefeller Plaza, Ste. 1420, New York, NY 10020,
Tel. (212) 265-6360, *Call toll-free* (U.S.only) 1-800-225-3998,
Fax (212) 265-6402
*All Other Countries:* Tijnmuiden 7, 1046 AK Amsterdam, The Netherlands.
Tel. ++ 31 (0)20 6114821, Fax ++ 31 (0)20 4472979
orders-queries@rodopi.nl                      www.rodopi.nl

# Health, Science, and Ordinary Language

Lennart Nordenfelt
With contributions by George Khushf and K. W. M. Fulford:

Amsterdam/Atlanta, GA 2001.XII,235 pp.
(Value Inquiry Book Series 110)
ISBN: 90-420-1306-0                     EUR 50,-/US-$ 47.-

This book is a contribution to the current philosophical discussion on the nature of health and illness. It contains a comparative analysis and reevaluation of four influential contemporary theories in this field. These are the biostatistical theory of Christopher Boorse which represents the mainstream thinking in medicine, and three versions of a holistic and normative understanding of health and illness which are the theories of Lawrie Reznek, K. W. M. Fulford, and Lennart Nordenfelt. In this unusual volume of assessment, Nordenfelt critically reexamines his own theory, and George Khushf and K. W. M. Fulford contribute critical responses.

Editions Rodopi B.V.
USA/Canada: One Rockefeller Plaza, Ste. 1420, New York, NY 10020,
Tel. (212) 265-6360,
Call toll-free (U.S. only) 1-800-225-3998, Fax (212) 265-6402
All other countries: Tijnmuiden 7, 1046 AK Amsterdam, The Netherlands.
Tel. ++ 31 (0)20 611 48 21, Fax ++ 31 (0)20 447 29 79
Orders-queries@rodopi.nl                         www.rodopi.nl

# Local Insights, Global Ethics for Business

Daryl Koehn

Amsterdam/Atlanta, GA 2001. XIII,272 pp.
(Value Inquiry Book Series 111)
ISBN: 90-420-1436-9                    EUR 50,-/US-$ 47.-

This book evaluates strategies for managing ethical conflict. Macro-approaches that attribute select values to entire peoples and claim supremacy for these values are suspect. A micro-approach, focusing on the ethics of individual thinkers, is better. The study uses the ethics of Confucius and Tetsuro Watsuji to derive a process-based universal ethic that respects local differences yet is not relativistic.

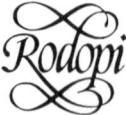
Editions Rodopi B.V.
USA/Canada: One Rockefeller Plaza, Ste. 1420, New York, NY 10020,
Tel. (212) 265-6360,
Call toll-free (U.S. only) 1-800-225-3998, Fax (212) 265-6402
All other countries: Tijnmuiden 7, 1046 AK Amsterdam, The Netherlands.
Tel. ++ 31 (0)20 611 48 21, Fax ++ 31 (0)20 447 29 79
Orders-queries@rodopi.nl                    www.rodopi.nl